T0297363

Future of AI in Medical Imaging

Avinash Kumar Sharma
Sharda University, India

Nitin Chanderwal
University of Cincinnati, USA

Shobhit Tyagi
Sharda University, India

Prashant Upadhyay
Sharda University, India

A volume in the Advances in Medical
Technologies and Clinical Practice (AMTCP) Book
Series

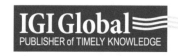

Published in the United States of America by
IGI Global
Medical Information Science Reference (an imprint of IGI Global)
701 E. Chocolate Avenue
Hershey PA, USA 17033
Tel: 717-533-8845
Fax: 717-533-8661
E-mail: cust@igi-global.com
Web site: http://www.igi-global.com

Library of Congress Cataloging-in-Publication Data

Names: Sharma, Avinash Kumar, 1982- editor. | Chanderwal, Nitin, 1978-
    editor. | Tyagi, Shobhit, 1996- editor. | Upadhyay, Prashant, 1991-
    editor.
Title: Future of AI in medical imaging / edited by Avinash Sharma, Nitin
    Chanderwal, Shobhit Tyagi, Prashant Upadhyay.
Other titles: Future of artificial intelligence in medical imaging
Description: Hershey, PA : Medical Information Science Reference, [2024] |
    Includes bibliographical references and index. | Summary: "This book
    will cover the transformative impact of medical imaging on healthcare,
    highlighting its evolution, core concepts, and various imaging
    modalities"-- Provided by publisher.
Identifiers: LCCN 2023056807 (print) | LCCN 2023056808 (ebook) | ISBN
    9798369323595 (hardcover) | ISBN 9798369323601 (ebook)
Subjects: MESH: Diagnostic Imaging--methods | Artificial
    Intelligence--trends
Classification: LCC RC78.7.D53 (print) | LCC RC78.7.D53 (ebook) | NLM WN
    180 | DDC 616.07/540285--dc23/eng/20240126
LC record available at https://lccn.loc.gov/2023056807
LC ebook record available at https://lccn.loc.gov/2023056808

This book is published in the IGI Global book series Advances in Medical Technologies and Clinical Practice (AMTCP) (ISSN: 2327-9354; eISSN: 2327-9370)

British Cataloguing in Publication Data
A Cataloguing in Publication record for this book is available from the British Library.

For electronic access to this publication, please contact: eresources@igi-global.com.

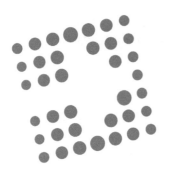

Advances in Medical Technologies and Clinical Practice (AMTCP) Book Series

Srikanta Patnaik
SOA University, India
Priti Das
S.C.B. Medical College, India

ISSN:2327-9354
EISSN:2327-9370

MISSION

Medical technological innovation continues to provide avenues of research for faster and safer diagnosis and treatments for patients. Practitioners must stay up to date with these latest advancements to provide the best care for nursing and clinical practices.

The **Advances in Medical Technologies and Clinical Practice (AMTCP) Book Series** brings together the most recent research on the latest technology used in areas of nursing informatics, clinical technology, biomedicine, diagnostic technologies, and more. Researchers, students, and practitioners in this field will benefit from this fundamental coverage on the use of technology in clinical practices.

COVERAGE

- Telemedicine
- Biometrics
- Clinical Data Mining
- Nutrition
- Biomechanics
- Nursing Informatics
- Medical imaging
- E-Health
- Diagnostic Technologies
- Clinical High-Performance Computing

IGI Global is currently accepting manuscripts for publication within this series. To submit a proposal for a volume in this series, please contact our Acquisition Editors at Acquisitions@igi-global.com or visit: http://www.igi-global.com/publish/.

Titles in this Series

For a list of additional titles in this series, please visit:
www.igi-global.com/book-series/advances-medical-technologies-clinical-practice/73682

Multisector Insights in Healthcare, Social Sciences, Society, and Technology
Darrell Norman Burrell (Marymount University USA)
Engineering Science Reference • © 2024 • 392pp • H/C (ISBN: 9798369332269) • US $545.00

Change Dynamics in Healthcare, Technological Innovations, and Complex Scenarios
Darrell Norman Burrell (Marymount University, USA)
Medical Information Science Reference • © 2024 • 331pp • H/C (ISBN: 9798369335550) • US $495.00

Intelligent Solutions for Cognitive Disorders
Dipti Jadhav (D. Y. Patil University (Deemed), Navi Mumbai, India & Ramrao Adik Institute of Technology, India)
Pallavi Vijay Chavan (D. Y. Patil University (Deemed), Navi Mumbai, India & Ramrao Adik Institute of Technolgy, India) Sangita Chaudhari (D. Y. Patil University (Deemed), Navi Mumbai, India & Ramrao Adik Institute of Technology, India) and Idongesit Williams (CMI, Denmark & Aalborg University, Copenhagen, Denmark)
Medical Information Science Reference • © 2024 • 411pp • H/C (ISBN: 9798369310908) • US $355.00

Intelligent Technologies and Parkinson's Disease Prediction and Diagnosis
Abhishek Kumar (Chitkara University Institute of Engineering and Technology, Chitkara University, Punjab, India) Sachin Ahuja (Chandigarh University, India) Anupam Baliyan (Geeta University, India) Sreenatha Annawati (University of New South Wales, Australia) and Abhineet Anand (Chandigarh University, India)
Medical Information Science Reference • © 2024 • 390pp • H/C (ISBN: 9798369311158) • US $355.00

Innovations, Securities, and Case Studies Across Healthcare, Business, and Technology
Darrell Norman Burrell (Marymount University, USA)
Medical Information Science Reference • © 2024 • 555pp • H/C (ISBN: 9798369319062) • US $360.00

Handbook of Research on Advances in Digital Technologies to Promote Rehabilitation and Community Participation
Raquel Simões de Almeida (CIR, ESS, Polytechnic of Porto, Portugal) Vítor Simões-Silva (CIR, ESS, Polytechnic of Porto, Portugal) and Maria João Trigueiro (CIR, ESS, Polytechnic of Porto, Portugal)
Medical Information Science Reference • © 2024 • 513pp • H/C (ISBN: 9781668492512) • US $480.00

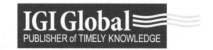

701 East Chocolate Avenue, Hershey, PA 17033, USA
Tel: 717-533-8845 x100 • Fax: 717-533-8661
E-Mail: cust@igi-global.com • www.igi-global.com

Editorial Advisory Board

Table of Contents

Detailed Table of Contents

Chapter 1
Sheelesh Kumar Sharma, ABESIT Engineering College, Ghaziabad, India

Artificial intelligence (AI) integration in medical image processing is a game-changing breakthrough in modern healthcare. This cutting-edge technology takes a multidimensional approach to diagnosis, treatment, and patient care, opening up significant prospects for improved medical outcomes and resource optimization. AI has proven its image analysis prowess in applications such as disease detection and diagnosis. Machine learning algorithms, combined with massive datasets of medical pictures, allow for precise and speedy detection of anomalies in radiological scans such as X-rays, CT scans, MRIs, and ultrasounds. Early diagnosis of diseases such as cancer, neurological disorders, and cardiovascular ailments has improved, allowing for earlier intervention and personalized treatment plans. Incorporation of AI in medical image processing is revolutionizing healthcare by boosting diagnosis speed and accuracy, optimizing treatment planning, and improving patient care.

Chapter 2
Amit Kumar Tyagi, National Institute of Fashion Technology, New Delhi, India
Shabnam Kumari, SRM Institute of Science and Technology, Chennai, India
Shrikant Tiwari, Galgotias University, Greater Noida, India

Internet of things (IoT) has emerged as a transformative technology in the healthcare sector, providing innovative solutions to enhance patient care, improve healthcare delivery, and optimize resource utilization. This chapter provides a comprehensive overview of the current state of IoT applications in smart healthcare. It provides the various aspects of IoT implementation, including device integration, data management, security, and privacy issues. This work begins by defining the key concepts of IoT and its relevance to healthcare, highlighting the potential benefits and challenges. It discusses several components of IoT-enabled smart healthcare systems, such as wearable devices, remote monitoring, and healthcare infrastructure integration. This work discusses the role of IoT in chronic disease management, telemedicine, and preventive healthcare, showcasing real-world examples and success stories. Moreover, this work outlines the critical role of data analytics and artificial intelligence in processing the vast amount of healthcare data generated by IoT devices.

  Jaspreet Kaur, Chandigarh University, India

The chapter explores the transformative impact of medical imaging on healthcare that prioritizes the needs and well-being of patients. It examines the influence of imaging technologies on the precision of diagnoses, the involvement of patients, and the results of healthcare, highlighting the revolutionary function of imaging modalities. This study examines the impact of medical imaging on patient empowerment by doing a thorough review of literature and analyzing empirical evidence. It demonstrates how visual representations offered by medical imaging enable people to better comprehend their health situations and promote collaborative decision-making with healthcare practitioners. The results emphasize the crucial significance of imaging in influencing a better-informed, involved, and empowered patient community within contemporary healthcare systems.

  Siham Moussaoui, Department of Electrical Engineering Systems, Systems and
      Telecommunications Engineering Laboratory, Boumerdes University, Algeria
  Sid Ali Fellag, Boumerdes University, Algeria
  Hocine Chebi, Faculty of Electrical Engineering, Laboratory Intelligent Control and
      Electrical Power System (ICEPS), Djillali Liabes University of Sidi Bel Abbes, Algeria

In general, blood pressure (BP) is measured using standard methods (medical monitors), which are widely used, or from physiological sensor data, which is a difficult task usually solved by combining several signals. In recent research, electrocardiogram (ECG) signals alone have been used to estimate blood pressure. The authors present a comparative study that evaluates ECG signal-based blood pressure estimation using complexity analysis to extract features, comparing the results obtained with a random forest regression model as well as with the combination of a stacking-based classification module and a regression module. It was determined that the best result obtained is a mean absolute error range of 3.73 mmHg with a standard deviation of 5.19 mmHg for diastolic blood pressure (DBP) and 5.92 mmHg with a standard deviation of 7.23 mmHg for systolic blood pressure (PAS).

  Harsh Vardhan, National Institute of Technology, Hamirpur, India
  Vijay Kumar, Dr B R Ambedkar National Institute of Technology, Jalandhar, India

The early prediction of diabetes mellitus may help improve the health of patients and cure them of this disease. In recent years, machine learning techniques have been widely used to predict diabetes in its early stages. In this chapter, an attempt has been made to analyse the performance of different machine learning techniques for diabetic prediction. Four well-known machine learning techniques, named as random forest, support vector machine, decision tree, and XGBoost are used. These techniques are evaluated on the Indian Diabetes dataset. Experimental results reveal that random forest algorithm achieved highest accuracy than the other techniques in terms of performance measures. These techniques will help to reduce diabetes incidence and health care costs. This work can be used to envisage diabetes in its early stages.

Chapter 6

Raghuraj Singh, School of Engineering and Technology, Sharda University, India
Kuldeep Kumar, National Institute of Technology, Kurukshetra, India

Counterfeit medicine is a major problem in the pharmaceutical industry that threatens public health. The fake drugs are often inefficient, toxic, and can even cause death. This chapter presents a counterfeit medicine detection system using blockchain that prevents counterfeit drugs from entering into the supply chain. The system uses blockchain to create a secure and transparent record of the entire supply chain of medicines, from manufacturer to distributor to the end consumer. It allows for real-time tracking of medicines, providing transparency and accountability at every step. Smart contracts automate the verification process, reducing the potential for human error and improving efficiency. When a medicine enters the supply chain, a smart contract is created with its unique identifier, manufacturer, and distribution details. It ensures that every medicine can be traced back to its origin, and counterfeit medicine can be easily identified and removed from the supply chain. The presented system also provides a platform for customers to verify the authenticity of their medicines.

Chapter 7

V. Hemamalini, SRM Institute of Science and Technology, Chennai, India
Amit Kumar Tyagi, National Institute of Fashion Technology, New Delhi, India
A. Rajivkannan, K.S.R. College of Engineering, KSR Kalvinagar, India

When it comes to the smart healthcare sector, blockchain technology presents several prospects. Aside from its usage in the financial industry, blockchain technology is now also utilised in the process of establishing trust, protecting privacy, and ensuring security. Within the scope of this work, we will provide an explanation of a new development in the healthcare business that strives to enhance the effectiveness and safety of the administration of healthcare data. We employ blockchain technology to construct a decentralised and tamper-proof network that facilitates safe data exchange among healthcare stakeholders such as patients, providers, and insurers. This technique is known as Blockchain-based Intelligent and Interactive Healthcare Systems (Blockchain-based IHS). The purpose of this chapter is to present an overview of BIIHS, including its advantages, disadvantages, and potential future paths. The BIIHS has the potential to enhance patient outcomes by facilitating personalised treatment plans, lowering the number of medical mistakes, and offering real-time access to vital and sensitive health data. Nevertheless, in order to fully realise the promise of BIIHS, it is necessary to solve problems such as regulation compliance, interoperability, and privacy concerns. Artificial intelligence and the internet of things are two examples of upcoming technologies that might be included into BIIHS in the future. This would allow for the healthcare sector to further improve its capabilities.

Chapter 8

Megha Bhushan, DIT University, India
Maanas Singal, DIT University, India
Arun Negi, Deliotte USI, India

Autism spectrum disorder (ASD) is a behavioural and developmental illness caused by brain abnormalities. Individuals with ASD have difficulty with limited or repeated acts, as well as social communication and participation. Additionally, people with ASD may learn, move, or pay attention in various ways. It should be remembered that some individuals without ASD may also experience some of these symptoms. However, these traits may render life very difficult for those with ASD. Since the trend of machine learning (ML) and deep learning (DL) techniques has been on an onset in every domain, the same is being actively utilized for diagnosis and treatment of this aliment. This chapter provides an in-depth insight into the efforts of researchers on diverse crowd for development and implementation of ML/DL models to assist the ailing individual along with their families and health caregivers. It provides the review of existing works in diverse directions in focus with ASD like prediction, segregation, correlation, etc. between parameters which would help the medical professionals.

Chapter 9
    Hariharan S., SASTRA University (Deemed), India
    Hemalatha Karnan, SASTRA University (Deemed), India
    Uma Maheshwari D., SASTRA University (Deemed), India

Electrocardiogram (ECG) acts as a symptomatic tool that routinely analyzes the functions of the heart. Till recently, most ECG records were kept on thermal paper. The evaluation of ECG charts needs considerable training and can be time-consuming and daunting process. The evaluation of ECG charts needs considerable training and can be time-consuming and daunting process. We can perform diagnosis and analysis with automation by digitizing the paper ECG. We can perform diagnosis and analysis with automation by digitizing the paper ECG. The main goal of this chapter is physical to-digital fusion of ECG signal and implement machine learning algorithm. This can be achieved by extracting the P, QRS, and T waves in ECG signals to demonstrate the heart's electrical activity using various techniques. The web-based application can make use of a machine-learning algorithm that analyzes and diagnoses cardiac disorders and normal conditions by uploading the ECG image. Thereby it reduces the time-consuming and daunting process for the analysis of ECG reports.

Chapter 10
    Pancham Singh, Ajay Kumar Garg Engineering College, Ghaziabad, India
    Mrignainy Kansal, Ajay Kumar Garg Engineering College, Ghaziabad, India
    Ayush Pratap Singh, Ajay Kumar Garg Engineering College, Ghaziabad, India
    Ayushi Verma, Ajay Kumar Garg Engineering College, Ghaziabad, India
    Snigdha Tyagi, Ajay Kumar Garg Engineering College, Ghaziabad, India
    Aditya Vikram Singh, Ajay Kumar Garg Engineering College, Ghaziabad, India

Early disease diagnosis is crucial for effective treatment, but current healthcare methods have limitations. Supervised machine learning algorithms, particularly deep learning networks, have proven effective in developing medical diagnostics and real-time applications for detecting high-risk diseases. This paper evaluates five algorithms: Multilayer perceptron (MLP), random forest, decision tree, Naive Bayes, and K-Nearest neighbours (KNN) for predicting diseases based on user-entered symptoms. MLP outperformed other algorithms, achieving an accuracy of 97.2%, which is 4-5% higher than existing disease prediction models. Notably, existing techniques account for only 94% accuracy on average. Highlighting the potential of MLP in early disease diagnosis, this paper concludes by summarizing its goals, challenges, and outcomes.

    Mrignainy Kansal, Ajay Kumar Garg Engineering College, Ghaziabad, India
    Pancham Singh, Ajay Kumar Garg Engineering College, Ghaziabad, India
    Prashant Srivastava, Ajay Kumar Garg Engineering College, Ghaziabad, India
    Radhika Singhal, Ajay Kumar Garg Engineering College, Ghaziabad, India
    Nishant Deep, Ajay Kumar Garg Engineering College, Ghaziabad, India
    Arpit Singh, Ajay Kumar Garg Engineering College, Ghaziabad, India

Social media has become a significant factor in the development of mental diseases, with the potential to significantly impact people's lives. This study explores the use of computational approaches and deep learning models to identify linguistic indicators suggestive of mental diseases such as depression, anorexia, and self-harm. The study also highlights the complex relationship between emotions and the underlying causes of mental diseases, emphasizing the need for understanding emotional triggers. The research demonstrates the effectiveness of machine learning models in detecting anxiety and depression on websites like Twitter, Facebook, and Reddit, particularly during the COVID-19 pandemic. The study highlights the potential of data mining techniques for automating the diagnosis of Social Network Mental Disorders among social media users, aiming to improve lives and address the rising incidence of mental illnesses in society.

    Shabnam Kumari, SRM Institute of Science and Technology, Chennai, India
    Amit Kumar Tyagi, National Institute of Fashion Technology, New Delhi, India
    Avinash Kumar Sharma, Sharda School of Engineering and Technology (SSET), Sharda
        University, India

In the recent decade, emerging, assistive, and digital technologies have revolutionized the field of telemedicine, enabling remote healthcare delivery, improving patient outcomes, and expanding access to medical services. This chapter provides an overview of the advancements and applications of these technologies in telemedicine systems. Today mobile apps provide convenient access to medical services, appointment scheduling, medication reminders, and health education. EHRs store and share patient information securely, enabling seamless collaboration and continuity of care across healthcare settings. Telemedicine apps provide intuitive interfaces for video consultations, remote examinations, and sharing of medical data, facilitating efficient remote diagnosis and treatment. Hence, emerging, assistive, and digital technologies have transformed telemedicine, enhancing healthcare delivery, patient engagement, and access to specialized medical expertise. These technologies have the potential to revolutionize healthcare systems, particularly in remote and underserved areas.

    Sachin Jain, Ajay Kumar Garg Engineering College, Ghaziabad, India
    Preeti Jaidka, JSS Academy of Technical Education, India

Abnormal growths in the lungs caused by disease. The classification of CT scans is accomplished by applying machine learning strategies. Classification methods based on deep learning, such as support vector machines, can categorize a wide variety of image datasets and produce segmentation results of the highest caliber. In this work, we suggested a method for deep feature extraction from images by altering SVM and CNN and then applying the hybrid model resulting from those modifications (NNSVLC). For this investigation, the Kaggle dataset will be utilized. The proposed method was found to be accurate 91.7% of the time, as determined by the results of the experiments.

Chapter 14

This study explores the economic implications of immediate magnetic resonance imaging (MRI) in treating suspected scaphoid fractures. Historically, conventional methods have been used, but recent advancements have introduced MRI into acute care settings, challenging established diagnostic paradigms. The study aims to close the empirical-economic evidence gap on the prompt use of MRI in cases with suspected scaphoid fractures, providing insight into cost-effectiveness, resource use, and overall healthcare efficiency. The literature study illuminates the evolution of diagnostic approaches for scaphoid fractures, highlighting the limitations of conventional methods. The findings underscore the pivotal role of MRI in scaphoid fracture management, demonstrating cost-effectiveness and enhanced healthcare outcomes, challenging traditional diagnostic pathways.

Chapter 15

In today's smart era, the healthcare landscape is rapidly evolving, driven by advancements in technology and the growing healthcare needs of an aging and increasingly interconnected society. To address these challenges, the concept of digital twins has emerged as a promising solution to transform healthcare services for the next generation. This work provides an overview of the key aspects and benefits of digital twin-based smart healthcare services and their potential to revolutionize the healthcare industry. DWT involves creating a digital replica or model of a physical entity, in this case, an individual's health and medical data. By harnessing real-time data from various sources, including wearable devices, electronic health records, and medical imaging, Digital Twins provide a holistic view of an individual's health status, treatment history, and predictive analytics for future health outcomes. This work provides information about data-driven approach enables healthcare providers to make more informed decisions and tailor personalized treatment plans/ improving patient outcomes.

Preface

In the rapidly evolving landscape of healthcare, the convergence of artificial intelligence (AI) has emerged as a transformative force, particularly in the realm of medical imaging. This book serves as an introduction to the comprehensive exploration of the future of AI in medical imaging, discussing about the revolutionary advancements, challenges, and ethical considerations that accompany this major shift. The intersection of AI and medical imaging holds immense promise, promising to enhance diagnostic accuracy, streamline workflows, and ultimately improve patient outcomes. As we embark on this journey into the future, it is important to understand the essential role that AI plays in reshaping the landscape of medical imaging.

This book project brings together the insights of experts, etc., at the forefront of AI and medical imaging, offering an important perspective on the ongoing developments and the potential trajectory of this dynamic field. From state-of-the-art image recognition algorithms to the integration of machine learning in radiology, the chapters within this book explore the various facets of AI applications in medical imaging (also including blockchain technology).

Note that with these revolutionary advancements come some serious issue like ethical, privacy and the need for responsible deployment or security. As we entrust AI with critical healthcare decisions, it becomes imperative to establish robust frameworks that ensure transparency, accountability, and patient-centric care. Hence, the Future of AI in Medical Imaging seeks to foster a dialogue among researchers, scientists, the wider public, aiming to demystify the complexities of AI in healthcare and encourage a collaborative approach to harnessing its potential. By exploring the challenges and opportunities presented by AI in medical imaging, this compilation strives to guide the trajectory of future research and development in the pursuit of a more efficient, accurate, and humane healthcare system. As we stand in a new era in medicine, let this compilation serve as a guiding beacon, explaining the path toward a future where the convergence between AI and medical imaging enhances our ability to diagnose, treat, and prevent diseases, ultimately improving the well-being of individuals and communities worldwide.

We hope that you will enjoy a lot in reading this book on this emerging topic.

Chapter 1
Use of AI in Medical Image Processing

Sheelesh Kumar Sharma
ABESIT Engineering College, Ghaziabad, India

ABSTRACT

Artificial intelligence (AI) integration in medical image processing is a game-changing breakthrough in modern healthcare. This cutting-edge technology takes a multidimensional approach to diagnosis, treatment, and patient care, opening up significant prospects for improved medical outcomes and resource optimization. AI has proven its image analysis prowess in applications such as disease detection and diagnosis. Machine learning algorithms, combined with massive datasets of medical pictures, allow for precise and speedy detection of anomalies in radiological scans such as X-rays, CT scans, MRIs, and ultrasounds. Early diagnosis of diseases such as cancer, neurological disorders, and cardiovascular ailments has improved, allowing for earlier intervention and personalized treatment plans. Incorporation of AI in medical image processing is revolutionizing healthcare by boosting diagnosis speed and accuracy, optimizing treatment planning, and improving patient care.

1. INTRODUCTION

Artificial intelligence (AI) integration in medical image processing is a game-changing breakthrough in modern healthcare. This cutting-edge technology takes a multidimensional approach to diagnosis, treatment, and patient care, opening up significant prospects for improved medical outcomes and resource optimization. AI has proven its image analysis prowess in applications such as disease detection and diagnosis. Machine learning algorithms, combined with massive datasets of medical pictures, allow for precise and speedy detection of anomalies in radiological scans such as X-rays, CT scans, MRIs, and ultrasounds. Early diagnosis of diseases such as cancer, neurological disorders, and cardiovascular ailments has improved, allowing for earlier intervention and personalized treatment plans. Incorporation of AI in medical image processing is revolutionizing healthcare by boosting diagnosis speed and accuracy, optimizing treatment planning, and improving patient care. This transition holds the possibility of more efficient healthcare systems and, most crucially, improved patient outcomes, and it represents a huge

DOI: 10.4018/979-8-3693-2359-5.ch001

step forward in the pursuit of enhanced medical excellence. This chapter provides a succinct review of the fundamental uses and consequences of artificial intelligence in medical image processing. Incorporation of AI in medical image processing is revolutionizing healthcare by boosting diagnosis speed and accuracy, optimizing treatment planning, and improving patient care. This transition holds the possibility of more efficient healthcare systems and, most crucially, improved patient outcomes, and it represents a huge step forward in the pursuit of enhanced medical excellence.

AI has found several uses in medical image processing, transforming how doctors diagnose, treat, and manage diseases. Here are some significant applications of AI in this field

- Disease Detection and Diagnosis: AI is able to recognize early indicators of breast, lung, or prostate cancer by analyzing mammograms, CT scans, and MRI pictures (Summers et al., 2016). *Artificial intelligence (AI)* may identify heart diseases such structural anomalies or ischemia by analyzing cardiac pictures, such as echocardiograms. *Neurological Disorders*; by examining brain MRIs, AI helps diagnose diseases like multiple sclerosis and Alzheimer's disease. *Diabetic Retinopathy*; by examining retinal images, AI is able to identify and classify the degree of diabetic retinopathy.
- Image Segmentation: AI algorithms can segment medical images to separate and identify particular regions of interest, such as organs, blood arteries, or tumors(Warfield et al., 2004).
- Image Registration: AI assists in the alignment and overlaying of various medical images for comparison, making it easier to monitor the course of a disease or the efficacy of a treatment (Viergever et al., 2016).
- Helping Pathologists and Radiologists: Artificial Intelligence (AI) gives pathologists and radiologist's tools to improve their diagnostic skills. It can shorten the time needed for picture interpretation, draw attention to anomalies, and make suggestions about possible diagnosis (Tang et al., 2018).
- 3D Reconstruction: AI is able to convert 2D medical pictures into 3D models, which is especially helpful for surgical planning and the visualization of intricate anatomical components.
- Treatment Planning: By offering information on tumor size, location, and closeness to vital structures, artificial intelligence (AI) assists surgeons and oncologists in planning their treatments.
- Real-time Image Analysis: By evaluating intra operative images and supporting surgeons in making decisions, artificial intelligence (AI) can offer real-time direction and information during surgery.
- Remote Diagnostics: AI is used in telemedicine to help doctors in far-off places by evaluating pictures and providing diagnostic assistance.
- Drug Discovery: By identifying possible therapeutic targets through the analysis of cellular and molecular pictures, artificial intelligence (AI) helps pharmaceutical companies discover novel medications.
- Predictive Analytics: AI can forecast the possibility of specific illnesses, the course of a disease, or patient outcomes using clinical data and past medical imaging(Simmons et al., 2011).
- Image Enhancement: AI may raise the clarity, boost contrast, and lower noise in medical photos to help with diagnosis.

Better patient outcomes could result from the application of AI in medical image processing (Figure 1), which has the potential to increase accessibility, efficiency, and accuracy in the field of medicine.

When applying AI solutions in the medical industry, it's imperative to take data protection, algorithm openness, and ethical and legal issues into account.

Figure 1. Uses of AI in medical image processing

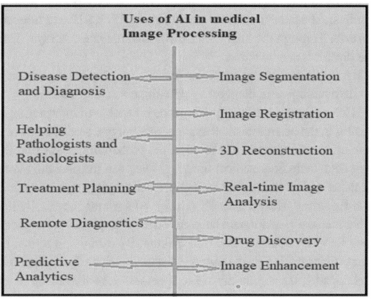

2. DISEASE DETECTION AND DIAGNOSIS

One of the most important uses of AI in healthcare, especially in the area of medical image processing, is the diagnosis and identification of diseases. A vast array of illnesses and medical disorders can be identified and diagnosed by healthcare practitioners with the help of AI technologies. Here's how AI is applied to the diagnosis and detection of diseases

- Medical Imaging Analysis: AI is utilized to analyze different types of medical imaging modalities, including CT, MRI, ultrasound, and X-rays. It can offer insights into disorders of the organs, tumors, and fractures as well as assist in identifying anomalies in these pictures. Histopathology slides are crucial for the diagnosis of diseases like cancer, and AI is capable of analyzing them. In addition to identifying malignant cells and assessing their severity, machine learning algorithms can also forecast patient outcomes.
- Cancer Diagnosis and Detection: Artificial Intelligence plays a critical role in the early diagnosis of cancer, particularly skin, lung, breast, and prostate cancers. Artificial Intelligence can detect possible tumors or lesions by examining dermatological photos, CT scans, and mammograms.
- Cardiovascular Disease: Echocardiograms, CT angiograms, and other cardiac imaging are analyzed by AI to aid in the diagnosis of heart-related disorders. It is capable of detecting symptoms of coronary artery disease, identifying anatomical abnormalities, and evaluating heart function.

- Neurological Disorders: AI is able to identify and diagnose neurological diseases including multiple sclerosis, Alzheimer's disease, and stroke by analyzing brain MRIs. It facilitates the detection of anomalies, lesions, and brain shrinkage.
- Ophthalmology: By examining retinal images, artificial intelligence in ophthalmology is able to diagnose diseases such as age-related macular degeneration and diabetic retinopathy. It has the ability to classify these illnesses' severity, which is essential for prompt action.
- Infectious disorders: AI can help with the diagnosis of COVID-19 and tuberculosis, among other infectious disorders. Through the analysis of CT scans and chest X-rays, distinctive patterns related to various disorders can be found.
- Dermatology: By examining photos of moles, rashes, or other anomalies on the skin, AI-driven tools can assist dermatologists in diagnosing skin ailments and diseases.
- Endoscopy and Colonoscopy: Artificial intelligence is capable of interpreting endoscopic pictures to detect anomalies in the gastrointestinal system, like polyps, ulcers, or tumors.
- Predictive Diagnostics: AI systems can forecast the probability of specific illnesses or ailments based on patient data, including medical imaging. They can forecast the likelihood of cardiovascular events or the course of diabetic retinopathy, for example.
- Integration with Electronic Health Records (EHR): AI systems may easily interface with EHRs, guaranteeing that medical practitioners have easy access to pertinent diagnostic information and medical imaging for more informed decision-making. By examining retinal images, artificial intelligence in ophthalmology is able to diagnose diseases such as age-related macular degeneration and diabetic retinopathy. It can classify these illnesses' severity, which is essential for prompt action.

AI in disease detection and diagnosis has many benefits, including better access to healthcare, especially in underserved areas, faster results, decreased diagnostic errors, and enhanced accuracy. To deliver the greatest patient care possible, it's crucial to make sure AI technologies are thoroughly examined, verified, and employed in concert with medical professionals. Using AI for disease detection and diagnosis also requires careful consideration of data privacy, transparency, and ethical and legal issues.

3. IMAGE SEGMENTATION

A key task in computer vision and medical image processing is image segmentation, which is breaking an image up into meaningful and discrete sections or segments. Applications like object recognition, computer-aided diagnostics, and medical picture analysis depend on this mechanism. Image segmentation is a critical step in medical image processing that helps isolate and identify particular structures or regions of interest in medical pictures(Okada et al., 2015). The following is an example of how picture segmentation is applied in medicine

- Tumor Detection and Localization: Image segmentation is used in radiology to locate and identify tumor in medical pictures, such as X-rays, CT scans, and MRIs. Precise tumor segmentation facilitates treatment planning, tumor growth tracking, and therapy efficacy evaluation.

- Organ Segmentation: In medical imaging, organs or other anatomical structures can be identified and highlighted using image segmentation. For an all-encompassing evaluation of these structures, it can be utilized, for instance, to isolate the liver, kidneys, heart, and lungs in CT images.
- Vessel Segmentation: The cerebral vasculature and coronary arteries are two examples of blood vessels that can be isolated using image segmentation in cardiovascular imaging. This is important for the diagnosis and treatment planning of vascular disorders, including the implantation of stents.
- Brain Segmentation: Various brain areas, including the white matter, grey matter, and cerebrospinal fluid, are segmented using image segmentation in neuro imaging. This holds significance in the field of brain mapping and neurological illness research.
- Cell Segmentation: On histopathology slides, individual cells or nuclei are isolated and identified via image segmentation in pathology. For the study of tissue samples and the detection of illnesses like cancer, this is essential.
- Lesion Segmentation: To identify and describe skin lesions, dermatologists utilize picture segmentation. This technique can be useful in the diagnosis of skin conditions, such as melanoma.
- Image Fusion: Data from various imaging modalities can be combined using image segmentation, for example, combining CT and MRI scans to provide more thorough information during treatment planning (Iglesias et al., 2015).
- 3D Image reconstruction: By using segmentation to create 3D models from 2D medical images, anatomical structures can be seen more clearly for surgical planning.
- Radiation Therapy Planning: To guarantee that the tumor receives an appropriate dose while minimizing damage to adjacent healthy tissue, radiation therapy planning for cancer treatment requires accurate tumor and organ segmentation.
- Endoscopy and Colonoscopy: To locate and emphasize problematic spots inside the gastrointestinal tract, like polyps or ulcers, image segmentation is performed to endoscopic pictures (Van et al., 2001).

Many techniques are commonly used to do image segmentation, including more sophisticated methods incorporating deep learning algorithms like convolution neural networks (CNNs) and more conventional methods like thresholding, edge detection, and region-growing. Recent years have seen a tremendous success of deep learning-based methods, especially in tasks requiring precise and sophisticated segmentation (LeCun et al., 2015).

For the purpose of increasing the accuracy of medical condition monitoring, treatment planning, and diagnosis, accurate picture segmentation is essential. Better patient outcomes and more effective healthcare delivery result from its ability to help medical practitioners concentrate on certain regions of interest within medical images(Park et al., 2003).

4. IMAGE REGISTRATION

Aligning and superimposing two or more medical photographs of the same patient or anatomical region is known as image registration, and it is a critical method in medical image processing. Assuring that the images are in the same coordinate system is the aim of image registration, as this enables precise information fusion, analysis, and comparison from various imaging modalities or time points. In the medical industry, image registration is utilized as follows

- Multi-Modal Imaging Fusion: Image registration allows data from many imaging modalities, such computed tomography (CT) and magnetic resonance imaging (MRI), to be combined. A more thorough understanding of the patient's anatomy and path physiology is provided by this fusion.
- Time-Series Analysis: Image registration is used in longitudinal studies to align images captured at various times in order to monitor the evolution of neurological disorders or the growth of tumors.
- Evaluation of Pre- and Post-Treatment: Image registration is essential for evaluating the efficacy of medical procedures like surgery or radiation therapy. It enables the evaluation of changes and the accuracy of the therapy by comparing photographs taken before and after the procedure.III
- Image-Guided Surgery: During minimally invasive surgeries, surgeons use image registration to guide them, ensuring exact targeting and the avoidance of important structures. By lining up pre-operative pictures with the patient's anatomy during surgery, it offers real-time advice.
- Respiratory Motion Compensation: To account for respiratory or cardiac motion in lung and cardiac imaging, image registration is utilized. This improves diagnosis and therapy planning.
- Functional Imaging: To pinpoint the precise location of functional abnormalities inside the body, image registration aligns functional pictures, such as PET and SPECT scans, with anatomical images, such as CT or MRI.
- Atlas-Based Analysis: By aligning patient pictures with a common anatomical atlas, image registration enables comparison analysis and helps spot outliers.
- 3D Image Reconstruction: Image registration is used to combine several 2D images to produce 3D models in radiation therapy and other applications. This facilitates understanding intricate anatomical structures.
- Interventional Radiology: By giving real-time feedback on needle placement, image registration is essential to image-guided treatments like percutaneous needle biopsies.
- Pediatric Medicine: Image registration is used in pediatric medicine to track changes in children's anatomical structures over time and to direct congenital condition therapies.

There are several ways to register an image: from simple translation, rotation, and scaling rigid (affine) transformations to more intricate non-rigid transformations that take local deformations into consideration. Additionally, sophisticated methods including deep learning and artificial intelligence have been developed to raise the precision and effectiveness of picture registration(Ferrante et al., 2017).

In medical image processing, image registration is a vital tool that minimizes patient harm while giving medical practitioners vital information for diagnosis, therapy planning, and intervention(Sharma et al., 2019).

5. ASSISTING RADIOLOGISTS AND PATHOLOGISTS

AI is a big help to pathologists and radiologists with their diagnosis and interpretation work. Artificial intelligence (AI) increases efficiency and improves the accuracy of medical image interpretation by automating repetitive and time-consuming tasks (Chartrand et al., 2017). AI helps radiologists and pathologists in the following ways:

5.1 Radiology

- Abnormality Detection: Artificial intelligence (AI) algorithms may be trained to recognize lesions, tumors, and fractures in medical images. They can identify possible trouble spots that radiologists should investigate further.
- Priority Triage: Radiologists can concentrate on the most urgent cases first by using AI algorithms to prioritize cases according to the severity of discovered anomalies.
- Second Opinion: By offering more insights, lowering the likelihood of missed diagnoses, and boosting diagnostic confidence, AI can act as a "second pair of eyes" for radiologists.
- Quantitative Analysis: Artificial Intelligence helps with quantitative analysis, which includes calculating the height and diameter of tumors and the degree of tissue damage caused by illnesses like multiple sclerosis.
- Tracking Disease evolution: By analyzing consecutive imaging studies, AI can assist in tracking the evolution of diseases over time, which is important for determining the efficacy of treatments and organizing patient care.
- Image Enhancement: AI can brighten, contrast, and reduce noise in images to improve their quality and make it easier for radiologists to interpret them correctly.
- Automatic Report Generation: By extracting important results and measures from medical pictures, AI can assist in the generation of preliminary radiology reports, saving radiologists' time on administrative duties.

5.2 Pathology

- Tissue and Cell Detection: Pathologists can find regions of interest more rapidly by using AI algorithms to recognize and distinguish particular tissues and cells on histopathology slides.
- Cancer Grading: AI can assign a grade to a malignant lesion based on its severity, giving pathologists more information to help with diagnosis and therapy planning.
- Cell Classification: AI is capable of classifying structures or cells on pathology slides. For example, it can distinguish between cancerous and healthy cells, which are essential for precise diagnosis.
- Accelerating Screening: AI can pre-screen pathology slides in screening programmers to find possibly problematic cases, freeing up pathologists to concentrate on situations that need more investigation.
- Data Organization: Pathologists may find and retrieve specific cases or patient histories more easily thanks to AI's assistance in indexing and organizing pathology slides.
- Quality Control: By spotting staining or preparation artifacts and guaranteeing the correctness of pathology slides, AI systems can help with quality control.
- Telepathology: Artificial intelligence plays a key role in telepathology, allowing pathologists to evaluate and diagnose patients from a distance. This is especially helpful in rural or disadvantaged areas.
- Prognostication and prediction: By examining pathology slides and patient data, AI can forecast patient outcomes or the severity of a disease.

The purpose of AI's assistance to radiologists and pathologists is to supplement human expertise rather than replace it. Artificial intelligence (AI) frees up healthcare workers to concentrate on complex situations and clinical decision-making by automating repetitive processes and offering assistance with data analysis and interpretation. Additionally, it enhances diagnostic precision, lowers diagnostic mistakes, and boosts productivity in medical environments(Sharma et al., 2019).

6. 3D RECONSTRUCTION

In the context of medical image processing, three-dimensional (3D) reconstruction is the process of building a three-dimensional model from a sequence of two-dimensional medical pictures, such as CT scans, MRIs, or X-rays, depicting anatomical structures or objects. This method has many uses and is frequently employed in the medical field. Here are some examples of how 3D reconstruction is used in medicine

- Surgical Planning: Surgeons can better see intricate anatomical structures in three dimensions thanks to 3D modeling. Examples of these structures include the heart and brain. This helps with surgical planning, choosing the best places to make incisions, and avoiding important structures.
- Orthopedics: To evaluate bone abnormalities, schedule orthopedic procedures, and create orthopedic implants or prostheses tailored to each patient, orthopedics uses 3D reconstructions.
- Dental Implants: 3D reconstruction is a crucial tool in dentistry as it helps with custom crowns and bridges as well as implant placement planning.
- Radiotherapy Planning: To precisely target tumors with radiation therapy while preserving healthy tissue, 3D reconstructions are utilized.
- Visualizing Complex Structures: Three-dimensional (3D) reconstruction offers a clear and comprehensive perspective for diagnostic and treatment planning for anatomical structures with complex geometries, such as the human airway or vascular system.
- Cardiovascular Imaging: To see the heart chambers and coronary arteries, cardiologists utilize 3D reconstructions. They support the process of locating obstructions, organizing actions, and evaluating valve performance.
- Visualization of Tumors: 3D tumor reconstructions facilitate the evaluation of a tumor's dimensions, form, and relationship to surrounding structures—information that is crucial for surgical planning.
- Educational Tools: To help medical professionals and student's better grasp anatomy and diseases, medical educators employ 3D reconstruction as a teaching tool.
- Tracking Disease Progression: 3D reconstructions are useful for tracking chronic diseases since they may be used to track changes in anatomical structures and disease progression over time.
- Interventional Radiology: During treatments like embolisation or catheter implantation, interventional radiologists can receive improved guidance thanks to 3D reconstructions.

The following steps are usually involved in the 3D reconstruction process

- Image Acquisition: Usually in the form of CT or MRI scans, a series of 2D medical pictures are obtained.

- Image Preprocessing: Artifacts, noise, and inconsistencies are corrected in the captured images by preprocessing.
- Image Registration: To make sure the photos are in the same spatial coordinate system, they are registered and aligned.
- Segmentation: The images are segmented or isolated to reveal the areas of interest, such as particular organs or structures.
- 3D Model Generation: Using the segmented photos, a volumetric representation of the item is created by stacking the 2D slices in the right order to generate a 3D model.
- Visualization and Analysis: Specialized software can be used to visualize and analyze the 3D model. It is able to be real-time altered and deconstructed for in-depth analysis.

Because 3D reconstruction offers a more comprehensive and intuitive representation of anatomical components, it has significantly increased the accuracy of diagnosis and treatment planning. Additionally, it makes it possible to build patient-specific models, which are very helpful for optimizing medical processes and delivering personalized treatment.

7. TREATMENT PLANNING

In the medical industry, treatment planning is the methodical process of creating a patient's unique treatment plan based on their medical condition, diagnostic data, and therapeutic objectives. In this process, medical imaging and related technologies are essential. The following describes the process of treatment planning and the function of medical image processing in this regard

- Patient Assessment: A thorough evaluation of the patient's medical history, clinical results, and diagnostic data including images from CT, MRI, X-ray, and ultrasound scans that is the first step in the process.
- Diagnostic Imaging: Radiologists and other specialists evaluate medical images to make crucial diagnostic choices. These images give comprehensive information about the anatomy of the patient as well as the location and severity of diseases or anomalies.
- Multidisciplinary Team: To develop a thorough treatment plan for complicated situations, a multidisciplinary team of medical specialists, comprising radiologists, oncologists, surgeons, and pathologists, works together.
- Image Segmentation and Analysis: Medicinal image processing methods define, measure, and segment areas of interest, such as organs, tumors, or other structures. This helps determine the treatment focus and neighboring vital buildings that need to be avoided.
- Quantitative Assessment: Treatment planning relies heavily on the quantitative measures obtained from medical pictures to determine the target's dimensions, volume, and other features. For instance, accurate tumor size assessments are necessary to determine dosage in radiation therapy.
- Selecting the Treatment Modality: Medical practitioners select the best course of action based on the features of the disease and the diagnostic data. This could involve immunotherapy, radiation therapy, chemotherapy, surgery, or a mix of these.
- Radiation Therapy Planning: A radiation treatment plan is created in radiation therapy using medical imaging as a reference. In order to provide the target area with the highest dose possible while

protecting healthy tissues, the treatment planner creates the radiation beams and determines the dosage.

- Surgical Planning: To guarantee accuracy during surgery, the incision, access locations, and approach are planned using 3D reconstructions of anatomical features from medical pictures.
- Chemotherapy and Drug Selection: Especially in oncology, medical imaging aids in determining the degree of tumor involvement and directs the choice of additional medications or chemotherapeutic agents.
- Monitoring and Follow-Up: Using medical imaging, treatment plans are modified as needed based on how the patient responds to treatment over time. Imaging follow-up aids in evaluating the efficacy of the selected treatment.
- Personalized Medicine: A growing component of treatment planning is personalized medicine, which combines imaging data with patient genetic and molecular information to customize medicines to each patient's unique requirements.
- Reducing Side Effects: Using medical imaging to precisely arrange treatments reduces harm to healthy tissue, lessens side effects, and enhances patient outcomes.
- Treatment Delivery: Medical personnel carry out the finalized treatment plan, which may include radiation therapy, chemotherapy, surgery, or other methods.

Medical image processing directs the entire treatment planning process in addition to helping with the initial diagnosis. It enables medical professionals to make well-informed choices, optimize the effectiveness of treatments, and reduce the negative effects on healthy tissue. Patients consequently receive more individualized and focused therapy, which eventually improves results.

8. REAL-TIME IMAGE ANALYSIS

In the medical domain, real-time image analysis refers to the instantaneous and automated evaluation of medical images as they are obtained. During medical treatments, this technique enables quick decision-making and gives medical experts vital information instantly. The following are some significant uses of real-time image analysis in the medical field

- Surgical Navigation: Surgeons can receive visual direction during operations thanks to real-time picture analysis. By superimposing preoperative pictures, like CT or MRI scans, onto the surgical field, it facilitates the surgeons' navigation and localization of vital structures.
- Image-Guided Interventions: Real-time image analysis in interventional radiology facilitates operations like embolisation, angiography, and catheter placement. It aids in providing direction for the insertion of medical equipment and therapy administration.
- Intraoperative Imaging: During surgery, real-time image analysis enables prompt evaluation of tissue health, abnormality detection, and procedure success confirmation. In orthopedics and neurosurgery in particular, intraoperative imaging can be quite significant.
- Endoscopy: In order to discover anomalies in the gastrointestinal tract, respiratory system, or other bodily cavities as soon as possible, real-time picture analysis is essential to endoscopic treatments.

- Ultrasound: During pregnancy, soft tissues, blood flow, and foetal development can all be seen using real-time ultrasound imaging. Tools powered by AI can assist in automating measurements and finding anomalies.
- Intravascular Imaging: Real-time image analysis is utilized during cardiology procedures to evaluate coronary artery health and direct the implantation of stents and other devices.
- Guidance for Radiation Therapy: Real-time imaging guarantees accurate tumor targeting during radiation therapy and reduces the amount of radiation that is exposed to healthy tissue. It is essential for both therapy efficacy and safety.
- Fluoroscopy: In processes like orthopedics, cardiology, and gastroenterology that call for continuous X-ray imaging, real-time picture analysis is employed.
- Telemedicine: During video consultations, remote healthcare providers can evaluate patient symptoms and offer prompt assistance thanks to real-time picture analysis via telemedicine.
- Point-of-Care Diagnostics: Handheld ultrasound equipment are used for brief assessments in emergency circumstances, and real-time image analysis is used for these examinations.
- Emergency Medicine: In cases of trauma, real-time picture processing helps ER doctors make quick decisions that enable prompt diagnosis and treatment planning.

Real-time image analysis can guide treatments, guarantee the precision and safety of medical procedures, and provide important information about the patient's state in various applications. Real-time image analysis is becoming more and more integrated with artificial intelligence and machine learning, enabling automated anomaly identification, picture improvement, and decision support. Better patient outcomes result from this technology, which also increases healthcare delivery's effectiveness and efficiency(Sharma et al., 2020).

9. REMOTE DIAGNOSIS

The use of artificial intelligence (AI) in remote diagnosis is a transformative application that leverages advanced technologies to facilitate accurate and timely healthcare assessments without the need for physical proximity between the healthcare provider and the patient. Here are several ways in which AI is employed in remote diagnosis.

- Store-and-Forward Telemedicine: Using photos or videos, people document symptoms like wounds or rashes and forward them to medical professionals for assessment. After looking over these pictures, the medical professionals recommend a course of action and a diagnosis.
- Medical Imaging Sharing: Patients can give distant healthcare practitioners access to their medical imaging, such as MRIs, CT scans, and X-rays. Radiologists and other experts examine these pictures in order to make diagnoses, including tumors and fractures.
- Dermatology Consultations: By examining pictures of rashes, moles, or other skin problems that patients send in, dermatologists can diagnose skin disorders from a distance. The identification and management of skin conditions can be aided by dermatological image analysis.
- Ophthalmology Consultations: Retinal imaging is frequently provided as part of remote ophthalmology services. Ophthalmologists can evaluate retinal photos taken by patients in order to diagnose eye diseases such as macular degeneration or diabetic retinopathy.

- Remote Monitoring: One of the features of remote diagnostics for patients with long-term medical disorders is the ongoing monitoring of vital signs including blood pressure, heart rate, and glucose levels. Healthcare professionals receive data from monitoring devices and can make necessary adjustments to treatment programmers.
- Pathology Consultations: To detect conditions like cancer, pathologists can remotely evaluate histopathology slides. The use of whole slide imaging technology enables in-depth tissue sample analysis.
- Emergency Remote Diagnostics: In an emergency, paramedics and emergency medical technicians can communicate with distant doctors via live video and picture sharing to evaluate vital conditions and provide prompt treatment.
- Imaging Teleradiology: The study and analysis of medical pictures from various geographic areas by remote radiologists. This is especially helpful for coverage during the weekends or at night in hospitals and other locations where radiologists are not readily available.
- Teleconsultations with experts: By using remote diagnostics, primary care doctors can confer with experts to guarantee that patients obtain professional advice without the need for in-person referrals.
- Second opinions: Before beginning significant therapies or for difficult medical issues, patients might get second views from distant healthcare providers. This aids in the validation of treatment strategies and diagnosis.
- Teledentistry: By using pictures or real-time video consultations, dental experts can evaluate dental problems and provide advice for therapy. the weekends or at night in hospitals and other locations where radiologists are not readily available.
- Teleconsultations with experts: By using remote diagnostics, primary care doctors can confer with experts to guarantee that patients obtain professional advice without the need for in-person referrals.
- Second opinions: Before beginning significant therapies or for difficult medical issues, patients might get second views from distant healthcare providers. This aids in the validation of treatment strategies and diagnosis.
- Teledentistry: By using pictures or real-time video consultations, dental experts can evaluate dental problems and provide advice for therapy.

Medical image analysis and other remote diagnostics have many benefits, including bettering healthcare access in underprivileged areas, lowering travel expenses, and facilitating prompt diagnosis and treatment. It does, however, present certain difficulties, such as protecting data privacy, security, and the requirement for top-notch imaging equipment. It is anticipated that remote diagnostics would keep contributing significantly to improving patient care and increasing access to healthcare.

10. DRUG DISCOVERY

The process of finding new drugs is difficult and time-consuming in the realm of pharmaceutical development. To produce drugs that can treat, cure, or prevent diseases, it entails the discovery of novel compounds or the repurposing of preexisting ones. Deep learning and machine learning are two types of artificial intelligence (AI) that have become indispensable for accelerating the drug discovery process. Using AI in drug discovery works like this

- Target Identification: By examining biological data, such as genomic and proteomic information, AI can assist in the identification of possible therapeutic targets. It helps identify compounds that can interact with these targets and comprehend the fundamental causes of disorders.
- Compound Screening: By identifying which compounds are most likely to have the intended biological effects, AI speeds up the screening of huge chemical compound libraries. As a result, fewer actual experiments are needed.
- Chemo informatics: AI analyses a compound's chemical attributes to help researchers find lead compounds and improve their structural integrity for increased safety and efficacy.
- Generative Chemistry: AI-powered generative models are able to suggest unique chemical structures that may be suitable for future pharmaceuticals. This method works very well for creating novel compounds with certain characteristics.
- Biological Assay Design: Artificial Intelligence can be used to optimize biological assay design, making sure that the tests are sensitive, specific, and economical when assessing possible therapeutic candidates.
- Data Analysis: To find biomarkers, possible treatment targets, and disease-relevant pathways, AI can process and analyze enormous volumes of omics data (such as genomes, transcriptomics, and proteomics).
- Drug-Drug Interaction Prediction: Artificial intelligence models are able to anticipate possible drug interactions and evaluate the safety of mixing various prescriptions.
- Toxicology Prediction: By predicting a compound's and its metabolites' probable toxicity, artificial intelligence (AI) lowers the possibility of unfavorable outcomes in clinical trials.
- Modeling Pharmacokinetics and Pharmacodynamics: Artificial Intelligence facilitates the understanding of drug absorption, distribution, metabolism, and excretion in the body. Additionally, it helps in dosage regimen optimization and modeling medication reactions.
- Patient Stratification: AI enables the development of personalized medical techniques by identifying patient subpopulations with unique genetic or clinical traits that are likely to benefit from a given medication.
- Repurposing Current Drugs: AI can find current medications that might work well for novel uses, which might save time and money.
- Clinical Trial Optimization: AI can help with the design of more effective and economical clinical trials, as well as better patient monitoring and recruiting.
- Natural Product Discovery: AI can identify bioactive molecules from natural sources for possible therapeutic development by analyzing natural chemicals.
- Drug Formulation Optimization: Artificial Intelligence can help optimize the composition and administration of medications to increase their effectiveness and patient adherence.

Because AI can make better decisions, it speeds up the process, lowers expenses, and raises the chance of success in drug discovery. It also aids in the creation of more specialized and potent therapies. Even though AI has showed promise, in order to guarantee medication safety and efficacy, AI-generated hypotheses must be rigorously validated through experimental and clinical testing. To further guarantee patient safety, regulatory organizations such as the FDA are actively engaged in assessing and overseeing AI-based drug discovery methodologies(Kraus et al., 2015).

11. PREDICTIVE ANALYSIS

Predictive analytics is a data-driven approach that determines the probability of future events based on past data by using statistical algorithms and machine learning. Predictive analytics is essential to the healthcare industry because it enhances patient care, resource allocation, and overall productivity. The following are some significant uses of predictive analytics in the medical field.

- Disease Prediction and Prevention: By analyzing patient data, including genetics and electronic health records (EHRs), predictive algorithms can identify people who are at risk of contracting particular diseases. This makes early treatments and preventative actions possible.
- Readmission Risk: Predictive analytics can be used by hospitals to evaluate the likelihood that patients will return after being discharged. This aids in lowering expensive readmission rates and giving follow-up treatment priority.
- Resource Allocation: By employing predictive models to estimate patient demand, healthcare organizations may optimize resource allocation, including staffing and inventory management.
- Patient Flow: By anticipating patient flow and streamlining bed management, hospitals can make sure that patients receive the right care and resources when they need them.
- Medication Adherence: Using predictive analytics, healthcare providers can identify patients who run the risk of not taking their drugs as directed. Then, in order to increase compliance, healthcare providers can provide assistance or interventions.
- Chronic Disease Management: By identifying individuals who are most likely to have problems or exacerbations of their disease, predictive models can be used to treat chronic diseases and enable prompt interventions.
- Cost Prediction: For financial planning and budgeting purposes, healthcare organizations can project expenses for specific populations or individuals.
- Telemedicine Triage: By determining which patients require urgent care, predictive analytics can help with the triage of patients for telemedicine visits.
- Appointment Scheduling: By anticipating appointment demand and modifying schedules appropriately, healthcare facilities can maximize appointment scheduling and minimize patient wait times.
- Resource Utilization: Predictive analytics aids medical professionals in making the best use of costly resources, such as operating rooms and imaging apparatus.
- Diagnostics: Predictive models driven by AI can help analyze medical pictures, improving the precision and speed of diagnosis.
- Pharmacovigilance: By examining enormous datasets of patient and clinical trial data, predictive analytics is utilized to track medication safety and detect adverse events.
- Public Health Surveillance: By examining data from sources like social media, medical claims, and online searches, predictive analytics can identify illness outbreaks and monitor the spread of infectious diseases.

- Genomic Medicine: By utilizing predictive analytics, medical professionals can better understand genetic risk factors and customize treatment plans based on a patient's genetic profile.
- Behavioral Health: Early intervention and support are made possible by predictive models that evaluate the likelihood of substance addiction and mental health problems.

In order to produce predictions and insights, predictive analytics uses big datasets along with statistical and machine learning approaches. When included into healthcare workflows, these projections facilitate improved patient outcomes, more effective resource allocation, and better decision-making. It is imperative to guarantee that the data utilized for predictive analytics is of superior quality and that ethical and privacy concerns are taken into account while managing patient data(Sharma et al., 2019).

12. IMAGE ENHANCEMENT

In the realm of medical image processing, image enhancement is a method used to raise the caliber, readability, and clarity of medical images. The precision of diagnosis and treatment planning can be greatly impacted by the quality of the images, which makes this technique very important in medical imaging. The following are the main facets of image enhancement in the healthcare industry.

- Noise Reduction: One of the main objectives of image enhancement is to lessen noise in images obtained from medical procedures including CT, MRI, ultrasound, and X-rays. Noise reduction techniques are vital because noise can mask important features.
- Contrast Enhancement: To enhance the visibility of subtle anatomical structures and anomalies, an image's contrast must be improved. To increase contrast, methods such as contrast stretching and histogram equalization can be applied.
- Brightness Adjustment: Increasing or decreasing an image's overall brightness can improve visualization, particularly in photos with underexposed or overexposed areas. Making the necessary brightness adjustments guarantees that no important information is lost because of excessive brightness.
- Sharpening: Techniques for sharpening images improve the image's fine details and edges. This is very helpful in locating tissue borders or minor anomalies.
- Artifact Removal: To guarantee the accuracy of the diagnosis, artifacts in medical pictures, such as motion artifacts in MRI scans or beam-hardening artifacts in CT scans, can be minimized or eliminated through image enhancement.
- Resolution Enhancement: By improving an image's effective resolution, many image processing methods make it possible to see finer details in the picture.
- Histogram Equalization: By redistributing pixel intensity values to create a more equal distribution, this approach improves image contrast and increases the visibility of details.
- Multi-Modality Image Fusion: Image enhancement can facilitate the fusion process and provide a composite image that is more informative when data from various imaging modalities (such as PET and CT) needs to be integrated.
- Adaptive Enhancement: Localized contrast modifications are possible by techniques such as adaptive histogram equalization, which adapt the enhancement process to different sections of the image.

- Structural Enhancement: Radiologists can more easily concentrate on important areas by using image enhancement to emphasize particular structures or features of interest.
- Color Mapping: Color mapping can be used in some medical imaging applications to improve the visualization of particular tissue characteristics, including blood flow in Doppler ultrasonography.
- Image Registration: Image improvement can help make several images more visually coherent and compatible when they need to be aligned.
- Techniques for enhancing images can be as basic as following rules or as complex as using deep learning and artificial intelligence. The imaging modality, the type of medical image, and the particular objectives of the image enhancing procedure all influence the technique selection. The ultimate goal is to give medical practitioners more lucid and insightful visuals so they can diagnose and arrange treatments more accurately.

13. CONCLUSION AND FUTURE SCOPE

The integration of Artificial Intelligence (AI) into medical image processing has undeniably transformed the landscape of healthcare, ushering in an era of unprecedented precision and efficiency. The amalgamation of advanced algorithms with medical imaging technologies has resulted in quicker, more accurate diagnostics, ultimately improving patient outcomes. AI's ability to detect patterns and anomalies in medical images has proven invaluable, aiding healthcare professionals in early disease detection and personalized treatment planning. This not only enhances the quality of patient care but also streamlines the decision-making process for clinicians and radiologists.

The future of AI in medical image processing holds immense promise and potential for further advancements. Ongoing research and development efforts are focused on refining existing algorithms, making them more robust and capable of handling diverse datasets. Additionally, the integration of AI with other emerging technologies, such as augmented reality and virtual reality, could revolutionize medical imaging interpretation and surgical planning.

Furthermore, the implementation of AI in real-time image analysis during medical procedures could become more commonplace, providing instantaneous feedback to surgeons and enhancing the precision of interventions. Continued collaboration between technologists, healthcare professionals, and regulatory bodies is crucial to address challenges related to data privacy, standardization, and ethical considerations.

As AI continues to evolve, its role in medical image processing is poised to expand beyond diagnostics and treatment planning. The development of AI-driven predictive models for disease progression and response to treatment represents a compelling avenue for future research. Ultimately, the ongoing integration of AI in medical image processing holds the promise of a more efficient, personalized, and accessible healthcare landscape.

REFERENCES

Chartrand, G., Cheng, P. M., Vorontsov, E., Drozdzal, M., Turcotte, S., Pal, C. J., Kadoury, S., & Tang, A. (2017). Deep learning: A primer for radiologists. *Radiographics*, *37*(7), 2113–2131. doi:10.1148/rg.2017170077 PMID:29131760

Ferrante, E., Dokania, P. K., Marini, R., & Paragios, N. (2017) *Deformable registration through learning of context-specific metric aggregation*. Machine Learning in Medical Imaging Workshop. MLMI (MICCAI 2017), Quebec City, Canada. 10.1007/978-3-319-67389-9_30

Iglesias, J. E., & Sabuncu, M. R. (2015). Multi-atlas segmentation of biomedical images: A survey. *Medical Image Analysis*, 24(1), 205–219. doi:10.1016/j.media.2015.06.012 PMID:26201875

Kraus, W. L. (2015). Editorial: Would you like a hypothesis with those data? Omics and the age of discovery science. *Molecular Endocrinology (Baltimore, Md.)*, 29(11), 1531–1534. doi:10.1210/me.2015-1253 PMID:26524008

LeCun, Y., Bengio, Y., & Hinton, G. (2015). Deep learning. *Nature*, 521(7553), 436–444. doi:10.1038/nature14539 PMID:26017442

Okada, T., Linguraru, M. G., Hori, M., Summers, R. M., Tomiyama, N., & Sato, Y. (2015). Abdominal multi-organ segmentation from CT images using conditional shape-location and unsupervised intensity priors. *Medical Image Analysis*, 26(1), 1–18. doi:10.1016/j.media.2015.06.009 PMID:26277022

Park, H., Bland, P. H., & Meyer, C. R. (2003). Construction of an abdominal probabilistic atlas and its application in segmentation. *IEEE Transactions on Medical Imaging*, 22(4), 483–492. doi:10.1109/TMI.2003.809139 PMID:12774894

Sharma, S. K., & Sharma, N. K. (2019). Text Document Categorization using Modified K-Means Clustering Algorithm. [IJRTE]. *International Journal of Recent Technology and Engineering*, 8(2), 508–511.

Sharma, S. K., & Sharma, N. K. (2019). Text Classification using Ensemble of Non-Linear Support Vector Machines. [IJITEE]. *International Journal of Innovative Technology and Exploring Engineering*, 8(10), 3170–3174. doi:10.35940/ijitee.J9520.0881019

Sharma, S. K., & Sharma, N. K. (2019). Unified Framework for Deep Learning based Text Classification. *INTERNATIONAL JOURNAL OF SCIENTIFIC & TECHNOLOGY RESEARCH*, 8(10), 1479–1483.

Sharma, S. K., & Sharma, N. K. (2019). Text Classification using LSTM based Deep Neural Network Architecture. *International Journal on Emerging Technologies.*, 10(4), 38–42.

Sharma, S. K., Sharma, N. K., & Potter, P. P. (2020). Fusion Approach for Document Classification using Random Forest and SVM. *Proceeding of SMART-2020, IEEE Conference ID: 50582, 9th IEEE Scopus Indexed International Conference on System Modelling & Advancement on Research Trends (SMART-2020)*. IEEE. 10.1109/SMART50582.2020.9337131

Simmons, J. P., Nelson, L. D., & Simonsohn, U. (2011). False-positive psychology: Undisclosed flexibility in data collection and analysis allows presenting anything as significant. *Psychological Science*, 22(11), 1359–1366. doi:10.1177/0956797611417632 PMID:22006061

Summers, R. M. (2016). Progress in fully automated abdominal CT interpretation. *AJR. American Journal of Roentgenology*, 207(1), 67–79. doi:10.2214/AJR.15.15996 PMID:27101207

Tang, A., Tam, R., Cadrin-Chênevert, A., Guest, W., Chong, J., Barfett, J., Chepelev, L., Cairns, R., Mitchell, J. R., Cicero, M. D., Poudrette, M. G., Jaremko, J. L., Reinhold, C., Gallix, B., Gray, B., Geis, R., O'Connell, T., Babyn, P., Koff, D., & Shabana, W.Canadian Association of Radiologists (CAR) Artificial Intelligence Working Group. (2018). Canadian Association of Radiologists white paper on artificial intelligence in radiology. *Canadian Association of Radiologists Journal, 69*(2), 120–135. doi:10.1016/j.carj.2018.02.002 PMID:29655580

Van Leemput, K., Maes, F., Vandermeulen, D., Colchester, A., & Suetens, P. (2001). Automated segmentation of multiple sclerosis lesions by model outlier detection. *IEEE Transactions on Medical Imaging, 20*(8), 677–688. doi:10.1109/42.938237 PMID:11513020

Viergever, M. A., Maintz, J. B. A., Klein, S., Murphy, K., Staring, M., & Pluim, J. P. W. (2016). A survey of medical image registration - under review. *Medical Image Analysis, 33*, 140–144. doi:10.1016/j.media.2016.06.030 PMID:27427472

Warfield, S. K., Zou, K. H., & Wells, W. M. (2004). Simultaneous truth and performance level estimation (STAPLE): An algorithm for the validation of image segmentation. *IEEE Transactions on Medical Imaging, 23*(7), 903–921. doi:10.1109/TMI.2004.828354 PMID:15250643

Chapter 2
Internet of Things for Smart Healthcare:
A Survey

Amit Kumar Tyagi

https://orcid.org/0000-0003-2657-8700

National Institute of Fashion Technology, New Delhi, India

Shabnam Kumari

SRM Institute of Science and Technology, Chennai, India

Shrikant Tiwari

https://orcid.org/0000-0001-6947-2362

Galgotias University, Greater Noida, India

ABSTRACT

Internet of things (IoT) has emerged as a transformative technology in the healthcare sector, providing innovative solutions to enhance patient care, improve healthcare delivery, and optimize resource utilization. This chapter provides a comprehensive overview of the current state of IoT applications in smart healthcare. It provides the various aspects of IoT implementation, including device integration, data management, security, and privacy issues. This work begins by defining the key concepts of IoT and its relevance to healthcare, highlighting the potential benefits and challenges. It discusses several components of IoT-enabled smart healthcare systems, such as wearable devices, remote monitoring, and healthcare infrastructure integration. This work discusses the role of IoT in chronic disease management, telemedicine, and preventive healthcare, showcasing real-world examples and success stories. Moreover, this work outlines the critical role of data analytics and artificial intelligence in processing the vast amount of healthcare data generated by IoT devices.

DOI: 10.4018/979-8-3693-2359-5.ch002

1. INTRODUCTION TO INTERNET OF THINGS BASED SMART HEALTHCARE

The healthcare sector is experiencing a technological revolution, propelled by the widespread adoption of the Internet of Things (IoT) (Shabnam Kumari, P. Muthulakshmi, 2023) (Amit Kumar Tyagi, V. Hemamalini, Gulshan Soni, 2023). IoT, a network of interconnected devices and sensors capable of communicating and sharing data over the internet, has significantly impacted healthcare, ushering in the era of "Smart Healthcare." This introduction provides a comprehensive overview of how IoT is reshaping the healthcare landscape, enhancing patient outcomes, and transforming the delivery and management of healthcare services.

1.1 The IoT Revolution in Healthcare

The advent of IoT technology has paved the way for improving the quality, efficiency, and accessibility of healthcare services. It integrates medical devices, wearables, data analytics, and connectivity to establish a secure and efficient healthcare ecosystem. Within this ecosystem, devices like wearable fitness trackers, remote patient monitoring devices, and hospital equipment are equipped with sensors and connectivity, allowing them to gather, transmit, and receive data in real-time. Here, we explore some key components of IoT-Based Smart Healthcare:

- Wearable Devices: Continuous monitoring of vital signs, including heart rate, blood pressure, and activity levels, is possible through wearable technology like smartwatches and fitness trackers. The collected data can be shared with healthcare providers for real-time assessment and prompt intervention.
- Remote Patient Monitoring: IoT enables remote monitoring of patients with chronic conditions. Devices like blood glucose monitors, ECG monitors, and medication dispensers can transmit data to healthcare professionals, allowing for proactive care management.
- Healthcare Infrastructure Integration: Hospitals and healthcare facilities can incorporate IoT into their infrastructure for improved patient care and operational efficiency. This includes smart beds, medication tracking, and asset management systems.
- Data Analytics and Artificial Intelligence: The massive amounts of data generated by IoT devices are processed and analyzed using AI-driven algorithms. This data-driven approach helps in early disease detection, treatment recommendations, and predicting healthcare trends.

1.2 Benefits of IoT in Healthcare

- Enhanced Patient Care: IoT allows for personalized and continuous monitoring of patients, leading to early detection of health issues and timely interventions.
- Efficient Resource Utilization: Healthcare providers can optimize resource allocation by using IoT for asset management, reducing waste, and improving operational efficiency.
- Telemedicine: The Internet of Things (IoT) supports telemedicine by enabling remote consultations, thereby reducing the necessity for in-person visits to healthcare facilities. This becomes particularly valuable during global health crises.
- Data-Driven Decision Making: Informed decisions by healthcare professionals, relying on real-time patient data, contribute to enhanced treatment outcomes and patient safety.

1.3 Challenges and Issues

- Despite its promise, IoT in healthcare comes with challenges, including data security and privacy issues, interoperability issues, and the need for regulatory compliance. Ensuring the security of patient data and compliance with healthcare regulations is paramount in IoT-based smart healthcare.

In summary, Smart Healthcare powered by IoT marks a revolutionary transformation in the healthcare industry. Through the utilization of interconnected devices, real-time data, and advanced analytics, healthcare is evolving to be more patient-centric, efficient, and effective. This work will delve into various facets of IoT in healthcare, examining its applications, benefits, challenges, and future trends to offer a comprehensive understanding of this dynamic and rapidly advancing field.

In the last, this work is summarized into 9 sections.

2. IOT FUNDAMENTALS

2.1 Definition, Key Components, Protocols Used of IoT Systems

The Internet of Things (IoT) encompasses a network of interconnected physical objects or "things" embedded with sensors, software, and connectivity features, allowing them to collect and exchange data with each other and central systems over the internet (Amit Kumar Tyagi, 2022). IoT systems are designed to offer real-time information, automation, and intelligent decision-making across diverse domains, such as healthcare, transportation, agriculture, smart cities, and industrial processes. Here, we explore some key components of IoT Systems:

- Sensors and Actuators: These form the foundational elements of IoT. Sensors acquire data from the physical world, capturing information like temperature, humidity, motion, or light. Actuators, on the other hand, enable IoT devices to carry out actions, such as turning on a light or adjusting a thermostat.
- Connectivity: To establish connections with the internet or other devices, IoT devices depend on diverse communication technologies. Standard connectivity options encompass Wi-Fi, cellular networks (2G, 3G, 4G, and 5G), Bluetooth, Zigbee, LoRaWAN, and RFID.
- Data Processing and Storage: IoT generates vast amounts of data, and processing and storage capabilities are essential. Edge computing, cloud computing, and fog computing are used to handle data processing and storage requirements.
- Communication Protocols: These protocols enable the exchange of data and communication between IoT devices and systems. Several widely used IoT communication protocols include MQTT (Message Queuing Telemetry Transport), HTTP/HTTPS, CoAP (Constrained Application Protocol), and AMQP (Advanced Message Queuing Protocol).
- IoT Platforms: IoT platforms offer tools and services for device management, data analytics, and application development, simplifying the deployment and oversight of IoT solutions. Examples include AWS IoT, Google Cloud IoT Core, and Microsoft Azure IoT.

- Security Mechanisms: Security is critical in IoT systems to protect data and devices from unauthorized access and cyberattacks. Security measures include encryption, authentication, access control, and regular software updates.
- User Interface: User interfaces in IoT solutions, such as mobile apps or web dashboards, enable users to interact with and control IoT devices, monitor data, and receive alerts.

Protocols Used in IoT Systems:

- MQTT (Message Queuing Telemetry Transport): MQTT is a lightweight publish-subscribe messaging protocol crafted for efficient communication in constrained environments. Widely employed for real-time data exchange in IoT applications, MQTT is recognized for its minimal overhead and low power consumption.
- HTTP/HTTPS (Hypertext Transfer Protocol): These protocols are widely used for web-based communication. While not as lightweight as MQTT, they are commonly used for RESTful API communication between IoT devices and cloud services.
- CoAP (Constrained Application Protocol): CoAP is tailored for resource-constrained devices and networks, rendering it well-suited for IoT applications. Resembling HTTP, CoAP stands out for its efficiency in terms of bandwidth and processing.
- AMQP (Advanced Message Queuing Protocol): AMQP is a resilient and efficient messaging protocol employed for transmitting messages between IoT devices and backend systems. It is frequently utilized in industrial IoT applications.
- DDS (Data Distribution Service): DDS is a communication protocol well-suited for real-time and mission-critical IoT applications, particularly in fields like aerospace and healthcare, where low-latency and reliability are imperative.
- Bluetooth and Bluetooth Low Energy (BLE): These wireless communication protocols find frequent use in consumer IoT devices, including wearables, smart home devices, and health monitoring devices.
- Zigbee and Z-Wave: These protocols are designed for low-power, short-range communication in smart home and industrial IoT applications, enabling devices to create mesh networks.
- LoRaWAN (Long Range Wide Area Network): LoRaWAN is a low-power, long-range wireless protocol used in IoT applications like smart agriculture, smart cities, and asset tracking.

It's important to note that the selection of a communication protocol relies on factors such as the particular IoT application, device constraints, power consumption requirements, and data exchange needs. Various protocols are optimized for specific use cases within the diverse IoT ecosystem.

2.2 IoT Security and Privacy Issues

Security and privacy stand as paramount concerns in the IoT ecosystem, given the substantial volume of sensitive data generated and transmitted by IoT devices (Amit Kumar Tyagi and Richa, 2023) (Meghna Manoj Nair and Amit Kumar Tyagi, 2023) (Sai Dhakshan Y., Amit Kumar Tyagi, 2023). It is imperative to address these issues to guarantee the trustworthiness and integrity of IoT systems. Here are some key security and privacy challenges in IoT:

A.   Data Privacy:
- Data Collection and Storage: IoT devices frequently gather sensitive personal information, including health data, location data, and user behavior. It is crucial to prioritize the secure and private collection, storage, and transmission of this data.
- Data Ownership: Deciding ownership and control of the data generated by IoT devices can be intricate, potentially giving rise to privacy disputes.

B.   Data Security:
- Unauthorized Access: Weak authentication mechanisms and default passwords can lead to unauthorized access to IoT devices and data. Malicious actors can exploit these vulnerabilities to compromise device security.
- Data Encryption: Ensuring data is encrypted during transmission and storage is important to prevent eavesdropping and data breaches.
- Firmware and Software Updates: Numerous IoT devices lack the capability to receive regular security updates, leaving them susceptible to known exploits. Ensuring that devices can undergo updates is essential for long-term security.

C.   Device Vulnerabilities:
- Insecure Hardware: Hardware vulnerabilities can be challenging to address once devices are deployed. These vulnerabilities can be exploited to compromise device security.
- Lack of Security by Design: Security issues are often an afterthought in IoT device development, leading to poorly designed security mechanisms.

D.   Network Security:
- Man-in-the-Middle Attacks: Hackers can intercept and modify data between IoT devices and the cloud or other devices, potentially compromising data integrity and security.
- DDoS Attacks: IoT devices can be hijacked and used to launch distributed denial-of-service (DDoS) attacks, disrupting networks and services.

E.   Identity and Authentication:
- Weak Authentication: Vulnerabilities such as weak or default passwords, absence of two-factor authentication, and inadequate identity management can result in unauthorized access to devices and data.

F.   Supply Chain Security:
- Counterfeit Devices: Fake or counterfeit IoT devices can introduce security risks into the ecosystem. Authenticating the source and integrity of devices is challenging.

G.   Lack of Standardization:
- Interoperability: The absence of standardization in IoT security practices and protocols can pose a challenge in implementing consistent security measures across various devices and platforms.

H.   Regulatory and Compliance Challenges:
- Privacy Regulations: IoT deployments need to adhere to privacy regulations, including GDPR and CCPA, necessitating informed consent, robust data protection, and transparency.

I.   Data Leakage:
- Data Leakage from Edge Devices: Edge computing in IoT can introduce risks if sensitive data is not adequately protected on local devices.

J.   Physical Security:
  ◦   Physical Tampering: Devices deployed in public spaces may be subject to physical tampering or theft, which can compromise their security.

Hence, these IoT security and privacy issues requires a multi-faceted approach involving device manufacturers, software developers, service providers, and regulatory bodies. Some recommended practices include:

- Implementing robust authentication and access control mechanisms.
- Employing encryption for data in transit and at rest.
- Regularly updating device firmware and software to patch vulnerabilities.
- Conducting security audits and penetration testing.
- Educating users about IoT security best practices.
- Ensuring compliance with privacy regulations.
- Promoting industry-wide standardization of security protocols.

Note that IoT security and privacy are ongoing issues as the technology continues to evolve. Stakeholders must remain vigilant in addressing emerging threats and vulnerabilities to maintain the trust and security of IoT systems.

3. SMART HEALTHCARE: AN OVERVIEW

3.1 Definition and Evolution of Smart Healthcare Technology

The evolution of smart healthcare technology, also known as digital health or eHealth, involves the integration of advanced technologies, data-driven solutions, and digital innovations into the healthcare sector (Nair & Tyagi, 2023) (Tyagi, 2023) (Adebiyi & Afolayan, 2023). This overarching concept aims to improve the quality, efficiency, and accessibility of healthcare services, ultimately enhancing patient outcomes. Smart healthcare technology encompasses diverse applications such as electronic health records (EHRs), wearable devices, telemedicine, IoT-based healthcare, artificial intelligence (AI) for diagnostics and treatment, and data analytics for healthcare management:

- Digital Health Records (DHRs): The journey towards smart healthcare began with the adoption of electronic health records (EHRs) to replace paper-based patient records. EHRs improved data accessibility, accuracy, and sharing among healthcare providers.
- Telemedicine: Telemedicine became widely embraced as a method for delivering remote healthcare consultations, enabling patients to receive medical services conveniently from their homes and diminishing the necessity for in-person visits to healthcare facilities.
- Wearable Health Devices: The widespread adoption of wearable devices, including fitness trackers and smartwatches, allowed for the continuous monitoring of vital signs and health metrics. These devices provided individuals with real-time health data, enabling early detection of potential health issues.

- IoT in Healthcare: The advent of IoT technology brought forth interconnected medical devices and sensors designed to collect and transmit real-time health data. Applications of IoT in healthcare encompass remote patient monitoring, medication adherence, and the development of intelligent healthcare infrastructure.

Artificial Intelligence (AI) in Healthcare: AI and machine learning have been integrated into healthcare for tasks like medical image analysis, disease diagnosis, and predictive analytics (Deekshetha, Tyagi,2023) (Tyagi, Kukreja, et al., 2022).

- AI-driven chatbots and virtual assistants also enhance patient engagement and support.
- Data Analytics and Healthcare Management: The use of big data analytics has transformed healthcare management by enabling better resource allocation, patient population management, and predictive modeling for disease outbreaks.
- Genomics and Personalized Medicine: Progress in genomics and molecular medicine has opened the door to personalized treatment plans tailored to an individual's genetic makeup. This approach enables the implementation of more precise and effective therapies.

Blockchain in Healthcare: Blockchain technology is being provided for securing medical records, enhancing data integrity, and enabling secure data sharing among healthcare stakeholders (Madhav A.V.S., Tyagi A.K. 2022) (Sheth, H.S.K., Tyagi, A.K. 2022) (A. K. Tyagi, S. Chandrasekaran and N. Sreenath, 2022) (A. Deshmukh, N. Sreenath, 2022) (Varsha Jayaprakash, Amit Kumar Tyagi,) (Amit Kumar Tyagi, Aswathy, et al., 2021) (Sai, G.H., Tripathi, K., 2023) (Shruti Kute; Amit Kumar Tyagi; et al., 2021) (Shruti Kute; Amit Kumar Tyagi; Meghna Manoj Nair, 2023).

- 5G Connectivity: The deployment of 5G networks assures swifter and more dependable connectivity, facilitating the real-time transmission of high-definition medical data. This advancement supports remote surgeries and enhances the performance of telehealth applications.
- Robotics and Automation: Robots are being used in surgery, rehabilitation, and patient care, enhancing precision and efficiency in healthcare delivery.
- Smart Hospitals and Infrastructure: Hospitals are adopting smart technologies for asset management, energy efficiency, and patient experience improvement.
- Consumer Health Apps: The proliferation of mobile health (mHealth) apps allows individuals to monitor their health, schedule appointments, and access medical information easily.
- Pandemic Response: Smart healthcare technologies played a important role in pandemic response efforts, including contact tracing, remote patient monitoring, and vaccine distribution management.

Hence, the evolution of smart healthcare technology continues to accelerate, driven by ongoing technological advancements, increasing demand for remote and personalized care, and the need for healthcare systems to become more efficient and patient-centric. As the healthcare industry embraces these innovations, it is poised to undergo significant transformations, ultimately leading to improved healthcare outcomes and experiences for individuals worldwide.

3.2 Benefits, Limitations, Issues and Challenges of Smart Healthcare

This section will discuss few benefits, limitations, issues and challenges of smart healthcare as:

A. Benefits of Smart Healthcare:
- ○ Improved Patient Outcomes: The utilization of smart healthcare technology allows for ongoing monitoring and early identification of health issues, resulting in timely interventions and improved patient outcomes.
- ○ Enhanced Patient Engagement: Patients can actively participate in their healthcare through wearable devices, mobile apps, and telemedicine, leading to increased engagement and better adherence to treatment plans.
- ○ Efficient Healthcare Delivery: Smart healthcare streamlines processes, reduces administrative burdens, and optimizes resource allocation, resulting in cost savings and more efficient healthcare services.
- ○ Remote Monitoring: Patients with chronic conditions can be remotely monitored, reducing hospital readmissions and healthcare costs while improving the quality of life.
- ○ Personalized Medicine: Smart healthcare uses data analytics and genomics to tailor treatment plans to individual patients, increasing treatment effectiveness.
- ○ Telemedicine: Telehealth services provide access to healthcare in remote or underserved areas and provide convenient options for consultations and follow-ups.
- ○ Preventive Care: Early detection and data-driven insights support preventive care, helping to reduce the prevalence of chronic diseases and the associated healthcare costs.
- ○ Data-Driven Decision Making: Informed decisions by healthcare providers, derived from real-time patient data, enhance treatment plans and healthcare management.

B. Limitations of Smart Healthcare:
- ○ Data Security and Privacy Issues: The collection and sharing of sensitive health data raise privacy and security challenges, including the risk of data breaches.
- ○ Interoperability Issues: Many healthcare systems and devices use proprietary protocols and standards, hindering seamless data exchange and interoperability.
- ○ Access Disparities: Not everyone has access to the necessary technology or internet connectivity, creating disparities in access to smart healthcare services.
- ○ Cost of Implementation: Implementing smart healthcare technology can be expensive, and not all healthcare systems have the resources for widespread adoption.
- ○ Reliability and Accuracy: The accuracy of data from wearable devices and IoT sensors can vary, potentially leading to false alarms or missed health issues.

C. Issues and Challenges of Smart Healthcare:
- ○ Regulatory Compliance: Adhering to healthcare regulations, such as HIPAA in the U.S., is crucial, and navigating intricate regulatory requirements can pose significant challenges.
- ○ Ethical Issues: Ethical issues surrounding data ownership, consent, and responsible use of patient data are complex and require careful handling.
- ○ Healthcare Workforce Adaptation: Healthcare professionals need training to effectively use and interpret data from smart healthcare technologies.

        ◦   Integration and Scalability: Integrating smart healthcare systems with existing healthcare infrastructure and ensuring scalability are significant challenges.

        ◦   Data Management: Handling and analyzing the enormous volume of data generated by smart healthcare devices require robust data management and analytics capabilities.

        ◦   Cybersecurity Threats: Healthcare systems are prime targets for cyberattacks, and IoT devices can be vulnerable without adequate security measures.

        ◦   Patient Trust: Building and maintaining patient trust in the security and privacy of their health data is essential for the widespread adoption of smart healthcare.

        ◦   Health Inequities: Smart healthcare can exacerbate health inequities if not implemented equitably, as vulnerable populations may have limited access to technology and resources.

Note that few other technical challenges towards IoT based smart healthcare are; IoT device reliability, battery life, and connectivity issues can pose technical challenges in smart healthcare implementations. In summary, while smart healthcare provides numerous benefits, it also presents a range of limitations, issues, and challenges that must be addressed to realize its full potential. Successful implementation requires a comprehensive approach that encompasses technology, regulation, ethics, and patient-centered care.

4. IOT APPLICATIONS IN SMART HEALTHCARE

Smart healthcare IoT applications are transforming the medical industry by enhancing patient care, optimizing operational efficiency, and lowering healthcare costs. Here are several key IoT applications in the realm of smart healthcare:

- Remote Patient Monitoring: Wearable fitness trackers, smartwatches, and medical sensors, among other IoT devices, have the capability to continuously monitor vital signs like heart rate, blood pressure, and glucose levels. These devices can transmit real-time data to healthcare providers, enabling professionals to remotely monitor patients with chronic conditions. In case of abnormal readings, timely interventions can be initiated, thereby reducing hospital admissions and enhancing patient outcomes.
- Telemedicine and Telehealth: The Internet of Things (IoT) supports remote consultations and telemedicine services, allowing patients to engage with healthcare providers through video calls, chatbots, or secure messaging apps. Telehealth applications improve access to healthcare services, especially in remote or underserved areas, and prove valuable during public health crises such as pandemics.
- Medication Management: Medication dispensers enabled by the Internet of Things (IoT) prompt patients to take their medications punctually and can issue alerts to caregivers or healthcare providers if doses are overlooked. Intelligent pill bottles can track medication usage and adherence, thereby boosting patient safety and the effectiveness of the treatment.
- Healthcare Infrastructure Optimization: IoT is used to improve the efficiency and management of healthcare facilities. Smart hospital beds, equipment, and inventory systems can streamline operations. Predictive maintenance of medical equipment reduces downtime, ensuring that critical devices are always available.

- Smart Home Healthcare: IoT-enabled devices in a patient's home, such as smart scales, blood pressure monitors, and glucometers, allow for proactive monitoring and reporting of health data. This setup empowers patients to manage their health more effectively and reduces the need for frequent clinic visits.
- Elderly Care and Fall Detection: IoT devices can detect falls or unusual activity patterns in elderly individuals living alone and automatically alert caregivers or emergency services. This application enhances the safety and well-being of elderly patients.
- Remote Surgery and Robotic Assistance: IoT and high-speed connectivity enable remote surgery with the assistance of robotic surgical systems. Surgeons can operate on patients located in different geographic locations. Surgical robots equipped with IoT sensors enhance precision and reduce the risk of human error.
- Chronic Disease Management: Individuals dealing with chronic conditions like diabetes or hypertension find value in IoT devices designed to monitor and manage their health. The data gathered from these devices can be analyzed to formulate personalized treatment plans and facilitate timely interventions.
- Preventive Healthcare: IoT helps in preventive care by collecting data on lifestyle, exercise, and diet habits. This information can be used to provide personalized recommendations for healthier living. Wearable devices often encourage individuals to adopt healthier behaviors.
- Emergency Response and Disaster Management: IoT sensors and devices play a important role in monitoring and responding to public health emergencies, such as tracking the spread of infectious diseases or assessing environmental conditions during natural disasters.
- Drug Temperature Monitoring: IoT sensors are used to monitor and ensure the proper storage and transportation of temperature-sensitive medications and vaccines, particularly relevant in the pharmaceutical supply chain and healthcare logistics.

Therefore, the potential of IoT applications in smart healthcare lies in enhancing patient care, reducing healthcare costs, and improving overall health outcomes. However, addressing crucial factors such as security and privacy concerns, interoperability issues, and regulatory compliance is imperative for the successful and widespread adoption of these technologies in healthcare. Some notable case studies in the realm of IoT for Smart Healthcare include Remote Patient Monitoring Solutions, Wearable Health Devices (e.g., Fitbit), and services like Telemedicine Platforms (e.g., Teladoc), Remote Patient Monitoring, Wearable Health Devices, Telemedicine and Virtual Health, Medication Adherence and Management, Healthcare Facility Management, and IoT in Public Health and Pandemic Response.

5. IOT DEVICES AND SENSORS IN HEALTHCARE

5.1 Types of IoT Devices in Healthcare

In the healthcare domain, IoT devices encompass a diverse array of technology and hardware explicitly crafted to monitor, gather, and transmit health-related data. These devices play a pivotal role in elevating patient care, facilitating remote monitoring, and augmenting the overall delivery of healthcare services. Below are some prevalent types of IoT devices employed in healthcare:

A.   Wearable Health Devices:
   - Smartwatches: These devices can track heart rate, activity levels, sleep patterns, and more. Some models include ECG and SpO2 sensors.
   - Fitness Trackers: These gadgets track physical activity, count steps taken, measure calories burned, and assess sleep quality.
   - Smart Clothing: Garments embedded with sensors can monitor vital signs and provide real-time health data.
   - Hearables: Ear-worn devices can monitor heart rate, body temperature, and provide audio notifications.

B.   Medical Sensors:
   - Blood Glucose Monitors: Glucose meters equipped with IoT capabilities can gauge blood sugar levels and send the collected data to smartphones or healthcare providers.
   - Blood Pressure Monitors: These devices monitor blood pressure and can provide readings to patients and healthcare professionals.
   - Pulse Oximeters: IoT pulse oximeters measure blood oxygen levels and heart rate and can send data to healthcare providers.
   - Temperature Sensors: Connected thermometers can provide real-time temperature readings for monitoring fever and illness.

C.   Implantable Medical Devices:
   - Cardiac Pacemakers: IoT-enabled pacemakers can transmit data on heart performance and battery status to healthcare providers.
   - Implantable Cardioverter-Defibrillators (ICDs): These devices can send alerts in case of arrhythmias or critical events.

D.   Medication Management Devices:
   - Smart Pill Dispensers: These gadgets prompt patients to adhere to their medication schedules and can notify caregivers or healthcare providers in the event of missed doses.
   - Connected Inhalers: IoT inhalers monitor inhalation technique and track medication usage for patients with respiratory conditions.

E.   Telehealth Devices:
   - Telemedicine Kits: These kits include cameras, microphones, and vital sign monitors to facilitate remote consultations with healthcare providers.
   - Digital Stethoscopes: IoT stethoscopes can transmit auscultation data for remote diagnosis.

F.   Smart Home Healthcare Devices:
   - Smart Scales: These devices can measure and track weight, BMI, and body composition.
   - Smart Blood Pressure Cuffs: IoT-enabled blood pressure cuffs can monitor and transmit blood pressure data.
   - Glucometers: Interconnected glucose meters aid individuals with diabetes in monitoring their blood sugar levels.

G.   Fall Detection and Elderly Care Devices:
   - Wearable Fall Detectors: IoT-enabled devices can detect falls and alert caregivers or emergency services.
   - Smart Home Monitoring Systems: These systems include motion sensors and cameras to ensure the well-being of elderly individuals living alone.

H. Connected Medical Equipment:
    ◦ IoT-Enabled Ventilators: These devices can transmit patient data to healthcare providers for remote monitoring.
    ◦ Infusion Pumps: IoT pumps can deliver medication and report usage data.
I. Environmental Sensors:
    ◦ Air Quality Monitors: These sensors can detect pollutants and allergens in indoor environments, relevant for individuals with respiratory conditions.
    ◦ IoT Tags for Asset Tracking: Healthcare facilities employ IoT tags to monitor the location and condition of medical equipment, ensuring effective asset management.
    ◦ Medical Imaging Devices: IoT can enhance the capabilities of medical imaging equipment, such as MRI machines and X-ray systems, by enabling remote monitoring and data sharing.

Therefore, these healthcare IoT devices contribute to remote patient monitoring, early disease detection, medication adherence, and personalized treatment plans. However, they also give rise to crucial issues concerning data security, privacy, interoperability, and regulatory compliance, which must be resolved for their successful implementation in the healthcare ecosystem.

5.2 Available Sensors and Actuators in Healthcare Systems

Healthcare systems employ a diverse array of sensors and actuators to monitor patient health, enhance medical procedures, and improve the overall quality of healthcare delivery (Kumari, S., Muthulakshmi, P., Agarwal, D., 2022) (Kute S.S., Tyagi A.K., Aswathy S.U, 2022) (Nair M.M., Kumari S., Tyagi A.K., Sravanthi K., 2021). Below are various types of sensors and actuators commonly utilized in healthcare systems:

5.2.1 Sensors in Healthcare Systems

Temperature Sensors:

*   Thermocouples: Measure temperature variations.
*   Thermistors: Detect temperature changes and are often used in thermometers.
*   Infrared (IR) Sensors: Non-contact sensors for measuring body temperature and monitoring fever.

Biometric Sensors:

*   Fingerprint Sensors: Used for patient identification and access control.
*   Iris Scanners: Verify patient identity.
*   Facial Recognition Sensors: Enable secure access and authentication.

Vital Sign Sensors:

*   Heart Rate Monitors: Measure the patient's pulse.
*   Blood Pressure Sensors: Monitor blood pressure.
*   Pulse Oximeters: Measure blood oxygen saturation levels.

- Respiratory Rate Sensors: Track breathing patterns.

Blood Glucose Sensors:

- Glucometers: Monitor blood sugar levels in diabetic patients.

Electrocardiogram (ECG) Sensors:

- ECG Electrodes: Record electrical activity of the heart for diagnostics.

Electromyography (EMG) Sensors:

- Measure electrical activity in muscles and are used in diagnostics and prosthetic control.

Electroencephalogram (EEG) Sensors:

- Detect electrical activity in the brain for diagnosing neurological disorders.

Imaging Sensors:

- X-ray Sensors: Capture X-ray images for diagnosing fractures and internal conditions.
- Magnetic Resonance Imaging (MRI) Sensors: Create detailed images of internal structures.
- Ultrasound Sensors: Use sound waves for imaging.

Motion Sensors:

- Accelerometers: Detect patient movement for tracking physical activity or monitoring sleep.
- Gyroscopes: Measure orientation and balance.

Environmental Sensors:

- Air Quality Sensors: Monitor indoor air quality for patients with respiratory conditions.
- Humidity Sensors: Control humidity in medical storage environments.

Chemical Sensors:

- Gas Sensors: Detect gases such as oxygen, carbon dioxide, and volatile organic compounds.
- pH Sensors: Measure pH levels in bodily fluids.

Biological Sensors:

- DNA Sensors: Analyze genetic material for diagnostics and research.
- Biosensors: Detect specific biological molecules, such as glucose or antibodies.

5.2.2 Actuators in Healthcare Systems

- Infusion Pumps: Administer medications, fluids, or nutrients at controlled rates.
- Ventilators: Assist patients with breathing by supplying oxygen and controlling airflow.
- Motorized Medical Beds: Adjust bed position for patient comfort and medical procedures.
- Surgical Robots: Assist surgeons in performing precise and minimally invasive procedures.
- Drug Delivery Systems: Dispense medications via controlled release mechanisms.
- Prosthetic Devices: Replace or augment missing or impaired body parts.
- Haptic Feedback Devices: Provide tactile feedback to surgeons during robotic surgeries.
- Hearing Aids: Amplify sound for individuals with hearing impairment.
- Visual Aids: Assist individuals with visual impairment through screen readers, braille displays, or magnification devices.
- Smart Pill Dispensers: Remind patients to take medications and dispense the correct doses.
- Exoskeletons: Assist patients with mobility impairments in walking and rehabilitation.
- Automated External Defibrillators (AEDs): Deliver electric shocks to restore normal heart rhythms in cardiac arrest cases.

Hence, these sensors and actuators, often integrated with IoT technology, help healthcare providers monitor patients, diagnose medical conditions, deliver treatments, and improve overall healthcare outcomes. They are vital components of modern healthcare systems that aim to provide personalized and efficient care.

5.3 Connectivity Technologies and Communication Protocols for Healthcare IoT Devices

Connectivity technologies and communication protocols are important components of healthcare IoT devices, ensuring that data is transmitted securely and efficiently within the healthcare ecosystem (Sajidha S. A, Rishik Kumar, 2023) (L. Gomathi, A. K. Mishra and A. K. Tyagi, 2023). Here are some common connectivity technologies and communication protocols used in healthcare IoT:

5.3.1 Connectivity Technologies

- Wi-Fi (Wireless Fidelity): Hospitals and clinics extensively employ Wi-Fi to connect IoT devices to local networks and the internet. Wi-Fi offers high-speed data transfer and is well-suited for applications demanding real-time data transmission.
- Bluetooth: Bluetooth is commonly used for short-range connections between IoT devices and smartphones or tablets. It is energy-efficient and suitable for wearables and medical sensors, such as blood glucose monitors.
- Zigbee: Zigbee is employed for low-power, short-range communication in healthcare settings, especially in smart homes and assisted living environments. It provides reliable, mesh network capabilities for connecting a large number of devices.
- Z-Wave: Z-Wave is a wireless technology used in home automation and healthcare applications for device control and monitoring. It provides low power consumption, making it suitable for battery-operated devices in smart healthcare.

- Cellular Networks (3G, 4G, 5G): Cellular connectivity is used in remote patient monitoring and telemedicine, allowing IoT devices to transmit data over long distances. It provides extensive coverage and high data speeds but may require higher power consumption.
- LoRaWAN (Long Range Wide Area Network): LoRaWAN is suitable for long-range IoT applications, such as tracking and monitoring patients in large healthcare facilities. It provides low power consumption and extended range, making it ideal for low-cost, large-scale deployments.
- NB-IoT (Narrowband IoT): NB-IoT is designed for low-power, wide-area IoT applications, including remote monitoring in healthcare. It provides extended coverage and deep indoor penetration with low power requirements.
- Satellite Communication: Satellite communication is employed for IoT devices in remote or rural areas with limited terrestrial network coverage. It provides global coverage, making it suitable for tracking and monitoring applications in remote regions.

5.3.2 Communication Protocols

- MQTT (Message Queuing Telemetry Transport): MQTT serves as a lightweight, publish-subscribe messaging protocol employed in real-time data communication within healthcare IoT. It excels in low-bandwidth, high-latency, or unreliable network conditions, showcasing efficiency.
- CoAP (Constrained Application Protocol): CoAP is designed for resource-constrained IoT devices and is suitable for applications like remote patient monitoring. It provides lightweight communication for constrained devices and is compatible with the HTTP protocol.
- HTTP/HTTPS (Hypertext Transfer Protocol/Secure): HTTP/HTTPS is utilized for web-based communication between IoT devices and cloud-based healthcare systems. This facilitates standard web communication, rendering it apt for interoperability with existing systems.
- AMQP (Advanced Message Queuing Protocol): AMQP is employed for efficient and reliable messaging between healthcare IoT devices and backend systems. It ensures message delivery and is suitable for mission-critical applications.
- DDS (Data Distribution Service): DDS (Data Distribution Service) is a protocol designed for real-time, data-centric communication, frequently applied in healthcare IoT for medical devices and patient monitoring. It delivers low-latency and high-reliability communication, crucial for critical healthcare applications.

The selection of connectivity technology and communication protocol hinges on factors such as device requirements, range, power consumption, and data volume. In healthcare IoT systems, a blend of these technologies is frequently integrated to cater to the distinct needs of various applications within the healthcare ecosystem.

6. EXISTED IOT PLATFORMS FOR SMART HEALTHCARE

There are several IoT platforms and solutions tailored for smart healthcare applications, providing a range of features and capabilities to support the deployment and management of healthcare IoT devices and services. Here are some of the notable IoT platforms used in smart healthcare:

- AWS IoT Core for Healthcare (Amazon Web Services): AWS IoT Core for Healthcare is designed specifically for healthcare applications, providing robust security, scalability, and device management capabilities. It facilitates the integration of medical devices with cloud services, analytics, and machine learning.
- Azure IoT (Microsoft Azure): Azure IoT provides a comprehensive platform for healthcare IoT, providing device provisioning, telemetry data ingestion, device management, and integration with Azure services like Azure IoT Central and Azure Machine Learning for data analytics.
- Google Cloud Healthcare API (Google Cloud): Google Cloud Healthcare API enables secure and compliant data exchange and storage for healthcare IoT applications. It supports FHIR (Fast Healthcare Interoperability Resources) standards for healthcare data interoperability.
- IBM Watson Health: IBM Watson Health provides a range of solutions for healthcare IoT, including IoT device management, data analytics, and AI-powered insights. It focuses on using AI and machine learning to improve patient care and outcomes.
- Cisco Kinetic for Cities (Cisco): Cisco Kinetic for Cities is used in healthcare applications within smart cities. It provides IoT data collection, processing, and analytics capabilities, enabling healthcare services like remote patient monitoring and telehealth.
- Siemens Healthineers Digital Ecosystem (Siemens Healthineers): Siemens Healthineers provides a digital ecosystem for healthcare, including IoT solutions for medical equipment and diagnostics. It enables data sharing, analysis, and integration with clinical workflows.
- Particle Health (Particle): Particle Health focuses on IoT connectivity for healthcare devices, providing a platform for device data collection, management, and secure transmission. It is suitable for remote patient monitoring and medication adherence solutions.
- Philips HealthSuite (Philips): Philips HealthSuite provides a cloud-based platform for connected healthcare solutions, including remote monitoring, telehealth, and data analytics. It supports interoperability with a wide range of medical devices.
- ThingWorx (PTC): ThingWorx is an IoT platform with applications in various industries, including healthcare. It provides device management, data analytics, and visualization tools for healthcare IoT solutions.
- Telit IoT Platform (Telit): Telit provides a platform for IoT device connectivity and data management, suitable for healthcare applications like remote patient monitoring and asset tracking.
- Bosch IoT Suite (Bosch): Bosch IoT Suite provides IoT solutions for various industries, including healthcare. It provides device management, data analytics, and security features for healthcare IoT deployments.

Therefore, these IoT platforms offer a variety of capabilities to meet the specific needs and requirements of smart healthcare applications. When choosing an IoT platform for healthcare, considerations such as data security, compliance with healthcare regulations (e.g., HIPAA), scalability, interoperability, and integration with existing healthcare systems and electronic health records (EHRs) must be taken into account.

7. DATA MANAGEMENT AND ANALYTICS IN HEALTHCARE

Data management and analytics play a critical role in healthcare, enabling healthcare organizations to make informed decisions, improve patient care, optimize operations, and advance medical research. Here's an overview of data management and analytics in healthcare:

A. Data Management in Healthcare:
- Data Collection: Healthcare organizations collect vast amounts of data from various sources, including electronic health records (EHRs), medical devices, wearable sensors, and patient surveys. Data can be structured (e.g., patient demographics, lab results) or unstructured (e.g., clinical notes, radiology images).
- Data Integration: Healthcare systems often consist of multiple data sources and formats. Data integration involves consolidating data from disparate sources into a unified and standardized format for analysis.
- Data Quality and Cleansing: Ensuring data accuracy and quality is important. Data cleansing processes identify and correct errors, duplicates, and inconsistencies in healthcare data.
- Data Storage: Healthcare data is typically stored in secure, compliant, and scalable databases or data warehouses. Cloud-based storage solutions are increasingly popular for their flexibility and accessibility.
- Data Security and Privacy: Healthcare data is governed by stringent regulations, such as HIPAA in the U.S. Effective data management involves implementing robust security measures, access controls, and encryption to safeguard patient information.
- Data Governance: Establishing policies and procedures for data access, sharing, and use, as well as assigning responsibility for data management within the organization.
- Data Lifecycle Management: Overseeing data across its lifecycle, from creation and storage to archival or disposal, while ensuring adherence to retention policies.

B. Analytics in Healthcare:
- Descriptive Analytics: Descriptive analytics entails scrutinizing historical healthcare data to derive insights into past events and trends, aiding healthcare organizations in comprehending what has transpired.
- Diagnostic Analytics: Diagnostic analytics aims to identify the causes of specific healthcare events or issues. It helps in diagnosing diseases, understanding readmission patterns, and identifying potential healthcare disparities.
- Predictive Analytics: Predictive analytics utilizes historical data to anticipate future events or trends. In healthcare, this can involve predicting disease outbreaks, patient readmissions, and the risk of complications.
- Prescriptive Analytics: Prescriptive analytics goes beyond prediction to suggest actionable recommendations. In healthcare, it can help with treatment planning, resource allocation, and personalized care plans.
- Clinical Decision Support (CDS) Systems: Clinical Decision Support (CDS) systems employ analytics to furnish healthcare professionals with evidence-based recommendations and alerts directly at the point of care, facilitating clinical decision-making.

      ○   Population Health Management: Analytics is used to monitor and improve the health of entire populations by identifying high-risk individuals, targeting interventions, and measuring outcomes.

      ○   Natural Language Processing (NLP): NLP techniques are applied to analyze unstructured clinical notes and free-text data, extracting valuable insights from clinical narratives.

      ○   Image Analysis: Machine learning and deep learning algorithms analyze medical images (e.g., X-rays, MRI scans) to aid in diagnosis, early detection, and treatment planning.

      ○   Genomic Data Analysis: Advanced analytics are applied to genomic data to understand genetic predispositions, identify biomarkers, and tailor treatment plans in precision medicine.

C.   Challenges and Issues:

      ○   Data Privacy and Compliance: Healthcare organizations must adhere to strict regulations governing patient data privacy and security (e.g., HIPAA, GDPR).

      ○   Interoperability: Facilitating seamless exchange and utilization of data among various healthcare systems and Electronic Health Records (EHRs) poses a significant challenge.

      ○   Scalability: As data volumes grow, healthcare systems must be scalable to handle the increasing data load efficiently.

      ○   Ethical Issues: Responsible and ethical use of healthcare data, especially in AI and machine learning applications, is a critical issue.

      ○   Data Literacy: Healthcare professionals need training in data analysis and interpretation to use analytics effectively.

      ○   Data Access and Governance: Striking the right balance between data access and governance is essential to ensure data is available for analysis while maintaining security and privacy.

Therefore, innovations in healthcare, driven by data management and analytics, are contributing to enhancements in patient outcomes, cost reduction, and advancements in medical research. As healthcare organizations increasingly leverage the potential of data, addressing these challenges becomes crucial to maximize the benefits of data-driven decision-making. Further exploration can include topics like Data Collection and Storage in Smart Healthcare, Big Data Analytics in Healthcare, and Privacy and Security of Healthcare IoT Data.

8. ISSUES, CHALLENGES AND FUTURE TRENDS TOWARDS IOT BASED SMART HEALTHCARE

Implementing IoT-based smart healthcare solutions presents various challenges and issues that need to be addressed to ensure successful deployment and maximize the benefits. Some of the key challenges and issues mentioned in table 1.

Hence, these challenges and issues require a collaborative effort among healthcare organizations, technology providers, regulators, and other stakeholders. By carefully addressing these issues, IoT-based smart healthcare solutions can provide significant benefits in terms of improved patient care, enhanced efficiency, and better health outcomes.

Table 1. Issues and challenges and future trends towards IoT based smart healthcare

Type	Issue	Challenges
Data Security and Privacy	Given the high sensitivity of healthcare data, concerns about data security and privacy breaches arise with the collection and transmission of patient information through IoT devices.	Implementing strong encryption, access controls, and ensuring compliance with healthcare regulations (e.g., HIPAA) is vital to safeguard patient data
Interoperability	Within the healthcare ecosystem, a multitude of devices, systems, and protocols frequently lack interoperability, posing challenges for seamless data exchange.	Establishing and embracing standards and protocols for interoperability is crucial to facilitate collaboration among various devices and systems.
Regulatory Compliance	Healthcare is subject to strict regulations, making it challenging to navigate compliance requirements for IoT-based solutions.	Ensuring that IoT systems comply with regulatory standards and obtaining necessary approvals are critical steps in the implementation process.
Reliability and Accuracy	IoT devices may not always provide accurate data due to sensor limitations or connectivity issues, leading to potential false alarms or missed health issues.	Ensuring the reliability and accuracy of IoT devices through rigorous testing and calibration is essential for patient safety
Scalability	As the number of IoT devices and data volume grows, healthcare systems must be scalable to handle the increasing workload efficiently.	Designing scalable infrastructure and ensuring network capacity are essential to accommodate the expanding IoT ecosystem.
Costs of Implementation	Deploying IoT-based smart healthcare systems can be expensive, requiring investments in devices, infrastructure, and personnel	Healthcare organizations must weigh the costs against the expected benefits and find sustainable funding models.
Data Overload	The sheer volume of data generated by IoT devices can overwhelm healthcare providers, leading to information overload.	Implementing advanced analytics and AI tools to filter and prioritize relevant data can help manage data overload.
Technical Challenges	IoT devices may face technical challenges, such as battery life limitations, connectivity issues, and device interoperability.	Addressing technical issues through ongoing maintenance, updates, and technological advancements is important for system reliability.
Patient Trust	Patients may be issueed about the security and privacy of their health data, leading to reluctance in adopting IoT-based healthcare solutions.	Building and maintaining patient trust through transparency, informed consent, and robust security measures is essential for successful adoption.
Health Inequities	Unequal access to technology and healthcare resources may exacerbate health disparities if not addressed in IoT implementations.	Implementing IoT solutions equitably and ensuring access for underserved populations is critical to avoid exacerbating healthcare inequalities.

8.1 Future Trends/ Innovations: AI and Machine Learning, Edge Computing, and Blockchain in Healthcare

AI and Machine Learning, Edge Computing, and Blockchain are transformative technologies that have found applications in healthcare, each addressing specific challenges and opportunities in the industry.

A.   AI and Machine Learning in Healthcare:
   ◦   Disease Diagnosis and Prediction: AI algorithms can examine medical images, such as X-rays and MRIs, aiding in the early detection of diseases like cancer and offering diagnostic support.
   ◦   Treatment Personalization: Machine learning models scrutinize patient data, genetic information, and treatment outcomes to formulate personalized treatment plans and identify the most effective therapies.

- Drug Discovery: AI expedites the drug discovery process by forecasting potential drug candidates, simulating molecular interactions, and pinpointing target molecules for specific diseases.
- Clinical Decision Support: Clinical decision support systems powered by AI assist healthcare providers in making evidence-based decisions by analyzing patient data, medical literature, and treatment guidelines.
- Remote Patient Monitoring: Clinical decision support systems powered by AI assist healthcare providers in making evidence-based decisions by analyzing patient data, medical literature, and treatment guidelines.
- Natural Language Processing (NLP): Natural Language Processing (NLP) techniques extract valuable insights from unstructured clinical notes, enabling sentiment analysis, trend detection, and automated coding.
- Predictive Analytics: Machine learning models predict patient readmissions, disease outbreaks, and resource utilization, helping hospitals allocate resources more effectively.
- Image and Speech Recognition: AI-powered speech recognition tools enhance medical transcription and simplify the documentation process. Image recognition aids in automating radiology report generation.

B. Edge Computing in Healthcare:

- Real-Time Data Processing: Edge computing positions computational power in proximity to the data source, enabling real-time processing of medical data from IoT devices and sensors.
- Low Latency: Reducing data transmission latency is important for applications like remote surgery and telemedicine, where split-second decisions are critical.
- Privacy and Security: Edge computing can process sensitive healthcare data locally, minimizing the risk of data breaches associated with centralized cloud processing.
- Offline Operation: In remote or underserved areas with intermittent connectivity, edge devices can operate offline and sync data when a connection is available, ensuring continuous healthcare services.
- Scalability: Edge devices can be easily deployed and scaled to accommodate the growing number of IoT devices in healthcare without overburdening centralized data centers.

C. Blockchain in Healthcare:

- Health Data Security: Blockchain guarantees the secure and tamper-proof storage of health records, safeguarding patient data from unauthorized access or alteration.
- Interoperability: Blockchain has the potential to enhance interoperability among diverse healthcare systems and Electronic Health Records (EHRs), enabling seamless data exchange and sharing.
- Consent Management: Patients can exercise increased control over their health data by granting granular consent for data access and sharing through consent management systems based on blockchain technology.
- Drug Traceability: Blockchain aids in monitoring the pharmaceutical supply chain, guaranteeing the authenticity and quality of medications while mitigating the risk of counterfeit drugs.
- Clinical Trials: Blockchain streamlines and secures the management of clinical trial data, ensuring transparency and integrity in research.

◦ Billing and Claims Processing: Smart contracts on the blockchain can automate and streamline billing processes, thereby reducing administrative overhead in healthcare finance.
◦ Healthcare Payments: Cryptocurrencies and blockchain-based payment systems provide secure, transparent, and cost-effective methods for healthcare payments.

Therefore, the implementation of these technologies in healthcare necessitates thoughtful consideration of regulatory compliance, data privacy, and interoperability. Nevertheless, when employed effectively, they hold the potential to revolutionize healthcare, contributing to improved patient outcomes, cost reduction, enhanced data security, and the facilitation of new and innovative healthcare services.

9. CONCLUSION

In today's era, IoT-based healthcare represents a transformative shift, redefining the way we deliver and experience healthcare services. Leveraging interconnected devices, data analytics, and real-time monitoring, IoT in healthcare aims to enhance patient care, streamline operations, and address industry challenges. Through the integration of IoT devices and sensors, healthcare providers can remotely monitor patients, track vital signs, and proactively intervene, especially for those managing chronic conditions. This not only improves patient outcomes but also alleviates the strain on healthcare facilities and reduces overall healthcare costs.

The application of AI and machine learning algorithms to healthcare IoT data unlocks unprecedented insights. From predictive analytics for disease outbreaks to personalized treatment plans and drug discovery, these technologies are revolutionizing healthcare, providing precise and efficient solutions. Furthermore, Blockchain technology ensures data security and integrity, enabling secure data sharing and consent management. It holds the potential to empower patients with greater control over their health data, fostering trust and transparency.

As technology continues to advance and healthcare providers embrace these innovations, a future is envisioned where healthcare services become more personalized, efficient, and accessible. This evolution is expected to significantly improve the lives of individuals and communities globally.

REFERENCES

Adebiyi, M. O., Afolayan, J. O., Arowolo, M. O., Tyagi, A. K., & Adebiyi, A. A. (2023). Breast Cancer Detection Using a PSO-ANN Machine Learning Technique. In A. Tyagi (Ed.), *Using Multimedia Systems, Tools, and Technologies for Smart Healthcare Services* (pp. 96–116). IGI Global. doi:10.4018/978-1-6684-5741-2.ch007

Deekshetha, H. R. (2023). Automated and intelligent systems for next-generation-based smart applications. Data Science for Genomics. Academic Press. doi:10.1016/B978-0-323-98352-5.00019-7

Deshmukh, A., Sreenath, N., Tyagi, A. K., & Eswara Abhichandan, U. V. (2022). Blockchain Enabled Cyber Security: A Comprehensive Survey. *2022 International Conference on Computer Communication and Informatics (ICCCI),* (pp. 1-6). IEEE. 10.1109/ICCCI54379.2022.9740843

Gomathi, L., Mishra, A. K., & Tyagi, A. K. (2023). *Industry 5.0 for Healthcare 5.0: Opportunities, Challenges and Future Research Possibilities.* 2023 7th International Conference on Trends in Electronics and Informatics (ICOEI), Tirunelveli, India. 10.1109/ICOEI56765.2023.10125660

Tyagi, A. (2023). Hemamalini, Gulshan Soni, Digital Health Communication With Artificial Intelligence-Based Cyber Security, in the book: AI-Based Digital Health Communication for Securing Assistive Systems. IGI Global. doi:10.4018/978-1-6684-8938-3.ch009

Kumari, S., Muthulakshmi, P., & Agarwal, D. (2022). Deployment of Machine Learning Based Internet of Things Networks for Tele-Medical and Remote Healthcare. In V. Suma, X. Fernando, K. L. Du, & H. Wang (Eds.), *Evolutionary Computing and Mobile Sustainable Networks. Lecture Notes on Data Engineering and Communications Technologies* (Vol. 116). Springer. doi:10.1007/978-981-16-9605-3_21

Kute, S. (2021). Building a Smart Healthcare System Using Internet of Things and Machine Learning. Big Data Management in Sensing: Applications in AI and IoT. River Publishers.

Kute, S. (2021). Research Issues and Future Research Directions Toward Smart Healthcare Using Internet of Things and Machine Learning. Big Data Management in Sensing: Applications in AI and IoT. River Publishers.

Kute, S. S., Tyagi, A. K., & Aswathy, S. U. (2022). Industry 4.0 Challenges in e-Healthcare Applications and Emerging Technologies. In A. K. Tyagi, A. Abraham, & A. Kaklauskas (Eds.), *Intelligent Interactive Multimedia Systems for e-Healthcare Applications.* Springer. doi:10.1007/978-981-16-6542-4_14

Kute, S. S., Tyagi, A. K., & Aswathy, S. U. (2022). Security, Privacy and Trust Issues in Internet of Things and Machine Learning Based e-Healthcare. In A. K. Tyagi, A. Abraham, & A. Kaklauskas (Eds.), *Intelligent Interactive Multimedia Systems for e-Healthcare Applications.* Springer. doi:10.1007/978-981-16-6542-4_15

Madhav, A. V. S., & Tyagi, A. K. (2022). The World with Future Technologies (Post-COVID-19): Open Issues, Challenges, and the Road Ahead. In A. K. Tyagi, A. Abraham, & A. Kaklauskas (Eds.), *Intelligent Interactive Multimedia Systems for e-Healthcare Applications.* Springer. doi:10.1007/978-981-16-6542-4_22

Nair, M. M., Kumari, S., Tyagi, A. K., & Sravanthi, K. (2021) Deep Learning for Medical Image Recognition: Open Issues and a Way to Forward. In: Goyal D., Gupta A.K., Piuri V., Ganzha M., Paprzycki M. (eds) *Proceedings of the Second International Conference on Information Management and Machine Intelligence. Lecture Notes in Networks and Systems.* Springer, Singapore. /10.1007/978-981-15-9689-6_38

Nair, M. M., & Tyagi, A. K. (2023). AI, IoT, blockchain, and cloud computing: The necessity of the future. Rajiv Pandey, Sam Goundar, Shahnaz Fatima (eds.), Distributed Computing to Blockchain. Academic Press. doi:10.1016/B978-0-323-96146-2.00001-2

Sai, G. H., Tripathi, K., & Tyagi, A. K. (2023). Internet of Things-Based e-Health Care: Key Challenges and Recommended Solutions for Future. In: Singh, P.K., Wierzchoń, S.T., Tanwar, S., Rodrigues, J.J.P.C., Ganzha, M. (eds) *Proceedings of Third International Conference on Computing, Communications, and Cyber-Security.* Springer, Singapore. 10.1007/978-981-19-1142-2_37

Sai Dhakshan, Y. (2023). Introduction to Smart Healthcare: Healthcare Digitization. 6G-Enabled IoT and AI for Smart Healthcare. CRC Press.

Sajidha, S. A. (2023). Robust and Secure Evidence Management in Digital Forensics Investigations Using Blockchain Technology. AI-Based Digital Health Communication for Securing Assistive Systems. IGI Global. doi:10.4018/978-1-6684-8938-3.ch010

Shabnam Kumari, P. (2023). *Muthulakshmi, Effective Deep Learning-Based Attack Detection Methods for the Internet of Medical Things, in the book: AI-Based Digital Health Communication for Securing Assistive Systems*. IGI Global. doi:10.4018/978-1-6684-8938-3.ch008

Sheth, H. S. K., & Tyagi, A. K. (2022). Mobile Cloud Computing: Issues, Applications and Scope in COVID-19. In A. Abraham, N. Gandhi, T. Hanne, T. P. Hong, T. Nogueira Rios, & W. Ding (Eds.), *Intelligent Systems Design and Applications. ISDA 2021. Lecture Notes in Networks and Systems* (Vol. 418). Springer. doi:10.1007/978-3-030-96308-8_55

Tyagi, A., Kukreja, S., Nair, M. M., & Tyagi, A. K. (2022). Machine Learning: Past, Present and Future. *NeuroQuantology: An Interdisciplinary Journal of Neuroscience and Quantum Physics*, 20(8). doi:10.14704/nq.2022.20.8.NQ44468

Tyagi, A. K., Chandrasekaran, S., & Sreenath, N. (2022). Blockchain Technology:– A New Technology for Creating Distributed and Trusted Computing Environment. 2022 International Conference on Applied Artificial Intelligence and Computing (ICAAIC), (pp. 1348-1354). IEEE.10.1109/ICAAIC53929.2022.9792702

Tyagi, A. (2021, October). Aswathy S U, G Aghila, N Sreenath "AARIN: Affordable, Accurate, Reliable and INnovative Mechanism to Protect a Medical Cyber-Physical System using Blockchain Technology". *IJIN*, 2, 175–183.

Tyagi, A. (2023). Decentralized everything: Practical use of blockchain technology in future applications. Distributed Computing to Blockchain. Academic Press. doi:10.1016/B978-0-323-96146-2.00010-3

Tyagi, A. (2023). Digital Twin Technology: Opportunities and Challenges for Smart Era's Applications. In *Proceedings of the 2023 Fifteenth International Conference on Contemporary Computing (IC3-2023)*. Association for Computing Machinery. 10.1145/3607947.3608015

Tyagi, A. (2022). Using Multimedia Systems, Tools, and Technologies for Smart Healthcare Services. IGI Global., doi:10.4018/978-1-6684-5741-2

42

Chapter 3
Insightful Visions:
How Medical Imaging Empowers Patient–Centric Healthcare

Jaspreet Kaur
Chandigarh University, India

ABSTRACT

The chapter explores the transformative impact of medical imaging on healthcare that prioritizes the needs and well-being of patients. It examines the influence of imaging technologies on the precision of diagnoses, the involvement of patients, and the results of healthcare, highlighting the revolutionary function of imaging modalities. This study examines the impact of medical imaging on patient empowerment by doing a thorough review of literature and analyzing empirical evidence. It demonstrates how visual representations offered by medical imaging enable people to better comprehend their health situations and promote collaborative decision-making with healthcare practitioners. The results emphasize the crucial significance of imaging in influencing a better-informed, involved, and empowered patient community within contemporary healthcare systems.

1. INTRODUCTION

The field of contemporary healthcare has seen a substantial transformation as a direct consequence of the discovery and development of capabilities related to medical imaging. Healthcare in the modern era has gotten significantly more advanced. It is possible to trace this growth back to the fact that medical imaging has developed into a key component in the processes of diagnosis and treatment planning as depicted in figure 1 below:

DOI: 10.4018/979-8-3693-2359-5.ch003

Copyright © 2024, IGI Global. Copying or distributing in print or electronic forms without written permission of IGI Global is prohibited.

Figure 1. Development of medical imaging technology over time

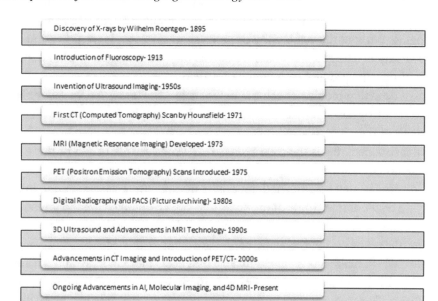

This progression is a consequence of the advancements that have been made in medical imaging recently. The advancement of medical imaging technology has led to the development of treatment models that are not only more customized but also more focused on the specific patient. The implementation of these treatment models has resulted in a significant impact on the outcomes and experiences of patients, which is a consequence of the fact that this has occurred. The outcomes and experiences of patients have been significantly altered as a consequence of this, which has brought about a significant impact (Aldamaeen et al., 2023).

In the year 1895, Wilhelm Roentgen made the groundbreaking discovery of X-rays, which initiated a new age in the field of medicine. This discovery had a profound impact on the entire world. Within the context of the time period in question, this discovery signified the beginning of a new era in the field of medicine. The method of observing and diagnosing persons who were suffering from diseases included the utilization of X-rays. This discovery is largely acknowledged to have been the impetus for the establishment of the scientific area of medical imaging.

In general, this is the widespread consensus. There have been significant advancements achieved in this area, beginning with the invention of X-rays and continuing through the development of modern imaging modalities like as computed tomography (CT), magnetic resonance imaging (MRI), ultrasound, and other imaging techniques. These advancements have been made possible by the introduction of X-rays. These developments are a direct result of the ongoing improvement of imaging technology, which has made them conceivable. These advances have been able to become a reality as a result of the ongoing development of the profession, which has been a driving force behind their occurrence (Caronongan et al., 2018).

Diagnostic capabilities are one of the most important aspects of the relevance of medical imaging. These capabilities are provided by medical imaging. Regarding the significance of medical imaging, there are a number of additional issues that should also be taken into consideration. These features are important and should be taken into account. Using imaging technologies, medical professionals are able to visually examine internal structures and identify anomalies or diseases that would not be obvious based only on the findings of physical examinations. This is made possible by the visualization capabilities of imaging technologies. Without the availability of imaging technology, it would be impossible to carry out this kind of evaluation. The broad availability of imaging technologies is what makes this promise a reality. Because of this, the promise may now be fulfilled.

The procedure of detecting problems such as malignancies, fractures, and vascular disorders is made significantly less difficult by the employment of computed tomography (CT) scans, which provide precise cross-sectional views of the affected area.

In this particular instance, this is the case because CT scans are the origin of these images. On the other hand, the technology known as magnetic resonance imaging (MRI) is able to effectively differentiate between soft tissues to a significant degree. It is possible to receive accurate images of a broad variety of places as a result of this. Some of the areas that can be obtained are the joints, the spinal cord, and the nervous system, among-st other areas. The manner in which patients are treated has undergone significant transformations as a consequence of the advantages that these technologies bring about. Imaging modalities, which make it possible to make a diagnosis more quickly and with more precision, frequently make it possible to carry out therapies in a timely way and contribute to the improvement of treatment possibilities. This is because imaging modalities make it possible to make a diagnosis quickly and with greater accuracy. Imaging modalities are responsible for this since they allow for earlier and more accurate diagnosis of illnesses.

This is the reason why this is the case. Imaging is of the utmost importance in the field of oncology since it plays a large role in defining the stage of cancer, creating treatment choices, and establishing whether or not therapy is therapeutically effective. In addition, imaging is used to generate possible treatment options. In light of this, imaging is of the utmost significance for the reason stated above. The final result is that patients who are hospitalized experience an improvement in their quality of life, as well as an increase in the percentage of patients who survive their disease. This is the ultimate consequence. This is the conclusion that can be reached having taken into account all that has been taken into consideration (Chalmers et al., 2017).

The development of medical imaging has not only resulted in an increase in the accuracy of diagnoses, but it has also made it possible for there to be an improvement in the efficiency of procedures. As a result of this development, there has been an improvement in the efficiency of treatments that only require techniques that are classified as minimally invasive. This is as a result of the fact that medical imaging has made it possible for there to be an improvement in the degree to which diagnostic procedures can be carried out with a higher degree of precision. Real-time imaging makes it possible to precisely identify certain regions of interest when it is used to the context of image-guided therapies or operations. This is made possible by the utilization of real-time imaging. An important benefit is that this is the case. Consequently, this results in a reduction in the pervasiveness of the treatments, a reduction in the amount of time that is necessary for recuperation, and a reduction in the consequences that these treatments have on the patients.

The field of medical imaging has not only been a significant contributor to the transformation that has taken place in the healthcare business, but it has also been a driving force behind the revolution that has taken place in the field of diagnosis and therapy. It has finally led to the transformation of the healthcare industry as a result of the fact that it has made the transition toward care models that are centered on the patient easier to accomplish. This is due to the fact that it has made the completion of the transfer much simpler. As a result of the utilization of these technologies, patients are able to play an active role in their own involvement in the process of getting medical care. This is because the utilization of these technologies makes it possible for patients to actively participate in the process from their own perspective.

This purpose is attained by providing patients with visual representations of the medical difficulties that they themselves are experiencing. This is the manner by which this objective is accomplished. The degree of communication that exists between medical personnel and patients can be improved via the employment of visual aids that are provided by imaging. This is something that is attainable. In the end, this results in decisions that are better informed, and it also contributes to the development of a method of treating patients that is based on teamwork (Chu et al., 2018).

Additionally, the development of imaging technology has been a driving force behind the change toward approaches to medical care that are adapted to the specific needs of each individual patient individually. This transition has been brought about by the growth of imaging technology. The growth of imaging technology is responsible for bringing about this change which has occurred. One of the options that is becoming more and more practical is the design of treatment regimens that are tailored to match the specific requirements of each and every individual patient. In order to accomplish this goal, it is absolutely necessary to take into account the specific characteristics of each individual participant in the study. The genetic make-up of the patients and the specific symptoms of their sickness that can be identified through the employment of imaging tools are both included in these characteristics. It is feasible to improve the efficacy of treatment while also minimizing the quantity of negative effects that are experienced by particular patients if a personalized strategy is implemented. This is something that can be accomplished.

The utilization of it is what makes this something that is possible. Patients report feeling a larger degree of pleasure or joy as a direct result of this, which ultimately leads to improved outcomes as a consequence of the particular conditions associated with the situation. On the other hand, in spite of these accomplishments, there are nonetheless challenges that need to be conquered. In particular, the worries regarding the availability of contemporary imaging technologies and the cost-effectiveness of these technologies continue to be a cause of concern, particularly in instances where there is an insufficient amount of services available.

Additionally, the medical community is continually placing a high priority on the right deployment of imaging technologies in order to, among other things, minimize the amount of radiation exposure and remove therapies that are not necessary. This is being done in order to improve patient safety. For the purpose of achieving both of these goals, this action is being taken in order to achieve them. This measure is being taken in order to provide patients with aid in avoiding therapies that are not suitable for their condition for the purpose of providing them with assistance (Ghonge, 2019).

In the end, the proliferation of medical imaging has had a significant influence on the businesses that are involved in healthcare as represented in figure 2 below:

This is due to the fact that technology has enhanced the precision of diagnoses, offered direction for medical treatments, and promoted care delivery systems that are based on the individual person receiving treatment. The field has been subjected to a fundamental change as a consequence of this enormous effect. It is anticipated that the ongoing development of these technical improvements will continue to be a driving force for innovation in the future. As a consequence of this, the use of individualized treatment will advance, which will ultimately result in better outcomes for patients. As we continue to make advances in this field of study, it is necessary to eliminate impediments and ensure that all patients have equal access to these technologies with the goal of achieving equal access for all patients. In order to achieve the objective of fully achieving the potential of medical imaging for the benefit of all patients, this is something that is required. One of the ways in which this objective might be accomplished is by ensuring that all patients have equitable access to the many technologies that are available (Jabarulla & Lee, 2020).

Figure 2. Influence of the proliferation of medical imaging on healthcare businesses

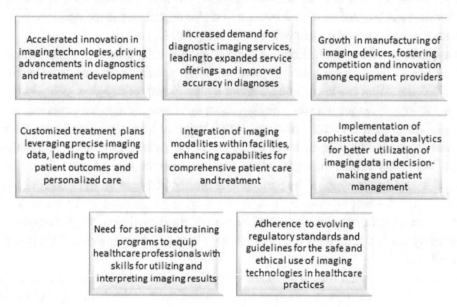

2. NUMERICAL APPROACHES AND ALGORITHMIC METHODS ON PATIENT-CENTRIST HEALTHCARE IN THE CONTEXT OF MEDICAL IMAGING

Early Detection and Diagnosis: Algorithms, through numerical methodologies, allow for the extraction of complex information from medical images that may be difficult for humans to see. This increased sensitivity enables the prompt detection of abnormalities, allowing for quick and proactive medical intervention. Early detection of diseases greatly enhances patient outcomes and promotes a patient-centered approach by emphasizing preventive interventions.

Tailored Treatment Planning: Algorithmic techniques analyze complex medical imaging data to detect subtle alterations in patients' situations. Such a high degree of accuracy enables the development of customized and individualized treatment strategies. Healthcare professionals can enhance therapeutic techniques by taking into account individual variations in anatomy, pathology, and treatment responses. This individualized approach not only improves the effectiveness of treatment but also adheres to the ideals of patient-centered care, recognizing the distinct attributes of each patient.

Precision Medicine: Numerical methodologies enhance the advancement of precision medicine by quantifying data obtained from medical imaging. Algorithms utilize genetic, environmental, and imaging-related aspects to assist clinicians in tailoring treatment regimens. This customized approach guarantees that therapies are in accordance with the distinct traits of each patient, promoting a patient-centered paradigm where healthcare is precisely adjusted to individual requirements and characteristics.

Remote Monitoring:Algorithmic surveillance of medical imaging data enables remote monitoring of patients' health condition. This live monitoring enables immediate intervention and modifications to treatment protocols without necessitating patients' actual presence at healthcare establishments. This not only improves patient convenience but also enables individuals to actively engage in their healthcare, fostering a patient-centrist approach that goes beyond typical healthcare facilities.

Improved Imaging Techniques:Numerical simulations and algorithmic modeling play a crucial role in enhancing imaging modalities by enhancing their precision and resolution. This not only facilitates more precise diagnoses but also improves the overall quality of medical imaging. These developments enhance patient-centrist care by furnishing healthcare personnel with precise and comprehensive information, thereby assuring that diagnostic processes are maximally informative and dependable.

Automated Image Analysis:Algorithmic image processing streamlines repetitive processes in the examination of medical images, hence diminishing the burden on healthcare practitioners. This enhancement in efficiency allows for expedited turnaround times in diagnostic outcomes, so promoting swift decision-making and ensuring that patients receive timely information regarding their health. The efficient workflow adheres to patient-centrist principles by emphasizing effectiveness and reducing any potential delays in the provision of healthcare services.

Data-Driven Insights: Applying numerical analytic to extensive datasets obtained from medical imaging tests yields useful insights into larger health patterns and treatment results. The utilization of data in decision-making in healthcare facilitates evidence-based practices, guaranteeing that therapies are led by thorough and current information. By integrating data-driven insights, patient-centrist care becomes better informed and more responsive to the changing field of medical knowledge.

Enhanced Workflow Efficiency:The productivity of medical imaging departments is enhanced through algorithmic optimization, which automates repetitive processes. This enables healthcare workers to spend additional time to patient engagement and individualized care. The enhanced operational effectiveness not only advantages healthcare professionals but also adheres to patient-centrist principles by highlighting the human element of healthcare delivery.

Overall, the use of numerical techniques and algorithmic methodologies in medical imaging has a profound effect on healthcare that prioritizes the needs of individual patients. By incorporating early detection, tailored treatment planning, remote monitoring, and data-driven insights, these methods collectively enhance the healthcare model, making it more accurate, effective, and responsive to the individual requirements of each patient.

3. LITERATURE REVIEW

The introduction of medical imaging, which is an essential component of modern healthcare, has resulted in a substantial change in the treatment and diagnosis of medical illnesses. Today, medical imaging is an essential component of modern healthcare. The development of medical imaging has been the driving force behind this shift in the industry. With the help of this study, we hope to shed light on the significant role that medical imaging plays in the creation of paradigms that are centered on the patient throughout the entirety of the healthcare system. The process of consolidation and evaluation will be utilized in order to attain this goal with the assistance of the existing body of material now available (Jabarulla & Lee, 2021).

The evolution of medical imaging processes has undergone a significant change over the course of the years that have passed since Wilhelm Roentgen made the accidental discovery of X-rays in the year 1895. This shift has occurred over the course of the years that have passed. There are many various factors that have had a role in the occurrence of this metamorphosis from beginning to end. These processes have resulted in the creation of a variety of advanced imaging modalities, some of which include nuclear imaging, computed tomography (CT) scans, ultrasound, and magnetic resonance imaging (MRI), to name just a few. These techniques are currently being applied in the contemporary medical practice that is being carried out. In the outset, the groundwork was laid by putting an emphasis on the diagnostic capacities of these modalities in the publications that were published, such as the ones that were written by Kanzaria et al (2015).

To emphasize the significance of imaging successes in transforming the detection and comprehension of diseases, it was mentioned that these discoveries have made correct diagnosis and treatment planning easier. This was discussed in order to highlight the value of imaging breakthroughs. All of this was done with the intention of highlighting the significance of imaging accomplishments. Our capacity to acquire a more profound grasp of diseases has been made possible as a result of the advancements that have been produced.

In addition, the findings of the research that was carried out by Khanna & Srivastava (2020) indicate that the application of artificial intelligence (AI) and machine learning in the field of medical imaging is the subject of research that is being carried out in the present day. This research is being carried out in the present day. When it comes to the interpretation of photographs, they place a considerable lot of emphasis on the part that algorithms driven by artificial intelligence serve to play. This helps to increase the accuracy of the diagnosis and speeds up the process to a larger extent than they would have been otherwise.

According to the findings of study that Kaur (2023) completed, the installation of technology that is powered by artificial intelligence in radiology departments is causing a revolution in the clinical operations that are generally carried out. Both the effectiveness of the procedure and the results for patients have been enhanced as a direct consequence of this integration, which has led to advances in both areas. All of these enhancements have been implemented.

One of the many recurring themes that can be found in the most recent medical imaging literature is the priority that is placed on delivering care that is centered on the patient. This is one of the numerous types of care that is provided. This body of literature also contains a variety of other subjects that can be found. Publications such as the one that Kaur & Sood (2018) published attract attention to the significance of patient involvement and the degree to which they are satisfied with the therapy that they are receiving when they are evaluated from a medical point of view. It is envisaged that developments in imaging technology will increase diagnostic capabilities and equip patients with more agency. This will be accomplished through the employment of visual representations and explanations of their diseases. By empowering patients to take an active role in their own healthcare journey, this objective will be satisfactorily realized. This goal will be accomplished through the utilization of imaging technology, which will be the way by which it will be accomplished.

An additional point of interest is that the accessibility and cost of imaging technology is a significant subject that has been addressed in a significant number of scholarly publications, such as the in-depth analysis that was carried out by Keikhosrokiani et al. (2018). This is a subject that has been explored in a substantial number of publications. This topic has been the subject of research that has been published in a significant number of documents. Not only does the subject matter include technological expertise, but it also takes into account socioeconomic disparities, obstacles to infrastructure, and the allocation of resources from a holistic point of view. In addition to that, the aforementioned subject area requires technological expertise. Patients are unable to obtain care that is truly centered on them because of the regularity with which these injustices occur. Consequently, this results in obstacles that must be conquered in order to give patients with the treatment that they are entitled to receive. Individuals who are in positions of legislative responsibility and those who are responsible for delivering medical treatment are required to spend a greater degree of attention to this subject matter as a result of this.

The most recent research literature review provides light on the significant impact that medical imaging has had on healthcare, which lays an emphasis on the needs and desires of patients that are being treated. This insight is supplied by the evaluation of the most recent research literature that has been conducted. This is done with the intention of providing a concise summary of the information that is available. According to the body of research that describes a landscape in which this potential for change exists, medical imaging has the ability to revolutionize diagnosis and treatment, as well as to improve patient experiences and results (Kaur, 2023). This potential for change is also likely to improve patient outcomes. It is also said in this body of literature that medical imaging has the potential to influence the outcomes for patients. Additionally, medical imaging has the ability to improve the treatment that patients get all during their course of treatment. Several factors, including the development of new technologies, the growing involvement of patients, and the imperative to address systemic problems, are all factors that contribute to this phenomena. This is the reason why this is the case. On the other hand, it also brings to light the necessity of lowering barriers associated with accessibility and affordability in order to ensure that healthcare is provided in a manner that is both unbiased and fair. This is done in order to ensure that adequate medical treatment is provided to patients (Mohsan et al., 2022).

4. RESEARCH METHODOLOGY

This era, which is characterized by rapid technological progress, has been distinguished by the inclusion of medical imaging into healthcare, which has had a big impact on treatment that is centered on the patient. This has been a significant development in contemporary medicine. In order to analyze the numerous effects that medical imaging has on healthcare models that put the requirements of patients first while providing care, a comprehensive research technique was utilized. This article offers a concise explanation of the approach that was applied in the process of carrying out the research.

Compilation of several approaches and methods that can be used to carry out research: A hybrid approach was chosen as the methodology of choice for the goal of merging the various features of medical imaging into patient-centered care (also known as PCC). Through the utilization of qualitative and quantitative research approaches, this methodology was able to provide a full knowledge of the subject matter that was being examined. This strategy was chosen as the ideal technique because it utilized triangulation of information, which ensured a comprehensive study into the myriad of effects that medical imaging can have. This was the aspect that led to the selection of this strategy as the appropriate technique.

Assortment of methods and sources: Scholarly publications, academic databases, and conference proceedings that were relevant to the subject matter that was being investigated were the primary sources of information that were employed. It was necessary to conduct a thorough search strategy in order to locate content that was pertinent to the topic that was being discussed at the time (the subject matter). Components of this strategy were the utilization of keywords, and the utilization of inclusion/

exclusion criteria. As a result of a careful screening approach that took into consideration the relevance of the publication, the study design, and the year in which the publication was released, contemporary research of the best possible quality was included in the collection. This was accomplished by included the research in the collection.

Method for carrying out a review of the previously published material that is relevant to the subject at hand: When it came to the process of data extraction and synthesis, it was very necessary to pay attentive and comprehensive attention to the particulars of the situation. The pertinent information was rigorously categorized according to themes in order to uncover repeating patterns, trends, and noteworthy insights that were extracted from the selected literature. This was done in order to discover these things. The recognition of these patterns and trends was made feasible as a result of this. It was possible to organize and analyze a large variety of scientific papers and studies in a methodical manner thanks to the employment of bibliographic software. The accomplishment of this was carried out in a manner that was not only organized but also organized.

Methodologies and Technologies of Research utilized for the Purposes of Researching and Analyzing: Both qualitative content analysis and quantitative synthesis were utilized as methods of analysis within the context of the study that was being conducted. The process of qualitative content analysis includes a number of important steps, one of which is the identification of subjects and themes that appear repeatedly across the body of text. In this way, the analysis is guaranteed to be as precise as it can possibly be. This approach makes it possible to get a thorough understanding of patient-centered care, which is made possible by medical imaging and takes into consideration minor alterations. This understanding may be obtained through the deployment of this strategy. The quantitative synthesis process also included the utilization of statistical analysis in order to recognize patterns, frequency distributions, and correlations that were present within the data.

When it comes to the methodology of the research, ethical considerations were of the utmost importance throughout the entirety of the investigation. A vigilant attention to ethical norms, an uncompromising regard for intellectual property rights, and a strong commitment to ethical standards were some of the fundamental principles. One of the essential principles was the assurance that all data sources would remain completely anonymous. The research was able to keep its ethical integrity because it first acknowledged the existence of potential biases, then put into action techniques to limit the influence of such biases, and lastly gained clearance from the institutional review board. All of these steps were taken in order to ensure that the research was conducted in accordance with ethical standards. There were intrinsic limits to the approach, such as the likelihood of publication bias and the limited capacity to generalize the findings due to changes in research populations and conditions. These limitations were made possible by the methodology. These constraints were a contributing factor to the limits of the technique. Because of the nature of the method that was being utilized, these limitations were inevitable. In order to improve the reliability and validity of the study approach, both the utilization of rigorous analysis procedures and the maintenance of transparency within the methodology were utilized. This was done in order to get the desired results. In nutshell, there are a few points to consider with relation to the approaches that were taken.

The study methodology that was applied resulted in the achievement of a comprehensive and nuanced understanding of the ways in which medical imaging contributes to the improvement of healthcare that is centered on the patient. The approach that was chosen made it possible to carry out a full examination into the multiple effects that medical imaging has on the procedures that are involved in the process of providing medical therapy. This was accomplished in spite of the fact that there were some constraints that were imposed on the method. The adoption of this methodology makes it easier to conduct research on outcomes, which in turn provides essential insights that can be utilized in the process of developing care patterns that are centered on the patient. This study presents a comprehensive research method that demonstrates how medical imaging contributes to the delivery of healthcare that is centered on the patient. The objective of this study is to present this method. The technique, the collection of data, the analysis, the ethical difficulties, the. Changes have been made in order to meet certain complexities or more particulars that are required for your research.

5. RESULTS AND DISCUSSION

Qualitative results: According to the findings of the qualitative research, the utilization of medical imaging in healthcare that is focused on the requirements of the person may result in an increase in the degree to which patients are empowered within the healthcare system. This study was carried out with the purpose of investigating the myriad of ways in which the utilization of medical imaging technology can result in enhancements to healthcare practices that are centered on the patient. The incorporation of qualitative data along with the completion of an exhaustive review of the academic literature resulted in the discovery of a number of notable patterns. In light of these trends, the relevance of the impact that medical imaging has on patient care and involvement is brought into sharper perspective. The improvement of the accuracy of diagnosis and the facilitation of a better understanding of the challenges that patients are facing will be one of the themes that will be covered during the meeting.

Throughout the entirety of the qualitative analysis, a consistent focus was placed on the crucial significance of medical imaging in terms of facilitating a more accurate diagnosis and enhancing patient comprehension for the purpose of improving patient comprehension. In order to bring attention to the significance of medical imaging, this was done specifically. The readers have been made aware of the fact that Naresh et al. (2021) have paid attention to the significance of utilizing imaging modalities in order to give patients with visual representations that are both clear and detailed. This information has been brought to the attention of the readers. These graphical representations are an essential component of the process of educating patients about complex medical conditions so that they can make informed decisions regarding their care. Radio-logical graphics serve two purposes: first, they help medical professionals improve their ability to explain diagnoses; second, they empower individuals by improving their comprehension of their own health problems, which in turn makes it easier for them to make decisions based on accurate information. Both of these functions are accomplished through the use of radiological graphics. The importance of both of these goals cannot be overstated (Park et al., 2016).

Examining a number of study studies, such as those written by Ploug & Holm (2020) and Roy et al. (2021) shed light on the major influence that medical imaging has on the degree to which patients are active in their own care. A number of these articles were examined. Within the community of professionals working in the healthcare industry, it was noted that the imaging results served as catalysts for substantial conversations between patients and their physicians. During the discussions that took place, the concept of shared decision-making, which describes the process by which patients actively participate in comprehending the results of their imaging and jointly designing treatment decisions, was the focal focus of the discussions that took place. The findings of the qualitative research highlighted the significance of medical imaging as a key component in the process of transitioning away from a paternalistic healthcare paradigm and toward one that places a higher emphasis on patient autonomy and active engagement in taking care of themselves. This transition is taking place in the context of the process of transitioning away from Paternalism in Healthcare (Price, 2016).

As a result of the findings of the qualitative synthesis, it was determined that the patient's experience also included an emotional component, and this emotional component was found to be associated with medical imaging. Patients experienced a sense of empowerment when they were given the option to view their own imaging data, as demonstrated by the findings of the study that was carried out by Singh et al. (2020).These findings were brought to light by the findings of the research. This was due to the fact that it provided them with a comprehensive awareness of their current state of health, which was the motivating factor behind this. Through the utilization of imaging tools that were implanted within their bodies, the patients were able to examine the internal structures of their bodies as well as any abnormalities that were present. The fact that they were able to comprehend the scale of their issues and that they were given a feeling of power as a consequence of this experience motivated them to take responsibility for the outcomes of their health-related circumstances. Furthermore, it was demonstrated that patients who had access to imaging data were able to ask questions that were well-informed and have the ability to request answers from healthcare practitioners. This led to an increase in the patients' sense of agency in the management of their health journey.

The findings of the qualitative research provide a deeper knowledge of the role that medical imaging plays in fostering confidence and assurance between patients and healthcare practitioners. This insight is provided by the findings of the research. As demonstrated by the findings of the research that was carried out by Spruit & Lytras (2018) those members of the medical staff who are able to successfully communicate imaging findings to patients are able to develop a sense of confidence in their patients. This is the case because they are able to convey the relevant information to their patients. The employment of medical imaging as a form of visual proof allowed patients to experience an increase in their trust in their healthcare professionals, which ultimately led to an improvement in the accuracy of diagnoses and recommendations for treatment. This was a direct effect of the utilization of medical imaging. The findings of the qualitative research, shed light on the numerous ways in which medical imaging contributes to the development of healthcare that is centered on the patient. Therefore, this is due to the fact that medical imaging becomes an essential component in the process of shifting paradigms in healthcare delivery toward models that are centered on the patient. The improvement of diagnostic accuracy, the stimulation of patient involvement, the empowering of emotions, and the creation of trust are the means by which this objective is attained (Zhuang et al., 2020).

Also included in this section of the study are the qualitative findings that were obtained from the prior research that was conducted. The purpose of this article is to demonstrate the various ways in which medical imaging helps to patient-centered healthcare. These ways include the improvement of diagnosis, the maintenance of patient engagement, the production of an emotional impact, and the establishment of trust. There is the possibility of making modifications in accordance with specific findings from the study or other patterns that were discovered throughout the evaluation. Certainly, this is something that is attainable.

Quantitative results: For the purpose of conducting an objective analysis of the patterns, frequency distributions, and correlations that are associated with the utilization of medical imaging in patient-centered care, the research project that was awarded the title "Medical Imaging Empowers Patient-Centrist Healthcare" made use of a number of different statistical techniques. This was done in order to accomplish the goal of conducting the analysis. It was necessary to carry out this action in order to achieve the objective of carrying out the analysis.

For the purpose of gaining an understanding of the frequency of particular imaging procedures and the order in which they were carried out over a wide range of patient demographics or medical conditions, we made use of frequency distributions. We were able to acquire this comprehension whenever we had the chance to do so as a result of this. It is feasible to undertake an analysis of the frequency of magnetic resonance imaging (MRI) scans across various age groups or the prevalence of computed tomography (CT) scans in the diagnosis of specific diseases in order to acquire valuable insight into the use patterns of imaging technologies. This research can be done in order to gain valuable insight into the use patterns of imaging technologies. One method for accomplishing this objective is to carry out an analysis of the data obtained.

For the purpose of determining whether or whether there had been any temporal shifts or adjustments in the utilization or effectiveness of medical imaging, a trend analysis was carried out. For the purpose of identifying any possible alterations that may have taken place, this was carried out. For the goal of shedding light on increasing patterns and improvements in medical imaging technology, the purpose of the study is to assess trends in the adoption of imaging modalities and changes in diagnostic accuracy rates over the course of several years. This will be done in order to throw light on these increasing patterns and improvements. To shed light on rising trends and improvements, this will be done in order to put things into perspective. This result will be accomplished through the collection of information concerning these fluctuations and trends, which will be the means by which this result occurs. The employment of medical imaging in conjunction with correlation analysis was utilized in order to build ties between the factors that are related with patient outcomes and the processes that are involved. This was done in order to develop connections between the variables. In an effort to build connections, this was carried out. For the purpose of gaining insights into the potential influence that imaging may have on therapeutic outcomes, it is conceivable to have a correlation between the frequency of imaging operations and the amount of time it takes for patients to recover or the percentage of treatment that is successful. A correlation would be beneficial for gaining insights into the potential influence that imaging may have on therapeutic outcomes. To acquire a better understanding of the possible impact that imaging could have on the results of therapeutic interventions, it would be helpful to establish a correlation. It would be done with the intention of acquiring a knowledge of the potential impact that imaging could have on the results of therapeutic operations, and this would be done in order to provide that insight.

On the other hand, it is likely that regression analysis was applied in order to analyze the predictive value of certain imaging modalities in connection to the outcomes of patients. The statement that this is something that was carried out is a possibility. The results of this study have the potential to be useful in establishing the amount to which specific imaging modalities contribute to the prediction of treatment responses or prognosis for patients. This might be determined by determining the extent to which these modalities contribute. Following that, this information could be utilized to have an effect on the formulation of treatment management strategies that are specifically targeted to the patient. There is a potential that statistical tests for significance, such as t-tests or chi-square tests, were applied in order to establish the significance of the changes or connections that were observed in the data. This is something that is possible. This would have been done with the intention of determining whether or not the changes or relationships that had taken place between the parties were relevant. In order to determine whether or not the correlations or differences that have been discovered between a numbers of different variables are statistically significant, or whether or not they might be attributed to random chance, these tests are being carried out. The goal of these tests is to establish whether or not the correlations or differences are statistically significant.

It was the objective of the quantitative synthesis to produce proof of this kind in order to fulfill the purpose of providing empirical data that substantiates the significance of medical imaging in promoting patient-centered healthcare. It was thought that this would be the best way to convey the evidence during the presentation. The purpose of this research was to shed light on the measurable influence and significance of imaging technologies in terms of improving patient outcomes, generating tailored therapy models, and strengthening diagnostic accuracy. The research was conducted with the intention of shedding light on these themes. A variety of statistical methodologies were applied in order to measure and assess the data, which ultimately resulted in the accomplishment of this task effectively accomplished. A better understanding of the part that medical imaging plays in patient-centered care was the objective of the study, which was aimed to achieve this understanding through the utilization of data. The target of the study was to achieve this understanding. This objective was intended to be achieved by the study. Through the employment of statistical analysis, which was applied as a means of complementing qualitative data and strengthening our comprehension of the connection, our awareness of the relationship between medical imaging technologies and the results of healthcare was enlarged. This was accomplished by utilizing statistical analysis.

6. CONCLUSION

Due to the development of medical imaging, which has ushered in a new era in the delivery of healthcare, there has been a substantial shift in the precision of diagnoses, the effectiveness of medicines, and the participation of patients. This has been the case because of the fact that medical imaging has ushered in a new era. This study's concluding portion presents a complete examination of the considerable impact that medical imaging technology has on the evolution of patient-centered healthcare. This analysis is offered in the final section of this study. A detailed review of a wide variety of literary sources, in addition to empirical data, serves as the basis for this analysis for its foundation. Beginning with its insignificant beginnings and continuing up to the present day, the evolution of medical imaging has demonstrated remarkable improvement. It is possible to follow this progression all the way back to the beginning of the field. Beginning with Wilhelm Roentgen's fortunate discovery of X-rays and continuing on to the development of more advanced techniques such as magnetic resonance imaging (MRI), computed tomography (CT) scans, and positron emission tomography (PET/CT), each new technical advancement has resulted in the establishment of new benchmarks for medical care. It was Roentgen who made the discovery of X-rays. As a direct result of technological breakthroughs, which have brought about these improvements, there have been substantial changes in the manner in which patient care is provided. Not only have these technical advancements made it possible to improve the quality of medical images, but they have also made it simpler to diagnose patients without the need for invasive procedures to be carried out.

Imaging for diagnostic purposes is a fundamental necessity in the field of medicine, since it is necessary for the accurate identification and classification of disorders. As a result of the fact that these imaging techniques show minute details, they make it possible for medical professionals to develop individualized treatment plans for their patients, which ultimately results in better outcomes for the patients. Imaging techniques have the ability to correctly identify subtle anatomical and pathological changes, which helps doctors to make judgments that are well-informed. At the end of the day, this eventually results in an improvement in the quality of therapy that patients receive. The results of the research lend credence to this interpretation. The application of medical imaging in the process of delivering care to patients is not limited to the areas of diagnosis and therapy; rather, its breadth encompasses a wider range of applications. Through the use of imaging modalities, patients and their families are given visual representations, which helps them better appreciate the complicated medical concerns that they are experiencing. For the purpose of making it simpler for patients to take part in their own treatment, it is vital to engage in conversations with them and to make decisions together. Imaging data can be used as teaching tools, which gives patients the opportunity to take an active role in their own healthcare experiences. This is made possible by the fact that utilizing imaging data is possible. The healthcare industry is undergoing a significant transformation as a result of the adoption of medical imaging apps that incorporate artificial intelligence (AI). This shift is being brought about by the confluence of these two technological advancements. It is possible for imaging modalities to improve their capabilities as a result of the implementation of algorithms that are driven by artificial intelligence. The diagnostic accuracy can also be improved with these methods, and analysis can be completed more quickly. The utilization of artificial intelligence (AI) in conjunction with imaging has resulted in an increase in the efficiency of workflow, as well as an expansion of the opportunities for predictive analytic. Personalized medicine has risen to the forefront of the medical field as a direct consequence of this development.

Because of the significant impact that it has, it is of the utmost importance to take into consideration the ethical challenges that are brought about by the utilization of medical imaging. In light of the fact that imaging technologies are continuing to grow in the direction of becoming more sophisticated, it is of the utmost need to carry out an exhaustive examination into problems around data privacy, equitable access, and excessive use. When it comes to the field of healthcare, it is of the utmost importance to solve these ethical challenges in order to ensure that imaging technology is implemented in a manner that is not only acceptable but also equitable. As a result, it is essential that these challenges be addressed. In the field of medical imaging, which is already playing a vital role in the advancement of healthcare that is centered on the patient, there is opportunity for additional innovation even if it is currently playing a crucial function. Innovative technologies, such as molecular imaging and advancements in hybrid imaging, have the potential to enhance disease characterization and tailor treatment regimens to the specific needs of individual patients. The utilization of these technologies could be the means by which this objective is attained. This holds the key to releasing the maximum potential that these technologies have to offer. Additionally, the utilization of imaging data in conjunction with other healthcare datasets helps to expedite the process of providing integrated and comprehensive patient care models. This is accomplished through the utilization of imaging data.

As a result of the introduction of medical imaging into healthcare, major development has been speed up, which has led to the development of healthcare models that place an emphasis on therapy that is centered on the patient. There has been a notable quickening of the forward movement of development. Accuracy, the active participation of patients, the inclusion of technology, and the consideration of ethical considerations are all essential components of medical imaging, which plays a significant role in the transformation of healthcare. The transformation is influenced by each of these components individually. If healthcare systems were to integrate these improvements with the appropriate amount of consideration, it would be possible for them to truly empower individuals. This would guarantee that patients receive treatment that is effectively customized to their needs while also demonstrating compassion. A comprehensive analysis of the ways in which medical imaging has had a significant impact on patient-centered healthcare is presented during the course of this essay. The improvements in technology, the engagement of patients, ethical issues, and the future direction of healthcare delivery are some of the topics that are discussed in this work. Other topics that are discussed include the future direction of healthcare delivery. There is a chance that the essay could be altered in order to accommodate certain scientific discoveries or an increased level of complexity that are associated with the subject of medical imaging.

REFERENCES

Aldamaeen, O., Rashideh, W., & Obidallah, W. J. (2023). Toward Patient-Centric Healthcare Systems: Key Requirements and Framework for Personal Health Records Based on Blockchain Technology. *Applied Sciences (Basel, Switzerland)*, *13*(13), 7697. doi:10.3390/app13137697

Caronongan, A., Gorgui-Naguib, H., & Naguib, R. N. (2018). The development of intelligent patient-centric systems for health care. *Theories to Inform Superior Health Informatics Research and Practice*, 355-373.

Chalmers, K., Pearson, S. A., & Elshaug, A. G. (2017). *Quantifying low-value care: a patient-centric versus service-centric lens.*

Chu, L. F., Shah, A. G., Rouholiman, D., Riggare, S., & Gamble, J. G. (2018). Patient-centric strategies in digital health. *Digital Health: Scaling Healthcare to the World*, 43-54.

Ghonge, N. P. (2019). Being a "Clinical Radiologist""Patient-centric approach" and "problem-solving attitude" in radiology. *The Indian Journal of Radiology & Imaging*, *29*(03), 336–337. doi:10.4103/ijri.IJRI_173_19 PMID:31741608

Jabarulla, M. Y., & Lee, H. N. (2020). Blockchain-based distributed patient-centric image management system. *Applied Sciences (Basel, Switzerland)*, *11*(1), 196. doi:10.3390/app11010196

Jabarulla, M. Y., & Lee, H. N. (2021, August). A blockchain and artificial intelligence-based, patient-centric healthcare system for combating the COVID-19 pandemic: Opportunities and applications. In Healthcare, 9(8). MDPI.

Kanzaria, H. K., McCabe, A. M., Meisel, Z. M., LeBlanc, A., Schaffer, J. T., Bellolio, M. F., Vaughan, W., Merck, L. H., Applegate, K. E., Hollander, J. E., Grudzen, C. R., Mills, A. M., Carpenter, C. R., & Hess, E. P. (2015). Advancing patient-centered outcomes in emergency diagnostic imaging: A research agenda. *Academic Emergency Medicine*, *22*(12), 1435–1446. doi:10.1111/acem.12832 PMID:26574729

Kaur, J. (2023). Robotic Process Automation in Healthcare Sector. In *E3S Web of Conferences* (Vol. 391, p. 01008). EDP Sciences.

Kaur, J. (2023, May). How is Robotic Process Automation Revolutionising the Way Healthcare Sector Works? In *International Conference on Information, Communication and Computing Technology* (pp. 1037-1055). Singapore: Springer Nature Singapore. 10.1007/978-981-99-5166-6_70

Kaur, N., & Sood, S. K. (2018). A trustworthy system for secure access to patient centric sensitive information. *Telematics and Informatics*, *35*(4), 790–800. doi:10.1016/j.tele.2017.09.008

Keikhosrokiani, P., Mustaffa, N., & Zakaria, N. (2018). Success factors in developing iHeart as a patient-centric healthcare system: A multi-group analysis. *Telematics and Informatics, 35*(4), 753–775. doi:10.1016/j.tele.2017.11.006

Khanna, S., & Srivastava, S. (2020). Patient-Centric Ethical Frameworks for Privacy, Transparency, and Bias Awareness in Deep Learning-Based Medical Systems. *Applied Research in Artificial Intelligence and Cloud Computing, 3*(1), 16–35.

Mohsan, S. A. H., Razzaq, A., Ghayyur, S. A. K., Alkahtani, H. K., Al-Kahtani, N., & Mostafa, S. M. (2022). Decentralized Patient-Centric Report and Medical Image Management System Based on Blockchain Technology and the Inter-Planetary File System. *International Journal of Environmental Research and Public Health, 19*(22), 14641. doi:10.3390/ijerph192214641 PMID:36429351

Naresh, V. S., Reddi, S., & Allavarpu, V. D. (2021). Blockchain-based patient centric health care communication system. *International Journal of Communication Systems, 34*(7), e4749. doi:10.1002/dac.4749

Park, G. W., Kim, Y., Park, K., & Agarwal, A. (2016). Patient-centric quality assessment framework for healthcare services. *Technological Forecasting and Social Change, 113*, 468–474. doi:10.1016/j.techfore.2016.07.012

Ploug, T., & Holm, S. (2020). The four dimensions of contestable AI diagnostics-A patient-centric approach to explainable AI. *Artificial Intelligence in Medicine, 107*, 101901. doi:10.1016/j.artmed.2020.101901 PMID:32828448

Price, M. (2016). Circle of care modelling: An approach to assist in reasoning about healthcare change using a patient-centric system. *BMC Health Services Research, 16*(1), 1–10. doi:10.1186/s12913-016-1806-7 PMID:27716188

Roy, S., Prasanna Venkatesan, S., & Goh, M. (2021). Healthcare services: A systematic review of patient-centric logistics issues using simulation. *The Journal of the Operational Research Society, 72*(10), 2342–2364. doi:10.1080/01605682.2020.1790306

Singh, A. P., Pradhan, N. R., Luhach, A. K., Agnihotri, S., Jhanjhi, N. Z., Verma, S., Kavita, Ghosh, U., & Roy, D. S. (2020). A novel patient-centric architectural framework for blockchain-enabled healthcare applications. *IEEE Transactions on Industrial Informatics, 17*(8), 5779–5789. doi:10.1109/TII.2020.3037889

Spruit, M., & Lytras, M. (2018). Applied data science in patient-centric healthcare: Adaptive analytic systems for empowering physicians and patients. *Telematics and Informatics, 35*(4), 643–653. doi:10.1016/j.tele.2018.04.002

Zhuang, Y., Sheets, L. R., Chen, Y. W., Shae, Z. Y., Tsai, J. J., & Shyu, C. R. (2020). A patient-centric health information exchange framework using blockchain technology. *IEEE Journal of Biomedical and Health Informatics, 24*(8), 2169–2176. doi:10.1109/JBHI.2020.2993072 PMID:32396110

Chapter 4
A Medical Comparative Study Evaluating Electrocardiogram Signal-Based Blood Pressure Estimation

Siham Moussaoui

Department of Electrical Engineering Systems, Systems and Telecommunications Engineering Laboratory, Boumerdes University, Algeria

Sid Ali Fellag

Boumerdes University, Algeria

Hocine Chebi

Faculty of Electrical Engineering, Laboratory Intelligent Control and Electrical Power System (ICEPS), Djillali Liabes University of Sidi Bel Abbes, Algeria

ABSTRACT

In general, blood pressure (BP) is measured using standard methods (medical monitors), which are widely used, or from physiological sensor data, which is a difficult task usually solved by combining several signals. In recent research, electrocardiogram (ECG) signals alone have been used to estimate blood pressure. The authors present a comparative study that evaluates ECG signal-based blood pressure estimation using complexity analysis to extract features, comparing the results obtained with a random forest regression model as well as with the combination of a stacking-based classification module and a regression module. It was determined that the best result obtained is a mean absolute error range of 3.73 mmHg with a standard deviation of 5.19 mmHg for diastolic blood pressure (DBP) and 5.92 mmHg with a standard deviation of 7.23 mmHg for systolic blood pressure (PAS).

DOI: 10.4018/979-8-3693-2359-5.ch004

1. INTRODUCTION

The electrocardiogram (ECG) records the electrical activity of the heart, which circulates blood throughout the body. The heart has four chambers, the two upper chambers called atria and two lower chambers called ventricles (Geselowitz, 1989). Among the most important factors to be monitored for the prevention of cardiovascular diseases (CVD) is blood pressure, which is defined as the force exerted by the blood flowing through the walls of blood vessels (Klabunde, 2005). CVD is one of the leading causes of death worldwide.

There is a risk of infection and pain associated with invasive (direct) blood pressure measurement using an intraarterial catheter (Pessana et al., 2019), and accurate blood pressure measurement using non-invasive methods such as Korotkoff sounds (Pickering et al., 2005) and oscillometry (Baker et al., 1997) is difficult, because certain parameters, including arrhythmia, obesity, and postural changes, tend to obscure arterial amplitude pulses detected with a cuff, resulting in errors in these measurements (Anastas et al., 2008; Sala et al., 2005). These are two traditional methods of measuring blood pressure. There have been several cuffless blood pressure methods proposed based on electrocardiograms (ECG) and photoplethysmograms (PPG), such as pulse transit time (PTT) and multiparameter approaches (Ding et al., 2016; He et al., 2015). An ECG and PPG can be used to calculate the pulse transit time (PTT), which measures how long it takes a pulse wave to propagate between two points in the cardiovascular system. In contrast, pulse wave velocity (PWV) is a very common method (Peter et al., 2014). In the tanks, pulse wave velocity (PWV) is the propagation speed of the pressure wave. It is based on the theory of wave propagation in elastic pipes.

There have been many attempts to fit regression models for BP estimation using PTT (Kumar, 2014; McCombie, 2006; Poon & Zhang, 2006), but none have met the standard criteria. According to (Gesche et al., 2012), this dependence could be eliminated by using a calibration procedure. Nevertheless, such calibrations are only reliable for a short period of time (Cattivelli & Garudadri, 2009). Calibration-based methods cannot be relied upon to replace conventional blood pressure measuring devices, but can be used to monitor blood pressure at short intervals (Kachuee et al., 2016). A robust and reliable method for non-invasive and continuous estimation of blood pressure is still a subject of research, leading researchers to develop other methods using machine and deep learning techniques using ECG signal only. Specifically, we compare two papers that estimate blood pressure via the ECG signal in terms of technique used for the extraction of statistical characteristics, complexity analysis, and machine learning modeling.

The reset paper is organized as follows, in section one we find the method, followed by results and discussion in the second section, and finally the conclusion.

2. METHOD

2.1 Data base

The method is trained and tested on data from CHARIS (Kim et al., 2016), plus three sets obtained from commercial ECG sensors, and MIMIC III waveforms with a wide range of blood pressure values (Moody et al., 2020).

2.2 Feature Extraction Sequence

Following preprocessing, both methods use statistical features to analyze the ECG signal's complexity. As input for the classification model, Simjanoska (2018) used six parameters: signal mobility, signal complexity, fractal dimension, entropy, autocorrelation, and age. In contrast, Wuerich (2022) defines 34 characteristics more than Simjanoska (2018), such as energy, Shannon entropy, signal mobility, C contrast, signal mean, standard deviation, asymmetry, kurtosis, signal complexity, multiple entropy, and correlation measures. Based on the feature importance (FI) calculation, which evaluates each feature's effect on prediction accuracy, the most useful measures were selected. The recursive feature elimination algorithm (feature selection algorithm) is therefore based on the FI ranking when eliminating features. Statistics used to describe ECG signals are listed in the table below.

3. CLASSIFICATION MODEL SEQUENCE

According to Simjanoska (2018), They used seven algorithms to train stacked machine learning (ML) algorithms using six parameters obtained from the complexity analysis of ECG signals. The results of each algorithm are combined into one meta-classifier (Random Forest), which predicts normal, prehypertensive, and hypertensive blood pressure. As a result of the meta-classifier, a new feature is added to the initial feature vector for regression analysis. A regression classification model is developed by adding the original BP class of a training subject and the classification result to the initial feature vectors. By contrast, Wuerich (2022) the output of the 13 features determined by the elimination of recursive features (RFR) was used as input to a random forest regression classification model to calculate SBP and DBP.

4. ORGANIGRAMMES

This diagram shows the grouping of two study methods:

As shown in the author's flowchart (Simjanoska, 2018), the raw ECG signals were inserted in the first section, the data was segmented and labeled in the second section and then was preprocessed using a pass band filter. The signals are then passed on to the complex analysis and feature extraction module in section three. In section four, two types of machine learning algorithms are used to classify features by stacking them into the ML module by using seven algorithms that return probabilities based on arterial tensor type (normal, prehypertensive, hypertensive) and group them into a single meta classifier. A regression module creates the BP estimate in the last section by combining the output of the meta classifier and the extracted features. Wuerich (2022) illustrates how raw ECG signals are inserted in the first section, and then data are pre-processed using a band pass filter in the second section. The third section involves calculating thirty-four statistical features. the fourth section is divided into two parts: the First, feature importance (FI) is calculated to assess the influence of each feature on prediction accuracy, and then recursive feature elimination (RFE) is applied to select only the most relevant features. To calculate systolic and diastolic blood pressure, the thirteen features obtained by recursive feature elimination are fed into a random forest regression (RFR).

Table 1. Feature extraction algorithms

The Authors	Statistical Characteristics	
Author's algorithm (Simjanoska, 2018)	Signal Mobility	$S_0 = \sqrt{\sum_{i=1}^{N} x_i^2 \Big/ N}$; $S_1 = \sqrt{\sum_{i=1}^{N} x_i^2 \Big/ N-1}$; $M = S_1 \big/ S_0$
	Signal Complexity	$S_2 = \sqrt{\sum_{k=3}^{N-2} g_k^2 \Big/ N-2}$; $C = \sqrt{S_2^2 \big/ S_1^2 - S_1^2 \big/ S_0^2}$
	Fractal Dimension	$L(k) = \dfrac{\left(\sum_{i=1}^{[N-m/k]} \lvert x(m+ik) - x(m+(i-1)k) \rvert (N-1) \right)}{\left(\left[\dfrac{N-m}{k} \right] \right) k}$
	Entropy	$E = \sum_{i=0}^{N-1} p_i \log\left(\dfrac{1}{p_i} \right)$
	Autocorrelation	$r_{xx}(\tau) = \int_{-inf}^{+inf} x(t) x(t-\tau) p_{xx}(x(t), x(t-\tau)) dt$
	Age	
Author's algorithm (Wuerich, 2022)	Energy	$E = \sum_{i=1}^{N} X_I^2$
	Shannon Entropy	$SE = \sum_{i=1}^{N} p_i \log\left(1 \big/ p_i^2 \right)$
	Signal Mobility	$S_0 = \sqrt{\sum_{i=1}^{N} X^2 \Big/ N}$; $S_1 = \sqrt{\sum_{i=2}^{N-1} [X_i - X_{i-1}]^2 \Big/ N-1}$; $SM = S_1 \big/ S_0$
	Contrast C	$C_d = \sum_{i=d}^{N} \sqrt{X_i * X_{i-d}^2}$
	Signal mean	
	Skewness	
	Kurtosis	
	Signal complexity	
	Entropy measures	
	multiple correlation measures	

5. RESULTS AND DISCUSSION

A comprehensive literature review of the two papers revealed that in Simjanoska (2018), three types of random forest regression models are constructed to predict SBP, DBP, and MAP values. As a result, the model is more complex than in Wuerich (2022), where computational effort was reduced to a single regression algorithm and more features were extracted.

Figure 1. A simple diagram combines the two approaches

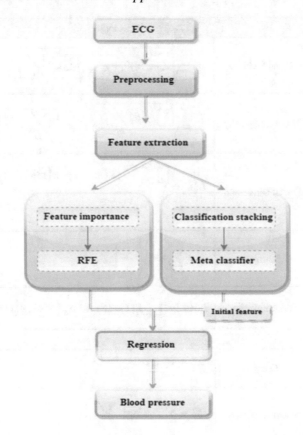

In terms of comparing model classifications, statistical characteristics, and complexity analysis, this refers to a comparison of models. The Table 2 below shows the comparison of mean absolute error (MAE), standard deviation, and root mean squared error (RMSE) results.

Table 2. Result study

Study	Matric	SBP	DBP
Simjanoska (2018)	MAE	7.72	9.45
	SD	10.22	10.03
	RMSE	10.50	11.07
Wuerich (2022)	MAE	5.92	3.73
	SD	7.23	5.19
	RMSE	9.35	6.39

6. CONCLUSION

Blood pressure is an important physiological parameter that needs to be monitored to prevent and detect cardiovascular disease. This article compares two different algorithms for estimating systolic and diastolic blood pressure from two authors. Both methods rely on the statistical characteristics of ECG signal feature extraction. In addition, the author's algorithm (Wuerich, 2022) presents an improvement to his algorithm that reduces the computational effort of parameter extraction and the classification model used. Wuerich's results are better than those of Simjanoska, who showed that blood pressure estimation using ECG signals can be highly accurate while providing continuous blood pressure monitoring in healthcare facilities and for portable devices.

REFERENCES

Anastas, Z. M., Jimerson, E., & Garolis, S. (2008). Comparison of noninvasive blood pressure measurements in patients with atrial fibrillation. *The Journal of Cardiovascular Nursing*, *23*(6), 519–524. doi:10.1097/01.JCN.0000338935.71285.36 PMID:18953216

Baker, P. D., Westenskow, D. R., & Kuck, K. (1997). Theoretical analysis of non-invasive oscillometric maximum amplitude algorithm for estimating mean blood pressure. Med. Biol. Eng. Comput, 35.

Cattivelli, F. S., & Garudadri, H. (2009). Noninvasive cuffless estimation of blood pressure from pulse arrival time and heart rate with adaptive calibration. *Wearable and Implantable Body Sensor Networks*. IEEE. 10.1109/BSN.2009.35

Ding, X. R., Zhao, N., Yang, G. Z., Pettigrew, R., Lo, B., Miao, F., Li, Y., Liu, J., & Zhang, Y.-T. (2016). Continuous Blood Pressure Measurement from Invasive to Unobtrusive: Celebration of 200th Birth Anniversary of Carl Ludwig. *IEEE Journal of Biomedical and Health Informatics*, *20*(6), 1455–1465. doi:10.1109/JBHI.2016.2620995 PMID:28113184

Gesche, H., Grosskurth, D., Küchler, G., & Patzak, A. (2012). Continuous blood pressure measurement by using the pulse transit time: Comparison to a cuff-based method. *European Journal of Applied Physiology*, *112*(1), 309–315. doi:10.1007/s00421-011-1983-3 PMID:21556814

Geselowitz, D. B. (1989). In the theory of the electrocardiogram. *Proceedings of the IEEE*, *77*(6), 857–876. doi:10.1109/5.29327

He, D., Winokur E., & Sodini, C. (2015). An Ear-Worn Vital Signs Monitor. *IEEE Transactions on Biomedica Engineering, 62*(11), 2547-2552.

Kachuee, M., Kiani, M. M., Mohammadzade, H., & Shabany, M. (2016). Cuffless blood pressure estimation algorithms for continuous health-care monitoring. *IEEE Transactions on Biomedical Engineering*, *64*(4), 859–869. doi:10.1109/TBME.2016.2580904 PMID:27323356

Kim, N., Krasner, A., Kosinski, C., Wininger, M., Qadri, M., Kappus, Z., Danish, S., & Craelius, W. (2016). Trending autoregulatory indices during treatment for traumatic brain injury. *Journal of Clinical Monitoring and Computing*, *30*(6), 821–831. doi:10.1007/s10877-015-9779-3 PMID:26446002

Klabunde, R. E. (2005). *Cardiovascular Physiology Concepts*. Williams & Wilkins.

Kumar, N. (2014). Cuffless BP measurement using a correlation study of pulse transient time and heart rate. *Int. Conf. Adv. Comp. Info. (ICACCI)*. IEEE. 10.1109/ICACCI.2014.6968642

McCombie, D. B. (2006). Adaptive blood pressure estimation from wearable PPG sensors using peripheral artery pulse wave velocity measurements and multi-channel blind identification of local arterial dynamics. *Annu. Int. Conf. Eng. Med. Bio. (EMBS)*. IEEE. 10.1109/IEMBS.2006.260590

Moody, B., Moody, G., Villarroel, M., Clifford, G. D., & Silva, I. (2020). MIMIC-III Waveform Database (version 1.0). *PhysioNet*. doi:10.13026/c2607m

Pessana, F. M., Lev, G., Mirada, M., Ramirez, A. J., Mendiz, O., & Fischer, E. I. C. (2019). *Central Blood Pressure Waves Assessment: A Validation Study of Non-Invasive Aortic Pressure Measurement in Human Beings*. Global Medical Engineering Physics Exchanges.

Peter, L., Noury, N., & Cerny, M. (2014). A review of methods for non-invasive and continuous blood pressure monitoring: Pulse transit time method is promising? *Ingénierie et Recherche Biomédicale : IRBM = Biomedical Engineering and Research*, *35*(5), 271–282. doi:10.1016/j.irbm.2014.07.002

Pickering, T. G., Hall, J. E., Appel, L. J., Falkner, B. E., Graves, J., Hill, M. N., Jones, D. W., Kurtz, T., Sheps, S. G., & Roccella, E. J. (2005). Recommendations for blood pressure measurement in humans and experimental animals—Part 1: Blood pressure measurement in humans: A statement for professionals from the subcommittee of professional and public education of the American Heart Association Council on high blood pressure research. *Hypertension*, *45*(1), 142–161. doi:10.1161/01.HYP.0000150859.47929.8e PMID:15611362

Poon, C., & Zhang, Y. (2006). Cuff-less and noninvasive measurements of arterial blood pressure by pulse transit time. *Annu. Int. Conf. Eng. Med. Bio. (EMBS)*. IEEE.

Sala, C., Santin, E., Rescaldani, M., Cuspidi, C., & Magrini, F. (2005). What is the accuracy of clinic blood pressure measurement? *American Journal of Hypertension*, *18*(2), 244–248. doi:10.1016/j.amjhyper.2004.09.006 PMID:15752953

Simjanoska, M. (2018). Non-invasive blood pressure estimation from ECG using machine learning techniques. *Sensors, 18*(4), 1160.

Wuerich, C. (2022). Blood Pressure Estimation based on Electrocardiograms. Current Directions in Biomedical Engineering, 8(2). doi:10.1515/cdbme-2022-1015

Chapter 5
Comparative Analysis of Machine Learning–Based Diabetes Prediction Approaches

Harsh Vardhan

National Institute of Technology, Hamirpur, India

Vijay Kumar

Dr B R Ambedkar National Institute of Technology, Jalandhar, India

ABSTRACT

The early prediction of diabetes mellitus may help improve the health of patients and cure them of this disease. In recent years, machine learning techniques have been widely used to predict diabetes in its early stages. In this chapter, an attempt has been made to analyse the performance of different machine learning techniques for diabetic prediction. Four well-known machine learning techniques, named as random forest, support vector machine, decision tree, and XGBoost are used. These techniques are evaluated on the Indian Diabetes dataset. Experimental results reveal that random forest algorithm achieved highest accuracy than the other techniques in terms of performance measures. These techniques will help to reduce diabetes incidence and health care costs. This work can be used to envisage diabetes in its early stages.

1. INTRODUCTION

Diabetes is a chronic disease that occurs either when the pancreas does not produce enough insulin or when the body cannot effectively use the insulin it produces. Insulin is responsible for regulating blood sugar levels in the human body. In the condition of diabetes, the body fails to regulate the amount of glucose in the blood (Saydah et al. 2004; Chhabra 2023). Hyperglycaemia, or raised blood sugar, is a common effect of diabetes and, over time, leads to serious damage to many of the body's systems, especially the nerves and blood vessels. If the diabetes is left untreated, then it can cause many health complications (Zimmet et al. 2016).

DOI: 10.4018/979-8-3693-2359-5.ch005

In recent years, diabetes mellitus has more than tripled. In 2021, about 537 million people were diabetic that is roughly about 7% of the entire world population. According to WHO, it is expected that about 800 million people will be diabetic by the end of 2045. The situation of diabetes in the world is in alarming condition. Hence, there is a need to take step before it gets out of control (Sartorius, 2022). Diabetes is still uncurable with the help of medical science (Mitratza et al. 2020). The treatment of diabetes is limited to prescribe the lifelong medicine that will help to halt the rate of damage done by diabetes. Therefore, the early detection of diabetes is even more useful for patients (Mir and Dhage 2018).

Machine learning techniques are used to detect the diabetes in a patient. In this paper, an attempt has been made to analyse the performance of machine learning techniques for the prediction of diabetes. The main contributions of this paper are

1. Machine learning techniques are used to predict diabetes from the patient data.
2. The techniques are tested on the Indian Diabetes dataset.
3. The performance of machine learning techniques is evaluated in terms of accuracy and F1-score.

The remaining structure of this paper is as follows. Section 2 discusses the brief description of machine learning models followed by related work done in the direction of diabetes prediction. The experimental results are presented in Section 3. Section 4 presents the discussion, followed by conclusions in Section 5.

2. METHODS

In this section, the machine learning models are briefly described followed by related work done in the direction of diabetes prediction.

2.1 Machine Learning Models

Four well-known machine learning models namely decision tree, support vector machines, random forest, and XG boost are briefly discussed in the preceding subsections.

2.1.1 Decision Tree

Decision tree comes under the category of supervised learning (Kamiński et al. 2018). In decision tree, decision is made by splitting the data into feature based splits. The decision tree works by forming a tree like structure that has multiple branches. This technique works for both regression and classification task. However, it is preferred for classification as compared to the regression. The formation of decision tree is complex for complex data. In decision tree, the splitting of data greatly affects the formulation of tree. The golden rule for splitting is to split tree in such a way that it will reduces the randomness present in the data.

2.1.2 Support Vector Machines

Support Vector Machines (SVM) is one of the most popular and powerful machine learning technique (Cortes and Vapnik 1995). SVM works for both classification and regression tasks. In SVM, the data points are classified by the formation of hyperplane in N-dimensional space. The main goal behind hyper plane is to differentiate the data into different classes and make prediction using that classes.

2.1.3 Random Forest

Random Forest algorithm is another famous machine learning techniques used for both regression and classification tasks (Piryonesi and El-Diraby, 2020). It gets its name 'forest' because a forest has trees. The trees, which are defined in random forest are actually decision trees. This technique is based on the concept of an ensemble learning. In ensemble learning, multiple classifies solve a given problem and improve the performance of a model. In random forest, many number of decision trees give their prediction and then the based-on majority votes of prediction. It predicts the final output. The greater number of decision tree may be responsible for higher model accuracy. This also help in tackling the problem of overfitting.

2.1.4 XG Boost

XG Boost stands for Extreme Gradient Boosting. It is developed by University of Washington. XG Boost is an open source library, which is written in C++ language (Sheridan et al. 2016). It works on Gradient Boosting Framework. XG Boost is very fast, accurate, efficient, and flexible. This library is one of the most popular of all libraries used in machine learning competitions. XG Boost is based on four pillars that are supervised learning, decision trees, ensemble learning, and gradient boosting.

2.2 Related Works

Many researchers are utilized machine learning techniques for prediction of diabetes.

Khanam and Foo (2021) noticed that other machine learning algorithms like Logistic Regression (LR) and Support Vector Machines (SVM) for predicting the diabetes. They built a neural network for prediction of diabetes, which contain different hidden layers. They found out that the model with 2 hidden layers provide them 88.6% accuracy. Hasan et al. (2020) proposed a robust technique for prediction of diabetes. Multilayer Perceptron (MLP), Naïve Bayes, Random Forest, and AdaBoost are used. These techniques were evaluated through accuracy under curve. Zou et al. (2018) performed a study to predict diabetes mellitus by using neural network, random forest, and decision tree. In their study, these techniques were validated through 5 fold cross-validation. Principal component analysis (PCA) was used to reduce the dimensionality.

Joshi and Dhakal (2021) performed an analysis on five main predictors of type 2 diabetes. They explored classification tree for validation of their analysis. The prediction accuracy obtained from classification tree was 78.26%. Sisodia and Sisodia (2018) utilized the classification algorithms such as Decision Tree, SVM, and Naïve Bayes to predict the diabetes in patient. The different performance measures were used to evaluate the performance of these classification techniques. Yahyaoui et al. (2019) proposed a direct support system for diabetes prediction. SVM, Random Forests and Convolution Neural Networks were used.

Xie et al. (2019) built machine learning model using weighted and univariate logistic regression to identify the potential risk of type 2 diabetes. Kopitar et al. (2020) utilized different machine learning based prediction models to predict Type 2 diabetes. They found out that Glmnet improved the prediction by 3.4% when more data provided to machine learning algorithms. Birjais et al. (2019) used Gradient Boosting Logistic Regression and Naïve Bayes to diagnosis the diabetes disease. The highest accuracy obtained from these model was about 86%. Haq et al. (2020) developed a technique for diabetes detection through machine learning approach. They implemented a filter method based on decision tree algorithm. They also utilized the concepts of Ada Boost and random forest techniques for developing the robust technique (Upadhyay and Chhabra, 2023).

It is observed from literature that the number of machine learning techniques were used for predicting the diabetes in patient.

2.3 Proposed Methodology

Fig. 1 shows the pipeline for machine learning model for predicting the diabetes. It consists of three main phases namely data pre-processing, model building, and evaluation. These phases are briefly described in the preceding subsections.

Figure 1. Pipeline for machine learning model

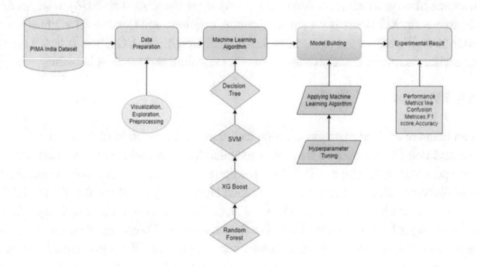

2.3.1 Data Pre-Processing

Data pre-processing is an extremely important because it helps in filling the missing values, removing outlies, scaling the values to fit into model easily, removing the duplicate, and inconsistent values increase the quality of data. Data cleaning and transformation are sub steps of data pre-processing. The main goal of data cleaning is to remove duplicate, inconsistent, irrelevant and improper data. By doing, the dataset becomes more sophisticated and results in better fitting on the machine learning model. Thereafter, data transformation converts data form one format to another to make it more useful for machine learning model. This process is used to make data more clean, efficient, and useful.

2.3.2 Model Building

Four machine learning models namely support vector machines (SVM), decision tree, random forest, and XG Boost are used. The processed data is decomposed into training and testing datasets. 70% of dataset is used for training set and the remaining 30% of dataset is used for testing set. The training set is used to train the machine learning models. Thereafter, the validation of these models is done through testing set.

2.3.3 Model Evaluation

The evaluation of these models is an important step for diabetes prediction. It gives an ability to improve the model by eradicating their shortcoming. There are many performance metrics that can be employed to measure how the machine learning model is performing. The performance matrices namely confusion matrix, accuracy, and F1-score are used in this paper. Confusion matrix is drawn to show how the model is actually performing (Stehman 1997). It is also known as error matrix because it clearly visualizes the errors of machine learning model. Fig. 2 depicts the confusion matrix. This matrix have actual values and predicted values as the labels.

Figure 2. Confusion matrix obtained from the machine learning models

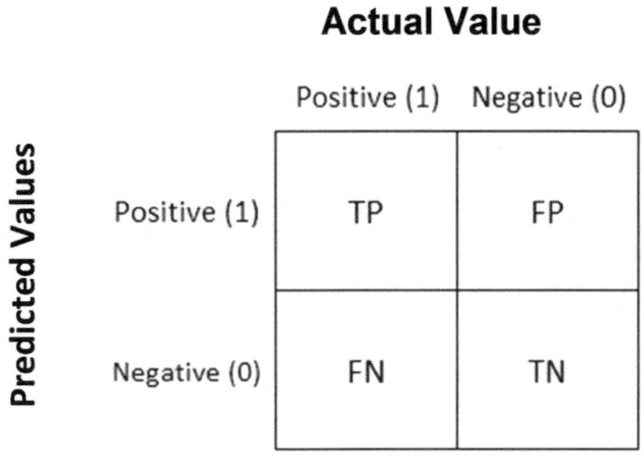

The accuracy in machine learning model is calculated by dividing the total number of correct prediction to the total number of predictions.

$$Acc = \frac{No. \ of \ correct \ predictions}{Total \ no. \ of \ predictions} \tag{1}$$

F1-score is a metric used in evaluation of machine learning modules (Sasaki 2007). It is a combination of precision and recall (Power 2020). The usage of F1 score provides a good balance between precision and recall.

$$F1 - score = 2 \times \frac{Precision \times Recall}{Precision + Recall} \tag{2}$$

3. EXPERIMENTAL RESULTS

This section describes the dataset description and results.

3.1 Dataset Description

In this paper, PIMA Indian diabetes dataset is used. This dataset is originated form National Institute of Diabetes and Digestive and Kidney Disease (http://archive.ics.uci.edu/ml/datasets/Pima+Indians+Diabetes). This dataset consists of information of total 768 female patients. It contains medical predictor variables to predict the final outcome whether the person is positive or negative for diabetes. The description of PIMA Indian Diabetes dataset is mentioned in Table 1.

Table 1. Description of PIMA Indian diabetes dataset

Sr. No	Column Name
0.	Pregnancy
1.	Glucose
2.	Blood Pressure
3.	Skin thickness
4.	Insulin
5.	BMI(Body Mass Index)
6.	Diabetes Pedigree Function
7.	Age
8.	Outcome

Starting from zero to seventh columns in this data. These are medical predictor variables. The medical predictors include number of pregnancies, glucose level, blood pressure level, skin thickness, insulin, BMI (Body Mass Index), Diabetes Pedigree Function, and Age. The eight column is for outcome. The values in this is either 0 or 1. The zero stands for negative and 1 stands for positive for diabetes respectively.

3.2 Data Analysis

The dataset is analysed through correlation matrix and bar chart. Correlation matrix is very helpful in telling insights about the data. Correlation matrix is used to find out the relation between different attributes in the dataset. By correlation matrix, it is observed that age and pregnancies are highly interlinked with each other. While, skin thickness and age are totally independent from each other. Insulin and Skin thickness are also highly linked with each other. Figure 3 shows the correlation matrix obtained from PIMA dataset.

Figure 3. Correlation matrix drawn from PIMA dataset

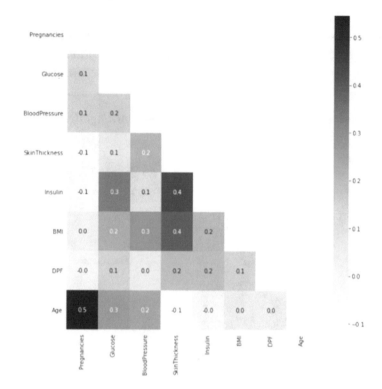

A bar chart is applied on diabetes dataset. This chart provides the information about the patients from PIMA dataset. It is observed from bar chart that about 500 patients are healthy and 268 patients of diabetic. This is case of imbalanced dataset. However, this dataset is slightly imbalanced data set. Hence, authors ignore this issue and do not employ any data augmentation on technique. The distribution of this dataset is illustrated in Figure 4.

Figure 4. Number of diabetic and healthy patients presented in PIMA dataset

3.3 Results

The confusion metric is used to evaluate the performance of machine learning techniques. Figure 5 shows the confusion metrics obtained from the different machine learning algorithms. It is observed from confusion metrics that the random forest outperformed the other machine learning algorithm.

Figure 5. Confusion metrics obtained from different machine learning algorithms

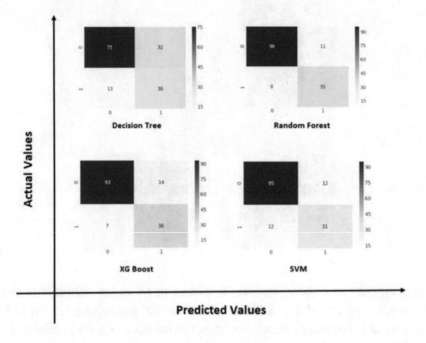

Figure 6. Accuracy and F1-score obtained from different machine learning models

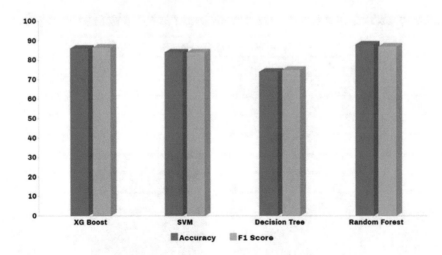

Figuer 6 shows the accuracy and F1- score obtained from machine learning models. Random Forest generates the accuracy of 88% and F1-score of 87%. While, the decision tree attained the accuracy of 74% and F1-score of 75%. For SVM and XG boost both produce the almost similar F1-score of about 84% and 86.5%, respectively.

Figure 7 shows the importance of features obtained from the random forest algorithm. It is observed from figure that the glucose is most important feature in PIMA dataset. According to the graph, glucose is most important feature with an importance score of about 28. For pregnancy, the importance score is 6. This makes it least important feature for random forest algorithm.

Figure 7. Importance of features obtained from random forest

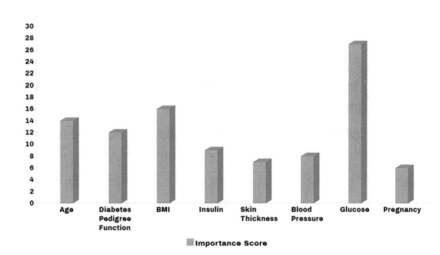

4. DISCUSSION

The random forest correctly predict the 96 instances as compared to SVM (95), decision tree (75), and XG Boost (93). However, decision tree provides less number of false prediction. The decision tree about 105 times it correctly predicts and 45 times it gives wrong outcome. It is observed from the results that random forest is the best among all other algorithms and decision tree is the worst. Whereas, both SVM and XG Boost is almost equal performers. With an importance value of around 28, glucose is the most essential element. The significance score for pregnancy is 6. As a result, it is the least essential element of the random forest algorithm.

5. CONCLUSION

In the last few decades, machine learning technique has made a significant contribution in healthcare. In this paper, the machine learning techniques have been used to tackle the diabetes problem in healthcare. A methodology is used to train the machine learning models for predicting the diabetes. Four well-known machine learning models have been used and evaluated on PIMA diabetes dataset. Results revealed that random forest algorithm outperformed the other models in terms of accuracy and F1-score.

The integration of machine learning algorithms with the existing healthcare technology will make them more efficient and accessible. This technology can be improved in future to match the clinical standards that will help the medical community to make better decision at the critical situations.

Authors' Contributions

Harsh Vardhan contributed to methodology, implementation, and writing original draft; Vijay Kumar contributed to data curation, writing review, editing and supervision. The authors read and approved the final manuscript.

REFERENCES

Birjais, R., Mourya, A. K., Chauhan, R., & Kaur, H. (2019). Prediction and diagnosis of future diabetes risk: A machine learning approach. *SN Applied Sciences*, *1*(9), 1–8. doi:10.1007/s42452-019-1117-9

Chhabra, M. (2023). Implications of Cloud Computing for Health Care. In *Cloud-based Intelligent Informative Engineering for Society 5.0* (pp. 41–59). Chapman and Hall/CRC. doi:10.1201/9781003213895-3

Cortes, C., & Vapnik, V. (1995). Support-vector networks. *Machine Learning*, *20*(3), 273–297. doi:10.1007/BF00994018

Haq, A. U., Li, J. P., Khan, J., Memon, M. H., Nazir, S., Ahmad, S., Khan, G. A., & Ali, A. (2020). Intelligent machine learning approach for effective recognition of diabetes in E-healthcare using clinical data. *Sensors (Basel)*, *20*(9), 2649. doi:10.3390/s20092649 PMID:32384737

Hasan, M. K., Alam, M. A., Das, D., Hossain, E., & Hasan, M. (2020). Diabetes prediction using ensembling of different machine learning classifiers. *IEEE Access : Practical Innovations, Open Solutions*, *8*, 76516–76531. doi:10.1109/ACCESS.2020.2989857

Joshi, R. D., & Dhakal, C. K. (2021). Predicting type 2 diabetes using logistic regression and machine learning approaches. *International Journal of Environmental Research and Public Health*, *18*(14), 7346. doi:10.3390/ijerph18147346 PMID:34299797

Kamiński, B., Jakubczyk, M., & Szufel, P. (2018). A framework for sensitivity analysis of decision trees. *Central European Journal of Operations Research*, *26*(1), 135–159. doi:10.1007/s10100-017-0479-6 PMID:29375266

Khanam, J. J., & Foo, S. Y. (2021). A comparison of machine learning algorithms for diabetes prediction. *ICT Express.*, *7*(4), 432–439. doi:10.1016/j.icte.2021.02.004

Kopitar, L., Kocbek, P., Cilar, L., Sheikh, A., & Stiglic, G. (2020). Early detection of type 2 diabetes mellitus using machine learning-based prediction models. *Scientific Reports*, *10*(1), 1–2. doi:10.1038/s41598-020-68771-z PMID:32686721

Mir, A., & Dhage, S. N. Diabetes disease prediction using machine learning on big data of healthcare. In *2018 fourth international conference on computing communication control and automation (ICCUBEA)* (pp. 1-6). IEEE. 10.1109/ICCUBEA.2018.8697439

Piryonesi, S. M., & El-Diraby, T. E. (2020). Role of data analytics in infrastructure asset management: Overcoming data size and quality problems. *Journal of Transportation Engineering. Part B, Pavements, 146*(2), 04020022. doi:10.1061/JPEODX.0000175

Powers, D. M. (2020). *Evaluation: from precision, recall and F-measure to ROC, informedness, markedness and correlation.* arXiv preprint arXiv:2010.16061. Oct 11.

Sartorius, N. (2022, April 1). Depression and diabetes. *Dialogues in Clinical Neuroscience.* PMID:29946211

Sasaki Y. (2007). The truth of the F-measure. *Teach tutor mater, 1*(5), 1-5.

Saydah, S. H., Geiss, L. S., Tierney, E. D., Benjamin, S. M., Engelgau, M., & Brancati, F. (2004). Review of the performance of methods to identify diabetes cases among vital statistics, administrative, and survey data. *Annals of Epidemiology, 14*(7), 507–516. doi:10.1016/j.annepidem.2003.09.016 PMID:15301787

Sheridan, R. P., Wang, W. M., Liaw, A., Ma, J., & Gifford, E. M. (2016). Extreme gradient boosting as a method for quantitative structure–activity relationships. *Journal of Chemical Information and Modeling, 56*(12), 2353–2360. doi:10.1021/acs.jcim.6b00591 PMID:27958738

Sisodia, D., & Sisodia, D. S. (2018). Prediction of diabetes using classification algorithms. *Procedia Computer Science, 132*, 1578–1585. doi:10.1016/j.procs.2018.05.122

Stehman, S. V. (1997). Selecting and interpreting measures of thematic classification accuracy. *Remote Sensing of Environment, 62*(1), 77–89. doi:10.1016/S0034-4257(97)00083-7

Upadhyay, P., & Chhabra, M. (2023). Personality Analysis using Edge Detection. In *International Conference on Artificial Intelligence and Smart Communication (AISC)* (pp. 151-155). IEEE.

Xie, Z., Nikolayeva, O., Luo, J., & Li, D. (2019). Peer reviewed: Building risk prediction models for type 2 diabetes using machine learning techniques. *Preventing Chronic Disease*, 16.

Yahyaoui, A., Jamil, A., Rasheed, J., & Yesiltepe, M. (2019). A decision support system for diabetes prediction using machine learning and deep learning techniques. *2019 1st International Informatics and Software Engineering Conference (UBMYK)* (pp. 1-4). IEEE. 10.1109/UBMYK48245.2019.8965556

Zimmet, P., Alberti, K. G., Magliano, D. J., & Bennett, P. H. (2016). Diabetes mellitus statistics on prevalence and mortality: Facts and fallacies. *Nature Reviews. Endocrinology, 12*(10), 616–622. doi:10.1038/nrendo.2016.105 PMID:27388988

Zou, Q., Qu, K., Luo, Y., Yin, D., Ju, Y., & Tang, H. (2018). Predicting diabetes mellitus with machine learning techniques. *Frontiers in Genetics, 9*, 515. doi:10.3389/fgene.2018.00515 PMID:30459809

Chapter 6
Counterfeit Medicine Detection Using Blockchain Technology

Raghuraj Singh

School of Engineering and Technology, Sharda University, India

Kuldeep Kumar

National Institute of Technology, Kurukshetra, India

ABSTRACT

Counterfeit medicine is a major problem in the pharmaceutical industry that threatens public health. The fake drugs are often inefficient, toxic, and can even cause death. This chapter presents a counterfeit medicine detection system using blockchain that prevents counterfeit drugs from entering into the supply chain. The system uses blockchain to create a secure and transparent record of the entire supply chain of medicines, from manufacturer to distributor to the end consumer. It allows for real-time tracking of medicines, providing transparency and accountability at every step. Smart contracts automate the verification process, reducing the potential for human error and improving efficiency. When a medicine enters the supply chain, a smart contract is created with its unique identifier, manufacturer, and distribution details. It ensures that every medicine can be traced back to its origin, and counterfeit medicine can be easily identified and removed from the supply chain. The presented system also provides a platform for customers to verify the authenticity of their medicines.

1. INTRODUCTION

The counterfeiting of drugs is currently becoming increasingly complex. The counterfeiting of pharmaceuticals poses a severe risk to public safety. Not only can fake medications negatively impact people's health, but they also cost real pharmaceutical manufacturing companies money. In the pharmaceutical sector, fake medications are also caused by a flawed supply chain structure (Alam et al., 2021). Drug counterfeiting has grown to be a worldwide problem that has to be addressed. The alarming statistic the World Health Organization provided indicates that around 10.5% of pharmaceuticals sold globally are counterfeit or of inferior quality. While most widespread medicine counterfeiting occurs in underdeveloped

DOI: 10.4018/979-8-3693-2359-5.ch006

and low-income countries, fraudulent or subpar drugs are also entering affluent countries, including the USA, Canada, and Europe (Pathak et al., 2023). The prevalence of fake medicines in the global market has become a serious and growing concern in recent years. Counterfeit drugs are intentionally made to look like genuine medicines, but they lack the efficacy and safety of original products. These fake drugs not only put patients' health at risk but also damage the pharmaceutical industry's reputation, which is supposed to be responsible for ensuring the safety and efficacy problem of counterfeit medicines. It is not limited to developing countries but also affects developed countries, where it is estimated that up to 1% of drugs in developed countries are fake. The World Health Organization reports that up to 10% of medicines in developing countries are counterfeit, reaching up to 30% in some cases (Siyal et al., 2019). India is a developing country and has a large population, which leads to counterfeit drugs as a significant concern for the health industry. As per the report of the World Health Organization, 25% of drugs sold in India are fake and lack efficacy, making it one of the world's largest markets for counterfeit drugs in the world (Singh, 2023).

These fake drugs pose a major threat to public health and our upcoming generation, leading to increased mortality rates, the spread of drug resistance, and loss of trust in the healthcare system (Kumar & Tripathi, 2019). There are several ways that counterfeit medications might enter the market, with local distributors and pharmacists playing a significant role. A pharmacy might profit handsomely by purchasing counterfeit medications from unlicensed sellers for less money. The major causes of the increase in productivity of counterfeit medicines are varied, ranging from the high cost of genuine drugs and the lack of regulation and corruption in some countries to the rise of online pharmacies. Due to the easy manufacture and distribution of these counterfeit drugs, along with the lack of regulatory authorities, makes it hard to control the prevalence (Ofori-Parku & Park, 2022). Now, the fight against the problem of fake medicines has become urgent and needs a powerful solution. Emerging technologies such as blockchain offer a promising solution to find counterfeit medicine. Blockchain provides a secure and transparent record of transactions. It helps to detect and prevent counterfeit drugs from entering the supply chain and ultimately protects people's health and safety (Keerthi et al., 2021).

1.1. Motivation and Contribution

Counterfeit medicines in India are often sold under the name of well-known and trusted brands, which makes it difficult for consumers to identify fake drugs because they look exactly like the original ones. Counterfeit medicines in India contain harmful ingredients, such as rat poison, floor wax, human sperm cells, and even human urine (Badhotiya et al., 2021). The prevalence of counterfeit medicines in India is a significant contributor to the rise of drug-resistant infections, which are estimated to kill more than 58,000 infants in India each year. The lack of an effective drug-tracking system is one of the contributors to the prevalence of fake medicines in the medicine market (Kumar & Tripathi, 2019). It gives the best opportunity for anyone to introduce fake medicine in the market because there is no way to trace the origin of the drug. Traditional methods of detecting counterfeit drugs are often ineffective. The supply chain for pharmaceuticals is complex, with multiple players involved, making it difficult to track and verify the authenticity of drugs. This lack of transparency and accountability in the supply chain creates opportunities for counterfeiters to introduce fake drugs (Anand et al., 2020)(Gökalp et al., 2018). Blockchain technology can be used to detect counterfeit medicine to ensure the safety and well-being of patients worldwide (Singh, 2023).

This chapter aims to explain the potential of blockchain technology to create a more transparent and secure supply chain, which will enable the stakeholders to detect and prevent the distribution of fake drugs effectively in the market. It explains how a blockchain-based application allows manufacturers, sellers, and customers to log in and track the shipments of medicines coming toward them in real-time. The application can also enable users to verify the authenticity of the medicines once they reach them, either using QR codes or the verification numbers printed on the shipment. It makes the application easy to use because using QR codes is easy to learn for everyone. In addition, in the application, an admin panel is implemented, which provides an overview of all the users, allows the admin to add new medicines to the database, and performs other administrative tasks such as verifying the user and medicine. Further, a user interface is designed, which is simple and fluent, providing a seamless experience for all the users. All the users have to do is just upload the QR code and click on a button. By providing a decentralized and tamper-proof system, the application can ensure the authenticity of medicines, helping to protect consumers and improve public health.

The rest of the chapter is organized as follows: Section 2 reviews the research on blockchain use cases and current pharmacy management techniques. The blockchain-based approach for counterfeit medicine detection is explained in Section 3. Section 4 describes the experimental setup used, and then it finally concludes in section 5.

2. RELATED WORKS

This section gives a brief overview of the various methods used to detect counterfeit medicines. Over the years, different methodologies came into the existence, different researchers proposed ways to prevent counterfeit drugs in the supply chain. A number of methods have previously been employed to track down fake medications in the medical supply chain. This overview explains the present patterns and effects of medicine counterfeiting on a worldwide scale, as well as the preventative actions proposed by various researchers that can play a role in combating this problem.

2.1 Different Methods of Counterfeit Medicine Detection

Over time, different methods have been applied to detect counterfeit medicines in the supply chain:

- **Barcode Scanning:** A software-based solution can be used to scan a barcode on the product against a database of known genuine products, and therefore can be used to authenticate original ones from the fake ones (Pham et al., 2019).
- **Blockchain Technology:** With the emergence of technology, blockchain has emerged as a trackable and transparent method to identify and prevent the entry of fake products into the supply chain, therefore eliminating threats and even providing transparency at various levels in the supply chain (Fei & Liu, 2016).
- **Data Analysis:** This method will use advanced algorithms and machine learning techniques to analyze the data collected from various sources to synthesize patterns to distinguish between counterfeit and original medicines (Anand et al., 2020).

- **Image Recognition:** Since most of the counterfeit medicines mimic the original packaging of the drugs, to establish the customer base on the existing image of the brand. Therefore, using sophisticated patterns on the packaging can differentiate the real ones from the counterfeit ones, and it can be authenticated using image recognition (Rodionova & Pomerantsev, 2010).
- **Spectroscopy:** As we know that counterfeit medicines do not share the same chemical composition as that of the original product. Therefore, samples of medicines can be taken from a suspicious domain of the supply chain and tested for their chemical composition, thereby leading to the identification of counterfeit medicines (Wilczyński et al., 2019).

The blockchain method is a transparent and a distributed ledger that will be used to keep a record of the supply chain, enabling the stakeholders to keep track of the movement of products to end customers from manufacturers (Reno et al., 2021). It increases trust and confidence in the authenticity of medicines. Additionally, blockchain is difficult to manipulate or hack, thereby making it an extremely secure and reliable method of verifying the authenticity of medicines. It makes blockchain one of the most efficient methods to solve the problem of counterfeit medicines (Sylim et al., 2018). Since it tackles most of the complex problems, it is surely one of the most reliable, transparent, and secure methods to ensure a better transparent supply chain in healthcare. Table 1 details a comparative analysis of various counterfeit medicine detection methods.

2.2 An Overview of Existing Blockchain-Based Methods

Anand et al. (Anand et al., 2020) developed a blockchain-based anti-counterfeit system for medicine products. The authors first discuss the necessity to prevent counterfeit medicines from entering the supply chain as they are harmful to patients and are a threat to the pharmaceutical industry. They proposed a system using blockchain to track and verify the authenticity of medicines from manufacturing to consumer. In order to provide the end users to verify the authenticity of the product, a QR code is provided which on scanning confirms that he is the first and the only receiver of that such product. The authors conducted a simulation of the proposed system using the Hyper Ledger Fabric blockchain platform, which showed promising results in terms of efficiency, transparency, and security. The simulation demonstrated that the proposed system could prevent the spread of counterfeit medicines by ensuring that every medicine product is verified and authenticated before it is sold to consumers.

Blockchain technology was used by Pandey and Litoriya (Pandey & Litoriya, 2021) to address the issue of fake medications in the e-health network. The authors draw attention to the substantial threat posed by counterfeit medications, which can put patient health at risk, cost healthcare providers money, and harm the industry's reputation. In order to trace and confirm the validity of medications across the supply chain, from the point of manufacturing to the point of consumption, the proposed solution uses a blockchain-based system. Every medicinal product in the system has a unique identifying code that is recorded on the blockchain and can be validated by parties involved at any point in the supply chain. The authors used a simulation to test the suggested system. The simulation demonstrated that the system offers a safe and transparent means to monitor and confirm the authenticity of pharmaceutical items, helping to ensure patient safety and avoiding financial losses for healthcare providers.

Table 1. Comparative analysis of various counterfeit medicine detection methods

Method	Description	Advantages	Disadvantages	Key Features	Scalability	Reliability	Security
Data Analysis	Analyzing data from various sources to synthesize patterns using advanced algorithms and machine learning techniques to distinguish between genuine and fake medicines	Can identify ways that may be difficult for humans to detect	It may require large amounts of data to be effective. Cannot track the supply chain	Detection Accuracy, Scalability, Cost, Data Requirements	It can be easily scaled up or down depending on the size of the dataset	May be less reliable if the algorithms used are not properly validated	May be vulnerable to hacking or unauthorized access to sensitive data
Image Recognition	Using image recognition technology to identify the packaging and labeling of medicines	Can identify counterfeit packaging that is designed to mimic genuine products	It may require a high-resolution image to be effective. It cannot work if the packaging is exactly the same, but the medicine under it is different.	Detection Accuracy, Scalability, Cost, Image Quality	It can be easily integrated into mobile applications or other software solutions	It may be less reliable if the image quality is poor or if there are variations in the appearance of the packaging or labeling	May be vulnerable to hacking or unauthorized access to sensitive data
Barcode Scanning	Scans the barcode of a medicine to verify its authenticity	Compares the barcode against a database of known genuine products to detect fakes. Easy operability, end customers can also verify the authenticity of medicines.	It can be difficult to verify the authenticity of the database used. Availability, Integrity, and security issues with the database	Detection Accuracy, Scalability, Cost, Database, Authenticity	It can be easily integrated into mobile applications or other software solutions	It may be less reliable if the barcode has been damaged or altered	May be vulnerable to hacking or unauthorized access to sensitive data
Blockchain	Using blockchain technology to track the supply chain of medicines and identify any counterfeit products that enter the supply chain	Can provide a secure and transparent way to track the supply chain of medicines. Data stored will be secure and distributed amongst various nodes; hence, there will be no central body failure issue.	Requires collaboration with pharmaceutical companies and regulatory bodies	Transparency, Traceability, Security, Efficiency, Collaboration	Can provide a scalable and flexible platform for tracking the supply chain of medicines	Provides a tamper-proof and secure record of the supply chain	Can be vulnerable to attacks
Spectroscopy		It can provide a highly accurate way to identify fake medicines. Can provide an exact chemical composition of medicines	Requires advanced equipment and expertise to be effective. It does not take into account reselling of the same medicine	Detection Accuracy, Scalability, Cost, Expertise Required	It can be used to identify fake medicines in real-time	It provides a highly accurate and reliable way to identify fake medicines	Requires advanced equipment and expertise to be effective, which may limit scalability

A realistic and practical anti-counterfeit system for managing pharmaceutical items is proposed by Pham et al. (Pham et al., 2019). The authors stress the significance of protecting the integrity and safety of pharmaceutical items, which might be jeopardized by the availability of fake goods on the market. The solution under consideration uses a blockchain-based platform to store and manage the records of pharmaceutical products, including details on production, transportation, and distribution. In order to confirm the legitimacy of the product, the system also makes use of a mobile application that enables consumers to scan the QR code located on the medicine packaging. The Ethereum blockchain platform was used by the authors to simulate the suggested system, and the findings were encouraging in terms of effectiveness, security, and usefulness. The simulation showed that the proposed system, which ensures that every medication product is validated and authorized before it is sold to consumers, may successfully stop the proliferation of counterfeit medications.

An overview of the potential uses for blockchain technology in the pharmaceutical sector was given by Schoner et al. (Schöner et al., 2017). To maintain patient safety, avoid the sale of substandard products, and improve medication distribution, the authors emphasize the necessity of a secure and transparent supply chain. The following use cases for blockchain technology in the pharmaceutical sector are covered in their paper: supply chain administration from the point of manufacture to the point of consumption, the movement of medications may be tracked using blockchain technology. By doing so, one can improve the distribution of medicines and assure their legitimacy and quality while also halting the proliferation of fake medications. Clinical studies: By offering a secure and transparent method to store and handle patient data, blockchain technology can be utilized to increase the transparency and dependability of clinical trials. The authors also cover technological difficulties, regulatory constraints, and the need for stakeholder cooperation as barriers to the adoption of blockchain technology in the pharmaceutical sector. Overall, the paper offers a thorough analysis of the potential blockchain applications in the pharmaceutical sector and emphasizes the necessity of a secure and transparent supply chain to guarantee patient safety and maximize the distribution of medications.

Mettler M. (Mettler, 2016) further explored the possible uses of blockchain technology in healthcare. To handle patient data efficiently, cut costs, and enhance patient outcomes, the author emphasizes the necessity for a secure and open healthcare system. Many application cases for blockchain technology in healthcare that are covered in the paper. Digital health records: The management of patient health records may be done in a safe and open manner using blockchain technology. In addition to lowering the danger of data breaches and giving patients authority over their own data, this can enhance the accuracy and accessibility of patient data. Clinical studies: By offering a safe and transparent method to store and handle patient data, blockchain technology may be utilized to increase the transparency and dependability of clinical trials. Management of the medication supply chain: Blockchain technology may be used to trace the flow of pharmaceuticals from the point of manufacturing to the point of consumption. This can assist in ensuring the legitimacy and caliber of pharmaceuticals, stop the proliferation of fake medications, and improve drug distribution. The author also covers the difficulties and restrictions associated with applying blockchain technology to the healthcare industry, including technological constraints, regulatory obstacles, and the requirement for stakeholder cooperation. The article, on its whole, offers a thorough analysis of the possible uses of blockchain technology in healthcare and emphasizes the need for a safe and open healthcare system that can efficiently handle patient data, cut costs, and enhance patient outcomes.

Clauson et al. (Clauson et al., 2018) investigated how blockchain technology may enhance hospital supply chain management. Using blockchain technology can help with issues in the healthcare supply chain, including fraud, traceability, and transparency. They discussed the salient characteristics of blockchain technology and how supply chain management in healthcare might benefit from it. The authors specifically discuss a decentralized, secure, and transparent supply chain that can follow goods from their place of origin to their point of consumption as a potential use for blockchain. The authors also provide a case study of a pharmaceutical supply chain management system that uses blockchain technology. The system tracks the flow of drugs along the supply chain, from the producer to the pharmacy, to assure the validity and quality of medications. According to the report, blockchain technology can boost the healthcare supply chain's effectiveness, openness, and security. By confirming that medications are genuine and of excellent quality, it can help increase patient safety. They also explain solutions to the problems of counterfeiting, traceability, and transparency that show the promise of blockchain technology to change healthcare supply chain management. Additionally, they offer a real-world illustration of how blockchain technology might be applied to the healthcare sector to enhance patient outcomes.

A blockchain-based system for managing the drug supply chain has been proposed by Tseng et al. (Tseng et al., 2018). According to the authors, the implementation of blockchain technology can address the problems associated with medicine fraud and enhance the effectiveness and transparency of the pharmaceutical supply chain. The notion of the Gcoin blockchain, a blockchain-based system for controlling the drug supply chain, is introduced in the paper. The application layer, the business layer, and the blockchain layer are the three levels that make up the Gcoin blockchain. The business layer administers the business logic and data storage, the application layer offers a user-friendly interface for stakeholders to access the system, and the blockchain layer guarantees the security and immutability of the data. Using a case study, the authors demonstrated how the Gcoin blockchain technology may be used to control the medication supply chain from the manufacturer to the final customer. The method ensures that every medicine is validated and monitored using a QR code and unique identification number. The system also incorporates smart contracts to automate the supply chain process and guarantee that all parties are held accountable. The advantages of the Gcoin blockchain technology are highlighted in the paper's conclusion, including enhanced transparency, less counterfeiting, and increased efficiency. The authors also cover the possibility of future research incorporating the Gcoin blockchain into further facets of healthcare, including the administration of patient data and medical equipment. Overall, the study illustrates how blockchain technology may be used to manage healthcare supply chains, handle difficulties like counterfeiting, and boost efficiency and transparency. By verifying that all medications are genuine and of the highest caliber, the Gcoin blockchain technology has the ability to completely alter the medical supply chain and enhance patient outcomes.

Reno et al. (Reno et al., 2021) presented a blockchain-based approach for detecting counterfeit medications. The application of blockchain technology, according to the authors, can solve the issue of fake medications and enhance patient safety. They presented a private blockchain based on the Hyperledger Fabric architecture. This blockchain is intended to trace the flow of medications throughout the supply chain, from the manufacturer to the final consumer, to assure the validity of medicines. Each medicine in the system has a distinct identification number and QR code, which are stored on the blockchain and may be used to trace the travel of the drug. To demonstrate how the Hyperledger-based system may be used to spot fake medications, the authors give a case study of its operation. The system analyzes supply chain data to spot counterfeit medications using a combination of machine learning and blockchain technologies. The system also incorporates smart contracts to automate the supply chain process and guarantee that all parties are held accountable. The advantages of the Hyperledger-based system, such as enhanced transparency, less counterfeiting, and increased efficiency, are highlighted in the paper's conclusion. The authors also discussed the system's potential expansion into other facets of healthcare, such as the administration of patient data and medical equipment. Overall, the study offers a real-world illustration of how blockchain technology may be used to control the healthcare supply chain in order to combat the problems caused by fake medications and raise patient safety. By assuring that all medications are real and of the highest caliber, the Hyperledger-based system has the ability to completely alter the drug supply chain and enhance patient outcomes. The authors also discuss the system's potential expansion into other facets of healthcare, such as the administration of patient data and medical equipment. Overall, the study offers a real-world illustration of how blockchain technology may be used to control the healthcare supply chain in order to combat the problems caused by fake medications and raise patient safety. Healthcare organizations may develop safe and open systems that help patients and healthcare providers by solving the problems and constraints with blockchain technology.

The possible use of blockchain technology in the pharmaceutical supply chain for the detection and prevention of fake medications is covered by Akhtar & Rizvi (Akhtar & Rizvi, 2021). They draw attention to the difficulties the pharmaceutical business faces, including the prevalence of fake drugs and the problem of tracking down items in the supply chain. To track and trace medications across the supply chain, from the producer to the end user, they suggested a blockchain-based architecture. A transparent, secure supply chain that can be tracked in real-time may be developed utilizing blockchain technology. This can increase the effectiveness of the supply chain and aid in preventing the entry of fake medications. The architecture comprises a consensus mechanism that maintains the data's integrity, a network of nodes that store and verify data, and a smart contract that streamlines some supply-chain procedures. The authors discuss the necessity for standardization, interoperability, scalability, and other issues. They discussed the drawbacks and difficulties of integrating blockchain technology into the pharmaceutical supply chain. They contend that the effective use of blockchain technology depends on cooperation among industry players in the pharmaceutical sector. The paper's main point is that blockchain technology has the ability to help the pharmaceutical supply chain identify and stop the distribution of fake medications. The pharmaceutical sector may boost efficiency, save costs, and improve patient safety by establishing a secure and transparent supply chain.

The possible benefits and drawbacks of using integrated blockchain technology in the healthcare industry are examined by Gokalp et al. (Gökalp et al., 2018). The authors describe how blockchain technology might help healthcare organizations handle data privacy and security issues, interoperability, and openness. They also identify several problems that these organizations face. To solve the issues of data security and privacy, clinical trials, supply chain management, and insurance claims, they suggested integrating blockchain technology into healthcare. The effectiveness of healthcare systems may be increased by employing blockchain technology to build a safe, open, and real-time-monitored system. They also covered the potential advantages of blockchain technology in the healthcare industry, including better data management, transparency, and inter-organizational cooperation. An electronic health record (EHR) system that is decentralized, secure, and allows for only authorized users to access patient data can be developed using blockchain technology. In addition to ensuring that patient data is accurate and current, this can assist in increasing patient privacy and security. They also discussed the drawbacks and difficulties of using blockchain technology in the healthcare industry, including scalability, interoperability, and legal concerns. The authors argue that further investigation is required before norms and laws guarantee blockchain-based healthcare systems' interoperability can be created. The study offers a thorough review of the opportunities and difficulties that integrated blockchain technology in healthcare may present. It could enhance healthcare results, offer patients better treatment, and lower healthcare costs by utilizing blockchain technology's security, transparency, and immutability.

Badhotiya et al. (Badhotiya et al., 2021) explored the potential use of blockchain technology in the pharmaceutical supply chain. The authors highlight the challenges faced by the pharmaceutical industry, such as the proliferation of counterfeit medicines and the difficulty of tracking and tracing products in the supply chain. The paper proposes the adoption of blockchain technology to improve the security and transparency of the pharmaceutical supply chain. By using blockchain technology, it is possible to create a secure and transparent supply chain that can be monitored in real-time. This can help to prevent counterfeit medicines from entering the supply chain and improve the efficiency of the supply chain. The authors conducted a survey of industry experts to assess the potential adoption of blockchain technology in the pharmaceutical supply chain. The survey found that blockchain technology is perceived as a promising solution to the challenges faced by the industry, with many experts predicting widespread adoption of the technology in the near future. The paper also discusses the limitations and challenges of implementing blockchain technology in the pharmaceutical supply chain, such as the need for standardization, interoperability, and scalability. The authors suggested that collaboration between stakeholders in the pharmaceutical industry is essential for the successful implementation of blockchain technology. Overall, the paper highlights the potential of blockchain technology in the pharmaceutical supply chain. By creating a secure and transparent supply chain, it is possible to improve patient safety, reduce costs, and increase efficiency in the pharmaceutical industry. The survey conducted by the authors provides insights into the potential adoption of blockchain technology in the industry. It highlights the need for collaboration and standardization to ensure the successful implementation of the technology.

The potential of blockchain technology to alleviate the issues faced by supply chain networks is investigated by Johnny and Priyadharsini (Johny & Priyadharsini, 2021). The authors stressed the significance of supply chain management while outlining how blockchain technology might enhance the effectiveness, openness, and security of supply chain networks. They provided a technical introduction of blockchain technology and discussed some possible applications in supply chain management. They investigated the use of blockchain technology in contract management, inventory management, and supply chain traceability. The authors also carried out a case study to look at how blockchain technology is applied in a supply chain network. They showed how blockchain technology may be used to monitor and trace items in a supply chain network, and increase the effectiveness and transparency of the network using a simulation model. The constraints and difficulties of applying blockchain technology in supply chain networks are also covered in the study, including technological difficulties, legal obstacles, and the requirements for stakeholder cooperation. The authors also employ a simulation model to show how blockchain technology might be used in a supply chain network. In conclusion, the article offers a helpful overview of the potential of blockchain technology in supply chain management. It emphasizes the need for more investigation and cooperation to enable its practical application.

2.3 Working Projects In the Same Domain

- **MediLedger** (https://www.mediledger.com/): This blockchain platform tracks and verifies the authenticity of prescription medicines in the pharmaceutical supply chain. It aims to prevent the distribution of fake medications by using a decentralized record-keeping system.
- **Blockpharma** (https://blockpharma.io/): This blockchain-based platform allows patients to verify the authenticity of their prescription medicines using their smartphones. The platform uses a com-

bination of blockchain and artificial intelligence (AI) technologies to track and verify the supply chain of medicines.

- **FarmaTrust** (https://www.farmatrust.com/): This blockchain-based platform uses AI and machine learning to track and verify the authenticity of prescription medicines in real-time. The platform aims to prevent counterfeit medicines' distribution by providing real-time supply chain tracking.
- **PharmaLedger** (https://pharmaledger.eu/): This collaborative project brings together leading pharmaceutical companies, technology companies, and academic institutions to develop a blockchain-based platform for the pharmaceutical industry. The platform aims to improve the transparency and efficiency of the pharmaceutical supply chain and prevent the distribution of fake medicines.
- **DAVA** (https://davascan.com/): This blockchain-based platform uses AI and machine learning to detect fake medicines in the supply chain. The platform allows patients to scan the QR code on their medicine packaging to verify its authenticity. The platform also provides real-time tracking of the supply chain to prevent the distribution of fake medicines.

3. THE BLOCKCHAIN-BASED APPROACH

Utilizing a typical Indian pharmaceutical distribution system as an example, the basic concept is described in this section. Each medicine will reach from the manufacturer to the end customer in the following manner as shown in Figure 1:

1. **Production:** The manufacturer will create the medicine and a unique identification ID for it. There will be a specific chain ID and shipment ID corresponding to each shipment.
2. **Packaging and Labeling:** Then, the manufacturer will package and label the medicine box. The label will have a QR code on it which will contain the unique identifier created in the previous step. The packaging will contain all the other information about the medicine, including the salts, side effects, dosage, etc. The QR data should also be printed on the box in case the QR scanner is not working in some specific shop.
3. **Transportation:** The next step would be transporting the medicine to the next node in the chain, be it a wholesaler, retailer, or the end customer itself.
4. **Distribution:** The distributor or wholesaler will receive the medicine and record its receipt on the blockchain network. They will then distribute the medicine to pharmacies or other healthcare facilities by creating a new shipment on the platform and printing a new QR on the box.
5. **Sale to Customer:** When the end customer purchases the medicine, he/she can scan the QR code to verify the medicine status and get the whole supply chain details. After scanning and verifying the medicine, a sold transaction will be recorded, so that medicine cannot be sold and verified again.

By recording each step of the medicine's journey on the blockchain network, this approach provides a secure and transparent solution for detecting and preventing the distribution of counterfeit medications, ensuring that only genuine medicines reach the end customers. All the stored data will be visible to the users, making a transparent system.

Figure 1. Block diagram of the approach used

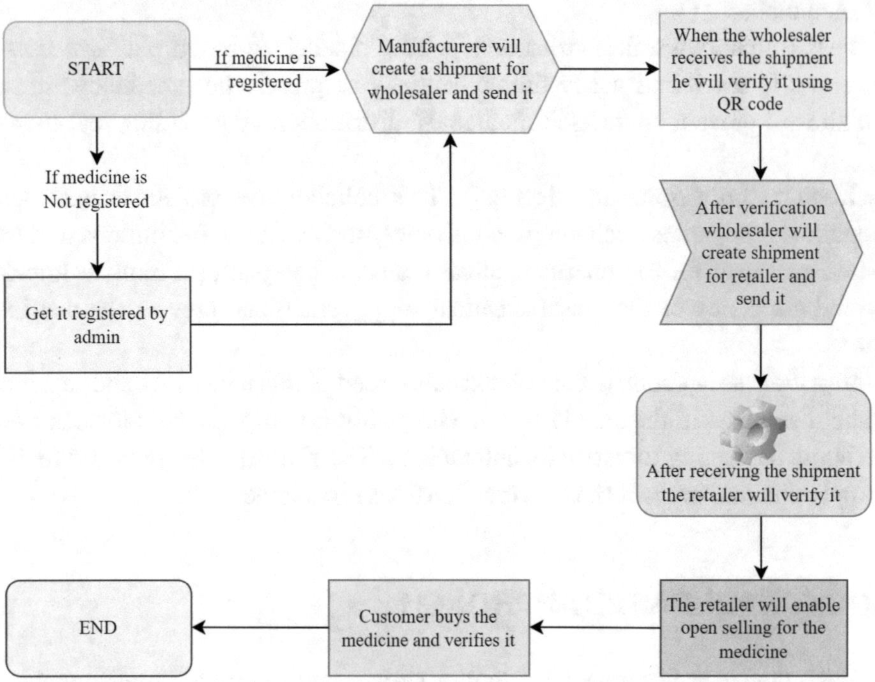

3.1 Algorithms

Algorithm 1 shows the pseudo code for creating a new shipment

Algorithm 1: Creating a new shipment
1. createShipment (bool newShipment, int chainID, int medicineId, receiver Address, deliveryStatus)
2. {
3. if (newShipment==true)
4. {
5. shipmentId = 1
6. chainId++
7. update list of shipments
8. }
9. else
10. {
11. shipmentId +=1
12. update list of shipments
13. }
14. }

Pseudo code for verifying result based on chain Id, shipment Id, shipment transaction status, shipment receiver address is given in Algorithm 2

Algorithm 2: Get Verification Results

```
1. getVerificationResult (int chainId, int shipmentId, account) {
2. shipment = get shipment from list
3. if (shipment. Receiver != account and shipment.receiver != address(0)) {
4. return 3 // Authentication error
5. }
6. else if (shipment.transactionStatus == true) {
7. return 2; // Shipment Already verified
8. }
9. else if (shipment.receiver == address(0)) {
10. return 1; // shipment does not exist
11. }
12. else {
13. return 0; // shipment original
14. }
15. }
```

Algorithm 3 presents the pseudo code for setVerified based on chain Id, shipment Id and transaction status

Algorithm 3: Set Verified

```
1. setVerified (int chained, int shipmentId)
2. {
3. shipment =get shipment from list
4. shipment.transactionStatus = true
5. }
```

Pseudo code for Complete Shipment Verification based on chain Id and shipment Id is given in Algorithm 4

Algorithm 4:Complete Shipment Verification

```
1. verifyShipment(int chainId, int shipmentId)
2. {
        3. web3 = initialize a new instance of the Web3 library, using the provider given by MetaMask or "http://localhost:7545"
4. shipmentListContract = create a new instance of the smart contract using its ABI and address
        5. accounts = await prompt the user to connect their Ethereum wallet, and retrieve the list of accounts associated with it
        6. account = select the first account from the list
        7. verificationResult = await call the "getVerificationResult" function of the smart contract, passing the chainId, shipmentId, and
account as arguments
        8. if (verificationResult is equal to 0) {
        9. await send a transaction to the "setVerified" function of the smart contract, passing the chainId and shipmentId as arguments,
and specifying the sender account and gas limit
10. }
11. return verificationResult
12. }
```

4. EXPERIMENTAL SETUP

This section explains the experimental setup that can be used to create the presented system using the VScode application framework, Javascript, and React JS. The blockchain network, smart contract, data source, scanning tool and web interfac modules are the main components of this prototype. Windows 10 operating system and local host are used to operate the proposed system.

4.1 Components

1. **Blockchain network:** To store the information on the medications, a blockchain network i.e., Ethereum blockchain needs to be put up.
2. **Smart contracts:** The conditions of the contract between the buyer and seller are directly encoded into code in smart contracts, which are self-executing contracts. To confirm the legitimacy of the medications, smart contracts will be employed. You must create deployable smart contracts for the blockchain network. In Solidity, smart contracts are being created.
3. **Data Sources:** Information about the medications, including their manufacturer, batch number, and expiration date, must be gathered. You can accomplish this by building a database or using one that an existing pharmaceutical business already has.
4. **Scanning Tools:** such as RFID readers or QR code scanners, to scan the medications and gather information on their legitimacy. To save the gathered data, these devices can be connected to the blockchain network.
5. **Web Interface:** A web interface will be necessary to communicate with the blockchain network and smart contracts. React JS library can be used to design the web interface. Web3 JS library helps to communicate with the frontend.

4.2 Software Requirements

The following are the software requirements:
    Backend:
    Ganache: A tool to run a local blockchain network
    Truffle: A set of tools for blockchain development
    Solidity: The language for writing smart contracts
    Frontend:
    React JS: The library for writing frontend using JavaScript
    MUI: Library for ready-to-use frontend components of material design
    npm: For package management
    Web3.js: Javascript library for web3 access using frontend
    Metamask Chrome Extension: for accessing the blockchain using frontend
    General:
    VSCode or any code editor
    Chrome or any other browser that supports Chrome extensions
    Git and GitHub: For version management

5. CONCLUSION AND FUTURE WORK

The use of blockchain technology in detecting fake medicines helps in enhancing the security and authenticity of the pharmaceutical industry. Because of the immutable nature of the blockchain, the presented system provides a tamper-proof record of the medicines' origin and supply chain, ensuring that patients or customers receive safe and genuine medications. Furthermore, integrating smart contracts enables the automatic verification of medicine authenticity, eliminating the need for manual inspections i.e., less corruption and reducing the risk of human error. While further research and development are required to optimize the system's performance, it is suggested that blockchain-based solutions have the potential to revolutionize the pharmaceutical industry's approach to medicine authentication and distribution.

The system presented in the chapter is just a prototype and not ready for market use. Many new features can be accommodated in it. Static data, like medicine data, could be stored in a distributed storage instead of the blockchain to reduce the number of transactions and hence the cost and energy consumption in performing the transactions, which is the biggest challenge with using blockchain technology in the application because once the user is out of Ethereum coins, he/she will have to buy more which is an overload on the consumer. The current experimental setup can be scaled up to accommodate more medicines and pharmacies. This will require the development of more sophisticated smart contracts and scanning devices that can handle the increased volume of data. We have used very limited attributes for the data models we are storing. To launch the application in the real world, we will need more attributes related to the user, medicines, and shipments. Collaborating with pharmaceutical companies will provide valuable insights into the challenges of medicine authentication and help to improve the system's accuracy. Pharmaceutical companies can also help to expand the system's reach by incorporating it into their supply chains. Further, to ensure the system's widespread adoption, it will be necessary to comply with regulatory standards like the FDA's Drug Supply Chain Security Act. It will require further research and development to ensure the system meets security and privacy requirements.

REFRENCES

Akhtar, M. M., & Rizvi, D. R. (2021). Traceability and detection of counterfeit medicines in pharmaceutical supply chain using blockchain-based architectures. In *EAI/Springer Innovations in Communication and Computing* (pp. 1–31). Springer Nature Switzerland. doi:10.1007/978-3-030-51070-1_1

Alam, N., Hasan Tanvir, M. R., Shanto, S. A., Israt, F., Rahman, A., & Momotaj, S. (2021). Blockchain based counterfeit medicine authentication system. *ISCAIE 2021 - IEEE 11th Symposium on Computer Applications and Industrial Electronics*, 214–217. 10.1109/ISCAIE51753.2021.9431789

Anand, R., & Khadheeja Niyas, S. G. and S. R. (. (2020). *Anti-Counterfeit on Medicine Detection Using Blockchain Technology* (pp. 1223–1238). *Springer Nature Singapore Pte Ltd., 2020.* doi:10.1007/978-981-15-0146-3_119

Anand, R., Niyas, K., Gupta, S., & Revathy, S. (2020). Anti-Counterfeit on Medicine Detection Using Blockchain Technology. *Springer Nature Singapore Pte Ltd., 2020*, 1223–1238. doi:10.1007/978-981-15-0146-3_119

Badhotiya, G. K., Sharma, V. P., Prakash, S., Kalluri, V., & Singh, R. (2021). Investigation and assessment of blockchain technology adoption in the pharmaceutical supply chain. *Materials Today: Proceedings, 46*(xxxx), 10776–10780. doi:10.1016/j.matpr.2021.01.673

Clauson, K. A., Breeden, E. A., Davidson, C., & Mackey, T. K. (2018). Leveraging Blockchain Technology to Enhance Supply Chain Management in Healthcare. *Blockchain in Healthcare Today*, 1–12. doi:10.30953/bhty.v1.20

Fei, J., & Liu, R. (2016). Drug-laden 3D biodegradable label using QR code for anti-counterfeiting of drugs. *Materials Science and Engineering C, 63*, 657–662. doi:10.1016/j.msec.2016.03.004 PMID:27040262

Gökalp, E.,, Mert Onuralp Gökalp, S. Ç., & Eren, P. E. (2018). Analysing Opportunities and Challenges of Integrated Blockchain Technologies in Healthcare. *Springer Nature Switzerland AG 2018*, 174–183. Springer. doi:10.1007/978-3-030-00060-8_13

Johny, S., & Priyadharsini, C. (2021). Investigations on the Implementation of Blockchain Technology in Supplychain Network. *2021 7th International Conference on Advanced Computing and Communication Systems, ICACCS 2021*, 1609–1614. 10.1109/ICACCS51430.2021.9441820

Keerthi, A. M., Ramapriya, S., Kashyap, S. B., Gupta, P. K., & Rekha, B. S. (2021). Pharmaceutical management information systems: A sustainable computing paradigm in the pharmaceutical industry and public health management. In EAI/Springer Innovations in Communication and Computing. Springer. doi:10.1007/978-3-030-51070-1_2

Kumar, R., & Tripathi, R. (2019). Traceability of counterfeit medicine supply chain through Blockchain. *2019 11th International Conference on Communication Systems and Networks, COMSNETS 2019, 2061*(1), 568–570. 10.1109/COMSNETS.2019.8711418

Mettler, M. (2016). Blockchain technology in healthcare: The revolution starts here. *Blockchain Technology in Healthcare, 2016 IEEE 18th International Conference on e-Health Networking, Applications and Services, Healthcom 2016*, (pp. 1–3). IEEE. 10.1109/HealthCom.2016.7749510

Ofori-Parku, S. S., & Park, S. E. (2022). I (Don't) want to consume counterfeit medicines: Exploratory study on the antecedents of consumer attitudes toward counterfeit medicines. *BMC Public Health, 22*(1), 1–13. doi:10.1186/s12889-022-13529-7 PMID:35650557

Pandey, P., & Litoriya, R. (2021). Securing E-health Networks from Counterfeit Medicine Penetration Using Blockchain. *Wireless Personal Communications, 117*(1), 7–25. doi:10.1007/s11277-020-07041-7

Pathak, R., Gaur, V., Sankrityayan, H., & Gogtay, J. (2023). Tackling Counterfeit Drugs: The Challenges and Possibilities. *Pharmaceutical Medicine, 37*(4), 281–290. doi:10.1007/s40290-023-00468-w PMID:37188891

Patil, P., & Karthikeyan, A. (2020). A survey on K-means clustering for analyzing variation in data. In Lecture Notes in Networks and Systems (Vol. 89). doi:10.1007/978-981-15-0146-3_29

Pham, H. L., Tran, T. H., & Nakashima, Y. (2019). Practical Anti-Counterfeit Medicine Management System Based on Blockchain Technology. *TIMES-ICON 2019 - 2019 4th Technology Innovation Management and Engineering Science International Conference*, 1–5. IEEE. 10.1109/TIMES-iCON47539.2019.9024674

Reno, S., Sadi, I., Karmakar, J., & Abir, M. (2021). Counterfeit medicine identification using hyperledger based private blockchain. *2021 2nd International Conference for Emerging Technology, INCET 2021*, (pp. 1–7). IEEE. 10.1109/INCET51464.2021.9456418

Rodionova, Y., & Pomerantsev, A. L. (2010). NIR-based approach to counterfeit-drug detection. *Trends in Analytical Chemistry*, *29*(8), 795–803. doi:10.1016/j.trac.2010.05.004

Schöner, M. M., Kourouklis, D., Sandner, P., Gonzalez, E., & Förster, J. (2017). Blockchain Technology in the Pharmaceutical Industry. *FSBC Working Paper, July*, 1–9. https://philippsandner.medium.com/blockchain-technology-in-the-pharmaceutical-industry-3a3229251afd

Singh, A. (2023). Combating Counterfeit and Substandard Medicines in India: Legal Framework and the Way Ahead. *Current Research Journal of Social Sciences and Humanities*, *6*(1), 101–111. doi:10.12944/CRJSSH.6.1.08

Siyal, A. A., Junejo, A. Z., Zawish, M., Ahmed, K., Khalil, A., & Soursou, G. (2019). Applications of blockchain technology in medicine and healthcare: Challenges and future perspectives. *Cryptography*, *3*(1), 1–16. doi:10.3390/cryptography3010003

Sylim, P., Liu, F., Marcelo, A., & Fontelo, P. (2018). Blockchain technology for detecting falsified and substandard drugs in distribution: Pharmaceutical supply chain intervention. *JMIR Research Protocols*, *7*(9), 1–13. doi:10.2196/10163 PMID:30213780

Tseng, J. H., Liao, Y. C., Chong, B., & Liao, S. W. (2018). Governance on the drug supply chain via gcoin blockchain. *International Journal of Environmental Research and Public Health*, *15*(6), 1055. Advance online publication. doi:10.3390/ijerph15061055 PMID:29882861

Wilczyński, S., Koprowski, R., Stolecka-Warzecha, A., Duda, P., Deda, A., Ivanova, D., Kiselova-Kaneva, Y., & Błońska-Fajfrowska, B. (2019). The use of microtomographic imaging in the identification of counterfeit medicines. *Talanta, 195*(October 2018), 870–875. doi:10.1016/j.talanta.2018.12.009

Chapter 7
Blockchain–Based Intelligent, Interactive Healthcare Systems

V. Hemamalini

SRM Institute of Science and Technology, Chennai, India

Amit Kumar Tyagi

🆔 https://orcid.org/0000-0003-2657-8700

National Institute of Fashion Technology, New Delhi, India

A. Rajivkannan

K.S.R. College of Engineering, KSR Kalvinagar, India

ABSTRACT

When it comes to the smart healthcare sector, blockchain technology presents several prospects. Aside from its usage in the financial industry, blockchain technology is now also utilised in the process of establishing trust, protecting privacy, and ensuring security. Within the scope of this work, we will provide an explanation of a new development in the healthcare business that strives to enhance the effectiveness and safety of the administration of healthcare data. We employ blockchain technology to construct a decentralised and tamper-proof network that facilitates safe data exchange among healthcare stakeholders such as patients, providers, and insurers. This technique is known as Blockchain-based Intelligent and Interactive Healthcare Systems (Blockchain-based IHS). The purpose of this chapter is to present an overview of BIIHS, including its advantages, disadvantages, and potential future paths. The BIIHS has the potential to enhance patient outcomes by facilitating personalised treatment plans, lowering the number of medical mistakes, and offering real-time access to vital and sensitive health data. Nevertheless, in order to fully realise the promise of BIIHS, it is necessary to solve problems such as regulation compliance, interoperability, and privacy concerns. Artificial intelligence and the internet of things are two examples of upcoming technologies that might be included into BIIHS in the future. This would allow for the healthcare sector to further improve its capabilities.

DOI: 10.4018/979-8-3693-2359-5.ch007

1. INTRODUCTION ABOUT INTELLIGENT AND INTERACTIVE HEALTHCARE

New healthcare systems called Blockchain-based Intelligent and Interactive Healthcare Systems (BIIHS) use blockchain technology to create a secure and decentralised network for healthcare data management. With its innovative approach to connecting patients, providers, and insurers, BIIHS might completely transform the way healthcare data is stored, managed, and shared. Among the many issues that have beset conventional healthcare systems are data breaches, an absence of interoperability, and inadequate data management. BIIHS proposes a solution to these problems by creating an unbreakable and transparent network that safeguards healthcare data and guarantees its complete integrity while also preventing tampering. Patients have more say over their healthcare data when they utilise BIIHS, which means they can trust their physicians and insurance providers with their sensitive information. Healthcare professionals may be able to access patient data in real-time and create personalised treatment plans with the aid of BIIHS. Insurance providers, meanwhile, may use the system to more accurately assess risks and provide better coverage to their customers. The use of blockchain technology in healthcare has the potential to revolutionise the industry, leading to safer, more accessible, and more effective healthcare for all. However, there are still challenges that must be overcome, including industry-wide concerns about privacy, interoperability, and regulatory compliance. Keep in mind that BIIHS is a groundbreaking novel finding with the potential to significantly alter the future of healthcare.

1.1 Smart and Secure Healthcare Systems is a Necessity of Modern Society: View from Industry 5.0's Perspective

Intelligent and secure healthcare systems are a need in modern society, and the Industry 5.0 viewpoint highlights the crucial role that technology can play in achieving this goal. Industry 5.0, the most current version of the manufacturing sector, integrates state-of-the-art technology such as blockchain, artificial intelligence (AI), and the Internet of Things (IoT) to create interconnected and smart systems. Smart and secure healthcare systems that boost patient outcomes, tighten data security and privacy, and enable more efficient and cost-effective healthcare delivery are within reach with the help of Industry 5.0 in the healthcare sector. Some of the most crucial parts of smart and safe healthcare systems, according to Industry 5.0, are:

- Using networked devices, sensors, and wearables to gather and send patient data in real-time is a key component of the connected devices idea within the framework of Industry 5.0. Doctors and nurses can now check in on their patients from afar and intervene quickly if issues emerge thanks to this technology.
- The importance of intelligent analytics is highlighted by the Industry 5.0 viewpoint as a means to decipher the massive amounts of data generated by interconnected devices. Healthcare providers can benefit from the use of AI and machine learning algorithms because these tools can identify patterns, predict results, and provide insights that improve decision-making.
- Blockchain Technology: From an Industry 5.0 point of view, blockchain has the ability to build trustworthy healthcare systems. By utilising blockchain technology, it is possible to generate a permanent and unchangeable record of patient data, ensuring the data's privacy and security. Furthermore, it may be used to ensure the authenticity and high quality of medical goods and devices by facilitating the transparent and safe management of supply chains.

- Elevating Patients' Agency: From an Industry 5.0 point of view, patient agency is paramount in healthcare. Intelligent and secure healthcare systems have the potential to enable patients to take a more active role in their own health management by giving them access to their own health records, encouraging transparency, and facilitating collaboration between patients and healthcare providers.

- The viewpoint of Industry 5.0 highlights the need of smart and safe healthcare systems that utilise new technology to improve patient outcomes, increase data security and privacy, and enable more efficient and cost-effective healthcare delivery. Embracing the promise of sector 5.0 and utilising technology is crucial for building a healthcare system that is smarter, more connected, and patient-centered. As long as healthcare is dynamic and ever-changing, this will be true.

1.2 Intelligent Systems

Artificial intelligence (AI) refers to computer systems designed to learn, reason, and solve problems at a human level, much like a human being. Artificial intelligence is another name for intelligent systems. These systems are built using techniques from data analytics, artificial intelligence (AI), and machine learning. Many different industries make use of intelligent systems, including medicine, finance, transportation, and the automotive industry. There is great promise for the application of intelligent systems in healthcare for tasks such as data analysis, accurate diagnosis, personalised treatment plan creation, and health monitoring. Intelligent systems may be used to detect fraud, provide investment recommendations, and assess market trends in the financial sector. The transportation industry may benefit from intelligent systems by optimising routes, reducing fuel consumption, and improving driver safety. The industrial sector may benefit from intelligent systems by automating production processes, streamlining supply networks, and improving quality control. The construction of intelligent systems has been driven by the demand for more efficient and effective techniques to assess and make decisions based on the ever-increasing amounts of data. With the continuous advancement of AI and machine learning techniques, intelligent systems are expected to see a significant increase in their capabilities in the next years. Because of this, our daily lives and the way we do business will be drastically altered.

1.3 Intelligent Healthcare System

Through the use of data analytics, machine learning, and artificial intelligence (AI), intelligent healthcare systems have the ability to completely transform the healthcare industry. These technologies aim to improve healthcare efficiency, accuracy, and quality by offering tailored treatment plans, real-time patient monitoring, and predictive analytics. Many different areas of medicine might benefit from intelligent healthcare systems, including diagnostics, medication discovery, patient tracking, and risk assessment. By utilising these technologies, doctors may examine patient records, which can contain results from imaging studies and lab work, to make accurate diagnoses and suggestions for possible treatments. Research into novel medicines and the improvement of current ones might benefit from the use of intelligent systems that can sift through mountains of data in search of promising leads. With the use of data analysis, these systems may detect and alert healthcare providers to any health issues in their patients before they escalate, making them ideal for patient monitoring. Intelligent healthcare systems might transform the healthcare industry by making personalised and efficient treatment more accessible, decreasing the number of preventable medical errors, and making better use of available healthcare resources. Problems with data security, privacy, and meeting regulatory requirements are just a few of the hurdles that must be overcome. The development of smart healthcare systems is an encouraging step towards improving people's health and well-being on a global scale. To sum up, this is encouraging news.

1.4 Interactive Healthcare System

An interactive healthcare system is a digital platform that allows patients and healthcare providers to communicate with each other in a way that is more efficient and productive. Among the many potential features of such a system are electronic medical records, patient portals, remote monitoring, virtual consultations, and real-time health alerts. By leveraging cutting-edge technologies like AI, ML, and NLP, an interactive healthcare system can provide patients with individualised treatment, raise diagnostic accuracy and speed, and boost patient engagement and satisfaction. In terms of major benefits, an interactive healthcare system's capacity to help close the gap between patients and healthcare providers stands out. When it's hard or impossible to meet in person, this becomes much more important. As an example, patients with mobility issues or who live in rural areas might benefit from consulting with their doctors remotely. They can get the treatment they need quickly without having to travel far. Finally, the way we provide and receive healthcare might be drastically altered by an interactive system. Healthcare providers would have the resources they need to deliver better, more efficient care, and patients would have easier access to treatment.

1.5 Intelligent and Interactive Healthcare

With the use of state-of-the-art technologies such as artificial intelligence (AI), machine learning (ML), and natural language processing (NLP), "intelligent and interactive healthcare" can streamline healthcare delivery, improve patient outcomes, and personalise treatment plans. One of the most crucial features of an intelligent and interactive healthcare system is its capacity to collect and evaluate large amounts of patient data instantly. The system uses machine learning algorithms to spot trends and patterns in patient data. This helps doctors make better diagnoses and treatment recommendations. Through an interactive and intelligent healthcare system, people may also receive personalised advice for their health. These recommendations are derived from the unique health information and medical background of each patient. Another crucial aspect of an intelligent and interactive healthcare system is its ability to empower patients to actively participate in their own treatment. For instance, individuals may monitor their symptoms, log their daily activities, and receive personalised recommendations for managing their health using an interactive health app. By taking this step, patients may have a better grasp of their health problems and be more equipped to help manage their therapy. In conclusion, healthcare professionals will be able to deliver more efficient and effective services to patients and offer more personalised treatment with the help of an intelligent and interactive healthcare system, which might completely transform the healthcare industry. By incorporating state-of-the-art technologies, this system has the potential to boost treatment quality and improve patient outcomes.

2. BLOCKCHAIN TECHNOLOGY IN HEALTHCARE

Blockchain technology has the ability to transform several industries, healthcare included. A distributed, secure, and transparent digital ledger, blockchain allows users to create, store, and trade data in an immutable way. By utilising blockchain technology, the healthcare business may enhance data security, privacy, interoperability, and transparency. An important benefit of blockchain technology for healthcare is its ability to create an immutable record of patient information. Using blockchain technology allows for a decentralised approach to medical record storage and access. This makes it harder for hackers to steal or alter the information. In addition to being able to choose who has access to their medical records, patients may work with their doctors to exchange information as needed. Blockchain technology has several potential uses in healthcare, one of which is the administration of clinical trials. By utilising blockchain technology, clinical trial data may be securely and transparently stored. As a result, this can aid in ensuring accurate data and preventing fraud. In the long run, this may lead to better patient outcomes and faster, more efficient clinical trials. Another potential area where blockchain technology might enhance healthcare supply chain management is in this sector. By adopting blockchain technology, pharmaceutical businesses can track their goods as they go from manufacturer to patient. This helps guarantee that the medications they manufacture are authentic and not outdated. In conclusion, healthcare organisations stand to gain from blockchain technology's capacity to increase openness, interoperability, privacy, and security, leading to better patient outcomes and more streamlined healthcare systems.

Blockchain technology might completely transform the healthcare industry by solving several problems associated with data security, interoperability, and trust. Here are the main points of blockchain technology as it pertains to healthcare, including its importance, features, characteristics, pros, and cons:

- Among the many traits and qualities are the following:

Distributed ledger technology, or blockchain, allows for the storing and processing of data without the intervention of a central authority. Among the several advantages of blockchain technology, this is one.

- Data added to the blockchain cannot be removed or altered after it has been added. The information's credibility and accuracy will be preserved in this way.

Blockchain relies on a consensus mechanism to verify and authorise transactions. Before any data is added to the chain, this technology makes sure that everyone in the network is on the same page.

- Contracts that automatically carry out predefined actions when certain circumstances are met are known as "smart contracts," and they are often enabled by blockchain technology. "Smart contracts" are another name for agreements that can execute themselves.

To secure data and provide anonymity for sensitive information, blockchain technology employs cryptographic algorithms. This restricts access to the data so that only approved individuals may view it. Here are a few benefits, then:

- Data Security and Integrity: Blockchain technology's decentralised and irreversible properties make healthcare data more secure and less vulnerable to data breaches and unauthorised changes.

- Blockchain technology enables disparate healthcare systems to communicate data in an easy and secure manner, facilitating interoperability. Better collaboration and more comprehensive patient care are now possible as a result of this.
- Procedures that are open and effective By providing an auditable and publicly shareable record of transactions, blockchain technology streamlines administrative processes, reduces paperwork, and boosts transparency.
- Patient Empowerment: When patients have greater say over their health records, they may more freely share information with doctors and participate in studies based on their interests. Access to information is one of the other advantages.
- Blockchain technology enables the secure sharing of data for research purposes, which facilitates the development of personalised medicine and insights into population health. This, in turn, benefits research and analytics.

Some of the restrictions are as follows:

- Because verifying and recording transactions requires a lot of computational power and time, blockchain technology is now facing scaling limitations.
- Compliance with laws governing data protection, privacy, and healthcare standards is essential when using blockchain technology in the healthcare sector, but doing so necessitates traversing many regulatory and legal frameworks.
- How advanced the technology is Because of the specific technical skills required for blockchain solution development and implementation, healthcare companies with limited resources or competencies sometimes struggle to establish and deploy blockchain solutions.
- Data Governance: Problems with data ownership, managing permission, and attribution arise as a result of blockchain technology. Therefore, in order to deal with these difficulties effectively, it is required to establish transparent governance systems.
- Achieving seamless integration of blockchain technology with current healthcare systems and infrastructure can be a daunting task that requires either the establishment of thorough interoperability standards or the execution of substantial modifications.

There is a lot of promise in blockchain technology, but before it can be used in healthcare, all of the pros and cons listed above must be carefully considered to ensure a smooth rollout and adherence to regulations.

3. EMERGING TECHNOLOGIES BASED INTELLIGENT AND INTERACTIVE HEALTHCARE

Using new technologies to boost patient satisfaction, enhance the healthcare experience, and cut costs is a prevalent practice in the healthcare business. Among the most exciting new developments in healthcare technology are intelligent and interactive systems. Improved patient engagement, individualised treatment plans, and healthcare professionals' ability to make well-informed decisions are all possible outcomes of these technological developments. Some examples of these technical manifestations are as follows:

- Healthcare providers may benefit from artificial intelligence (AI) in a number of ways, including the ability to track and analyse massive volumes of patient data, spot trends and patterns, and provide predictive analytics. Patients' unique traits, including their genetic composition, lifestyle choices, and medical history, can be considered when designing personalised treatment programmes with the help of AI.

- Augmented and Virtual Reality (VR/AR): By combining the two technologies, medical practitioners may build massive training environments where they can practise challenging procedures in a controlled environment. Patients with pain, anxiety, or depression may find relief via the use of virtual or augmented reality, which provides them with a wealth of distractions and methods to unwind.

- Internet of Things (IoT): Patients' vitals, activity levels, and medication adherence may be tracked in real time using IoT-enabled devices, such as wearable sensors and remote monitoring systems. One possible use of this data is the delivery of personalised therapies, such medication reminders and health lifestyle coaching.

- One potential use of chatbots is providing patients with individualised health information and support. Medication schedules, diet, and exercise planning are just a few of the many areas in which they are knowledgeable and can answer questions. Additionally, chatbots may triage patients, directing them to the appropriate care based on their symptoms.

- Medical personnel may access a patient's medical history and treatment plan in real time, no matter where they are in the globe, thanks to blockchain technology that securely stores and transmits patient data. The implementation of blockchain technology enables this.

- Healthcare professionals and patients alike stand to benefit from smart and engaging technology that may streamline processes, save expenses, and boost quality of life. To sum up, these advantages may be yours for the taking if you use these technological solutions.

4. BACKGROUND WORK

In their quest to become sophisticated platforms for healthcare delivery, traditional healthcare institutions are heavily investing in the use of new technologies. This shift is being propelled primarily by the consumer-centric priorities of ease of use and convenience. Several problems with data and user security, transparency, and privacy persist even with SHS. The research presented by (Tripathi, Gautami, Ahad, and Paiva., 2020) examines the social and technological barriers to the broad adoption of SHS by analysing user perception and the views of contemporary experts. Furthermore, it suggests a blockchain-based SHS architecture to ensure the system's inherent integrity and security. Future research directions and blockchain applications in the healthcare industry are discussed at the end of the session. Blockchain technology has already found acceptance in several academic disciplines, and its applications are expected to skyrocket in the next years. To expand the number of contracts that can be executed simultaneously and remove the need for intermediaries, Blockchain may run small scripts of prepared code called smart contracts. Blockchain and smart contracts are discussed in the paper "Sharma, Ashutosh, et al., 2020."

The authors also discuss how these technologies may be used in electronic healthcare within the context of the Internet of Medical Things (IoMT). This article presents a novel architecture and examines the future of the Internet of Medical Things (IoMT) in electronic healthcare in relation to decentralisation and smart contracts. It also discusses the pros, cons, and forthcoming trends related to this combination.

Among the irregular ailments that are leading to the fastest increase in the global death rate, diabetes is one such condition. The methodology for allowing the identification of diabetic sickness using the utilisation of Blockchain technology is presented in a recent publication (Mengji, Malook, Ateeq, et al., 2021). It uses a variety of machine learning classification methods to better understand the illness and safeguard patients' electronic health records (EHRs). Our EHR sharing platform incorporates several technologies such as interplanetary file system (IPFS), Blockchain technology, and symptom-based disease prediction. Data about patients' health is also gathered by means of wearable sensor devices. Once the EHR manager receives this data, they use a machine learning model to analyse it further and extract the results. Research by Jie and Xue (2019) indicates that Healthchain is an encrypted system built on the blockchain that aims to safeguard patients' personal health data. In order to establish granular access control, this system encrypts health information. User transactions allow users to effectively cancel or add approved doctors for important management purposes. Another way Healthchain prevents medical disputes is by making it difficult to alter or remove data or diagnosis from the internet of things. The suggested Healthchain is well-suited for integration into AI healthcare systems, as proven by security assessments and experimental data. An intelligent Blockchain Manager (BM) utilising Deep Q-Learning and its modifications was proposed by Al-Marridi, Abeer, and others (2021). In order to maximise the real-time behaviour of the Blockchain network, this intelligent Blockchain Manager (BM) considers the demands of medical data, such as the level of security and urgency. With the goal of optimising the trade-off between cost, latency, and security, the suggested BM attempts to intelligently alter the blockchain's network architecture. Three distinct machine learning-based methodologies are used to effectively solve the optimisation model, which is a Markov Decision Process (MDP). This article focuses on three methods: Deep Q-Networks (DQN), Double Deep Q-Networks (DDQN), and Duelling Double Deep Q-Networks (D3QN). Then, two heuristic approaches are compared with the suggested strategy in detail.

A proposed study by Khatoon and Asma (2020) would examine the current landscape of blockchain research and its applications in healthcare. Furthermore, this study provides a variety of blockchain-based procedures for healthcare organisations to improve data management efficiency. The Ethereum blockchain technology has been instrumental in the development and implementation of several medical procedures, including complex surgery and clinical trial processes. Several medical procedures are a part of these therapies. This package also includes the power to retrieve and manage a large amount of medical data. As part of the feasibility study that has been extensively covered in this paper, we have estimated the cost of this system. This budget goes towards the execution of medical smart contract system-related procedures for healthcare management. By 2020, healthcare data is expected to reach over 23,141 exabytes, according to Amit Kumar Tyagi 2022. The development of better data collection and networking tools is to blame for this. Health data is a valuable resource, and hackers are investing a lot of time, energy, and money into finding ways to use and profit from it. Despite this threat, experts predict that the healthcare cybersecurity industry would grow to 27.10 billion USD by 2026. It is feasible to build a unified database that safeguards patients' privacy while collecting data for clinical research using blockchain technology. According to Quasim, Tabrez, Fahad, and others (2020), a secure architecture built on blockchain technology should be used to guarantee the confidentiality of healthcare records. Technology like wearable sensors, the Internet of Things, and processing power should all be considered. When it comes to managing patient data and medical devices, Pham and Luan (2018) suggest using smart contracts built on blockchain technology to safeguard personally identifiable information and data produced by these devices. Patients, doctors, and healthcare providers (such hospitals) may all be a part of a remote healthcare system built using blockchain technology based on the Ethereum protocol. As soon as sensors detect changes in a patient's vitals, the data is instantly posted to a blockchain. Data processing that makes it possible to save medical records from patients in a way that is both efficient and sparing.

Note that 64 papers on blockchain-based healthcare systems were critically assessed by Leili, Reza, et al. (2020) between 2016 and January 2020. There were a total of 33 journals, 21 conferences, and 10 internet sites that published these publications. With that in mind, we will be concentrating on resolving three major concerns. How can blockchain technology be integrated into healthcare systems, and what are the steps, obstacles, and frameworks for using blockchain technology in a particular healthcare industry? Various blockchain applications are now in the development phase for use in healthcare. When considering these uses, how do we account for time, space, and technology? How relevant are blockchain-based healthcare system development and implementation to the third and fourth potential research directions? Our discussion also covers other avenues for further study, including blockchain's integration with AI, cloud computing, and parallel blockchain design. Safeguarding private patient information from prying eyes is a top priority for modern sophisticated healthcare systems. Consequently, secure data access procedures are crucial for ensuring that patients' medical records may be accessed by approved individuals only. Therefore, blockchain technology is deemed by the research to be a distributed method for safeguarding patient data. Vidhya, Tanesh, and others (2018) provide a secure and efficient method for patients and doctors to access data inside a particular healthcare system using blockchain technology. Furthermore, the proposed approach can safeguard the privacy of patients' records. Our design has been through extensive security testing, and the findings show that it can survive popular attacks without compromising the system.

The healthcare industry is experiencing a period of transition due to blockchain technology, which may cause a major shift in the current state of services. The healthcare industry, pharmaceutical businesses, and insurance corporations are all touched with in relation to the topic of healthcare system establishment and modification. The foundation for safeguarding healthcare data is laid up by (Khubrani, Mousa Mohammed., 2021). Proposed system foundational ideas include public and private ledgers, smart contracts, and context-based access control. In addition, the offered solution provides secure storage, dependable access to patient data, and interoperability with various interfaces. To safeguard sensitive medical records, a large-scale system based on blockchain technology employs encryption to implement granular access control. Adding or removing approved doctors from rosters is a breeze using user transactions for key management. Healthchain also makes it hard to delete or change data from IoT devices or diagnoses made by doctors, which helps keep medical disagreements at bay. According to Son, Ha, et al. (2021), a management system for emergency access control should be put in place to guarantee the security of patient information. The system is built on top of Hyperledger Fabric, which is developed for permissioned blockchains. An overwhelming amount of laws will be defined as a consequence of the proposed system's use of smart contracts and time length to handle emergency scenarios. In cases when the situation is critical, patients can also choose a time limit for when they can view the information. To further aid readers in understanding the offered management system, a plethora of algorithms describing the system's operation are also provided.

Healthcare 4.0 may make use of wearable sensors to implement remote patient monitoring (RPM), a more efficient and flexible method of patient surveillance. The most specific area of use for RPM is in the medical field, where doctors may use wireless communication technologies to remotely access real-time patient data. Clinicians have access to this feature. Because of this, RPM helps patients save both time and money. The care that the patient receives is also of the highest quality. The article's authors (Hathaliya, Jigna, et al., 2019) talk about a permissioned blockchain-based healthcare architecture that aims to make patient data more secure and private. We have also addressed the problems and how to fix them. The various applications of blockchain technology have already been discussed. In addition, we discussed the possible effects of blockchain and AI on the medical field. An intelligent healthcare system built on the blockchain that provides granular privacy protection to enable users to trust one other while sharing and exchanging data was presented in 2021 by Wu, Guangjun, and others. By integrating Local Differential Privacy (LDP) approaches with blockchain technology, we can build a framework for dynamic access control that provides attribute-based privacy protection in transaction processing. The system generates four different kinds of smart contracts to meet the needs of anonymous transactions, dynamic access control, beneficial matching decisions, and evaluation of public data in an open network. Ring Signature is a method for retrieving private information that is based on the blockchain and requires authorization (Aitizaz, Muhammad, et al., 2022). In order to aid in the improvement of privacy preservation inside the intelligent healthcare system, this approach is offered. To optimise appointment supplies based on accessibility, transparency, and security, the suggested approach first uses a more complex multi-transaction mode consortium blockchain. The healthcare providers are notified of this by receiving requests of varying volumes. If implemented, our proposed approach would greatly improve data retrieval across many fields. The suggested Scheme works quite well, according to the simulation findings, in terms of maximising patient privacy while reducing processing and transmission costs.

The paper (Sharma, Pratima, et al., 2022) suggests a blockchain-based Internet of Things architecture that uses the Identity-Based Encryption (IBE) algorithm to improve the security of healthcare data. In this case, everyone benefits from the smart contract's outlines of all the essential healthcare system processes. In order to determine the efficacy of the suggested approach, many tests are executed. Findings from the study suggest that the suggested system outperforms the popular approaches used at the moment. Blockchain technology is expected to make a significant impact on the healthcare business, among other notable application fields. The current healthcare systems are opening up a wide range of choices and possibilities as a result of this. Consequently, Kumar, Vidhya, and colleagues (2018) set out to study how blockchain technology could be integrated into current healthcare systems and what conditions are necessary for these systems to function well. Healthcare systems that are both trustless and transparent are part of these needs. Along with this, the paper explores the problems that must be solved before healthcare systems can effectively implement blockchain technology. On top of that, they supply the smart contract, an essential tool for establishing the beforehand-decided terms among the many participants in healthcare systems that rely on blockchain technology. Research done in 2022 by Le, Hai, and others suggests using the Patient-Chain platform, a control and management system, to keep patient data safe. Using Blockchain technology, this platform provides a healthcare system focused on the patient. The Patient-Chain system is constructed on the approved Blockchain platform, Hyperledger Fabric. Using smart contracts, it lays out a number of rules and regulations and gives a timeline for handling emergencies. Additionally, patients can set time limits on data access, which is useful for cases where time is of the essence. For the benefit of the readers, the suggested management system is accompanied with a plethora of algorithms that demonstrate its performance.

5. PROBLEM DEFINITION FOR DESIGNING A SECURED, PRIVACY PRESERVED, TRUST INTELLIGENT AND INTERACTIVE HEALTHCARE

- In order to create a healthcare system that is reliable, smart, engaging, secure, and private for patients, it is important to understand all the obstacles and problems that come with it. Some of the most crucial problem definitions to keep in mind are that which follows:
- When it comes to data security: It is critical to protect healthcare data from unauthorised access, modification, or theft since it is highly sensitive and valuable. To ensure the constant protection of patient information, an extensive set of security mechanisms must be included into the smart and participatory healthcare system.
- Ensuring the privacy of patients It is imperative that the intelligent and interactive healthcare system be designed in a way that protects patients' right to privacy when it comes to their health information. Ensuring that patient data may be accessed only by approved individuals and that patients can select who can access their data is of utmost importance.
- The success of the smart and interactive healthcare system depends on patients' trust in it. Building a trustworthy and accountable system and outlining clear guidelines for data exchange, access, and usage are essential steps in this direction.
- Integration: The smart and engaging healthcare platform should have the capability to connect with preexisting healthcare platforms. Medical equipment, electronic health records, and other healthcare-related technology are all part of these systems. This is why making sure the system works with the current procedures and technology requires a lot of preparation and cooperation.
- Factors related to ethics: Many moral questions arise from the integration of AI into healthcare systems, including issues around autonomy, informed consent, and the potential for bias in AI algorithms. If we want to make sure the system is created and implemented with ethics and responsibility in mind, we have to answer these questions.
- Remember that these problem definitions are critical to building a reliable, smart, and engaging healthcare system that safeguards patients' privacy, is safe, and can improve patient outcomes while keeping data secure and private to an absolute minimum. We need blockchain technology to fix issues like this.

6. ISSUES FACED IN DEVELOPING A BLOCKCHAIN BASED INTELLIGENT AND INTERACTIVE HEALTHCARE

Creating an intelligent and interactive healthcare system that uses blockchain technology is an intricate process fraught with technical and non-technical challenges (Singh, Suruchi, et al., 2022). Among the many difficulties that could arise in creating such a system are:

- Keeping information private and secure: Health information is very private and delicate. Consequently, a major obstacle to building a blockchain-based healthcare system is ensuring the privacy and security of data. It is critical that the system be built in a way that prevents unauthorised persons from accessing patient information and guarantees the data stays confidential.
- Accessing and integrating healthcare data may be a huge challenge since it is often spread out across different healthcare providers. This is where interoperability comes in. Building a health-

care system that integrates with many healthcare providers and systems and is rooted on blockchain technology is no easy feat.

- Because of the massive amounts of data generated by the healthcare system, scalability is a major issue. The blockchain-based healthcare system must be capable of handling massive amounts of data with ease and without compromising its overall performance.

- Health Insurance Portability and Accountability Act (HIPAA) compliance is critical since the healthcare industry is subject to stringent regulations. If the blockchain-based healthcare system is serious about protecting patients' privacy and security, it must follow these guidelines.

- Knowledge in technical areas: Building a blockchain-based healthcare system calls for experts with knowledge in data analytics, healthcare systems, and blockchain technology. The creators of the system must possess an in-depth understanding of these domains to build an efficient and effective system.

- Usability and adoption: The potential for adoption and use determines the efficacy of any healthcare system. For this reason, it is critical to build a healthcare system that utilises blockchain technology and is user-friendly and well-received by everyone involved.

- Data privacy and security, interoperability, scalability, regulatory compliance, technical competency, acceptance, and usability are some of the challenges that must be overcome in order to create an intelligent and interactive healthcare system based on blockchain technology. In the next steps, we will address all of the issues, including the somewhat less technical ones.

6.1 Technical Issues

Building an intelligent, interactive healthcare system on top of blockchain technology could be a challenging and intricate process. A few examples of potential technological issues are as follows:

- The establishment of a blockchain-based healthcare system faces several formidable challenges, not the least of which is scalability. The blockchain network must be able to efficiently and rapidly handle a large number of transactions. As a result of their current architecture, most blockchain systems may have limited scalability, which might lead to slow transaction processing times.

- In order to keep patient information private, all healthcare records must be protected from prying eyes. However, it may be difficult to safeguard one's privacy with blockchain technology due to its features, such as the decentralised and transparent nature of all data maintenance. We need to create mechanisms that can restrict access to the data so that only allowed individuals may access it.

- Interoperability: Ensuring that varied systems and technologies can interact with one another is vital, since blockchain-based healthcare systems may need the integration of several systems and technology. Problems arise while trying to build a seamless data flow due to the fact that various systems may use different standards and protocols.

- Safety: The safety of any healthcare system is of paramount importance, and blockchain-based solutions are no different. Blockchain technology is secure, but it may still be compromised. It is critical to construct reliable security measures in order to ward off hackers and other security threats.

- Construction of Electronic Contracts: Particularly challenging and intricate might be the process of developing smart contracts for a healthcare system based on blockchain technology. The details of the purchase and sale agreement are instantly codified into computer code in smart contracts.

There is an automated renewal process for certain contracts. Developing these contracts requires a thorough familiarity with the healthcare industry as well as the use of blockchain technology.

- Having an in-depth understanding of blockchain technology as well as the healthcare business is crucial for building a healthcare system that utilises this technology. On top of that, it calls for robust security measures, the ability to offer scalability, privacy, interoperability, and the generation of smart contracts.

6.2 Non- Technical Issues

In addition to technological hurdles, there are a plethora of other non-technical issues that must be overcome in the course of developing a blockchain-based intelligent and interactive healthcare system. Among these issues are:

- **Adherence to regulations:** Building a blockchain-based system in the healthcare industry necessitates adhering to several government regulations and industry standards, and the industry as a whole is subject to heavy regulation. It is critical to ensure the system meets all relevant regulatory requirements in order to prevent any financial and legal risks.
- **Moral Deliberations** Many moral questions arise when healthcare organisations use blockchain technology, such as who owns the data, how to regulate permission, and patients' right to privacy. It is necessary to develop ethical frameworks and standards for the collection, use, and sharing of healthcare information.
- **Price:** Considering the system's cost-benefit analysis is essential, since developing a healthcare system based on blockchain technology might be rather expensive. Finding a happy medium between the system's costs and its potential benefits—which can include better patient outcomes, lower expenditures, and more energy efficiency—is essential.
- **Acceptance:** Many obstacles, such as resistance to change, confusion, and worries about data privacy and security, may slow the healthcare industry's adoption of blockchain technology. The best way to get people on board with the system is to highlight its benefits and solve any issues that crop up.

Finally, it is critical to address both the technical and non-technical challenges that have arisen throughout the development of the blockchain-based healthcare system if it is to be a success. If you want to make sure the technology is deployed effectively, you need to build adoption plans, cost-benefit analyses, ethical frameworks, stakeholder engagement, and regulatory compliance.

6.3 Legal Issues

Greater interoperability, improved data security, and more patient control are just a few of the potential advantages that could result from developing an intelligent and interactive healthcare system based on blockchain technology. However, that is not all that must be considered; there are also challenges and legal issues. The following are examples of major legal issues that could arise while creating such a system:

- Ensuring Data Privacy and Security: Due to the sensitive nature of healthcare data, any use of blockchain technology must adhere to data protection regulations like the General Data Protection

Regulation (GDPR) or comparable statutes. Maintaining the privacy and security of patients' records is of the utmost importance when using blockchain technology. Developers must implement appropriate security measures and obtain informed consent from patients before collecting and processing their data.

- Consent management is an ongoing activity, and patient consent is a crucial component of healthcare data processing. Mechanisms for efficient consent management should be present in any system built on blockchain technology. The ability for patients to grant or withdraw permission for specific data uses is important for patients' right to privacy and for healthcare providers to follow the law.

- Intellectual Property: New healthcare systems built on the blockchain may necessitate the development of IP-protected innovations. Developers should think about ways to protect their intellectual property so that their ideas are safe and that they meet all the requirements for patents, copyright, and trademarks. If you want to incorporate preexisting patents or use technology that was provided by other parties, you may need to get a licencing agreement.

- Users, healthcare providers, and developers are just a few of the many parties involved in blockchain-based healthcare systems, which raises important questions about accountability and liability. In the case of a data breach, incorrect diagnosis, or other system-generated harm, it may be difficult to ascertain responsibility and liability. Developers can help alleviate these issues by including clear disclaimers, limitations of liability, and terms of use in their products.

- Standards and Interoperability: Achieving interoperability between the different blockchain platforms and healthcare systems is crucial to guarantee the uninterrupted transmission of data. To ensure compatibility and conformity with industry standards, developers should consider already established healthcare interoperability standards like FHIR and HL7.

- Difficulty in various legal contexts A number of jurisdictions may find it challenging to ensure legal compliance with blockchain technology due to the fact that it operates across international boundaries. The developers should be informed about the legal requirements and constraints of the many countries where the system could be used.

- Data storage, data transfer across borders, and data collection from all over the globe are areas where this is of paramount importance.

- Legal complications may emerge depending on the particular implementation and jurisdiction, so please keep that in mind. With the help of attorneys specialising in healthcare, data protection, and blockchain technology, these legal hurdles can be efficiently navigated and applicable rules and regulations can be assured.

7. CHALLENGES FACED TOWARDS BLOCKCHAIN BASED INTELLIGENT AND INTERACTIVE HEALTHCARE

Using blockchain technology to build a decentralised healthcare system is the goal of the relatively new idea of intelligent and interactive healthcare. Before this kind of system can be implemented, several hurdles must be surmounted (Dasaklis, Fran, et al., 2018). This is so even though such a system might have huge positive effects. Here are a few of these challenges:

- Patient privacy concerns: safeguarding patient privacy ranks high among the many obstacles to blockchain-based healthcare. Despite its promise of a safe and transparent way to store medical records, blockchain technology might leave patient data more vulnerable to threats if not applied properly. Also, maintaining patients' privacy by ensuring that only approved persons may access their sensitive medical information can be challenging.
- Another major obstacle is interoperability, which arises when various blockchain systems cannot communicate with one other. There needs to be a way for different systems to connect with each other smoothly for blockchain-based healthcare to be a success.
- Any new technology introduced to the highly regulated healthcare sector must adhere to all relevant rules and regulations. There are several difficulties that regulatory bodies face because of this. Blockchain technology still faces several regulatory hurdles before it can find widespread use in healthcare. This is also true with blockchain technology.
- Challenges in implementation: Blockchain-based healthcare is no different from the healthcare industry as a whole in that it has been sluggish to embrace new technology. Healthcare practitioners and patients alike need greater information and understanding in order to boost adoption rates.
- Accurate and full data is essential for blockchain-based healthcare to function properly. Healthcare data is frequently dispersed across several systems and may have variable quality, making data quality assurance a formidable problem.

Blockchain technology's slowness and inefficiency provide a problem for healthcare applications that rely on real-time data access in terms of scalability. The effective scalability of healthcare systems built on the blockchain is an important issue that needs fixing.

Finally, despite the great potential of blockchain-based intelligent and interactive healthcare, achieving this goal would need substantial work and cooperation among all parties involved.

7.1 Security Challenges Faced Towards Blockchain Based Intelligent and Interactive Healthcare

According to Abou-Nassar, Eman, et al. (2020), there are several security concerns with blockchain-based intelligent and interactive healthcare systems. These concerns include the following:

- Confidentiality: Protecting patient information is essential since it is sensitive. The inherent immutability and transparency of blockchain technology raises concerns about its suitability for protecting sensitive healthcare data.

Secure identity management solutions must be implemented in blockchain-based healthcare systems to guarantee that only allowed individuals may access patient data. This can be particularly problematic in healthcare settings because to the high volume of healthcare professionals that may need access to patient records.

- Smart contracts' safety: Automated contract execution is the capability of "smart contracts," which are recorded on the blockchain. Many healthcare-related interactions and transactions might be mechanised with the use of these contracts. However, smart contracts may be attacked, and malicious actors can take advantage of any flaws or weaknesses in the smart contract's code.

- Consensus procedures: Healthcare systems that rely on blockchain technology rely on these to ensure the data is accurate. Attacks on these procedures are not out of the question, especially on less secure and smaller networks.
- To ensure the safe and effective interchange of patient information, blockchain-based healthcare systems must be able to interface with other systems. This is called interoperability. Conversely, interoperability may be challenging to attain, especially in cases when many healthcare systems utilise a variety of distinct protocols and standards.

Finally, top-notch security solutions are required to ensure the privacy and integrity of patient data in blockchain-based smart and interactive healthcare systems. Some of the components that come under this category include the creation of strong consensus procedures, secure smart contract code, and robust identity management systems.

7.2 Privacy Challenges Faced Towards Blockchain BASED INTELLIGENT and Interactive Healthcare

Prabadevi, Natarajan, and colleagues (2021) state that there are several privacy issues with intelligent and interactive healthcare systems that are built on the blockchain. Here are some of the difficulties:

- **Transparency and immutability:** Patients' personal information might be at risk if they use blockchain technology, which makes maintaining anonymity a priority. While patient identities can be concealed via pseudonyms or other means, complete anonymity for those patients may remain elusive.
- **Breach of data security:** Healthcare systems built on the blockchain are not immune to data breaches; this is true of all healthcare systems. Blockchain technology's decentralised design, on the other hand, may make it harder to detect and react to security breaches.
- Patients must provide their informed consent before any data may be transferred to a healthcare system that is based on blockchain technology. But it's not always easy to make sure patients fully understand the risks and repercussions of giving their consent.
- **Laws:** Few laws have been passed that explicitly address the proper use of blockchain-based healthcare systems, perhaps due to the fact that these systems are still in their early stages. Because of this, it could be hard to ensure that patient data is being handled correctly.
- **Interoperability:** Healthcare systems built on the blockchain must be able to talk to each other for patient data to be transferred securely and efficiently. But interoperability may be tough to accomplish, especially when separate healthcare systems use distinct protocols and standards. Because of this, it could be hard to ensure that patient data is being handled correctly.

To ensure the security and privacy of patient information, it is necessary to develop strong privacy solutions when using blockchain technology in intelligent and interactive healthcare systems. Among these, you may find rules that are clear about their usage, safe ways of data storage and transfer, and durable anonymization techniques.

7.3 Trust Challenges Faced Towards Blockchain Based Intelligent and Interactive Healthcare

Several trust issues arise with intelligent and interactive healthcare systems built on blockchain technology. These include:

- **The complexity of the system:** Due to its complexity and specific expertise requirements, blockchain technology is challenging to implement and maintain. There may be miscommunication and distrust between patients and doctors because of this, which might make it hard for anybody to fully grasp how the system works.

One potential advantage and one potential disadvantage of blockchain-based healthcare systems is their intended transparency. This might end up being an advantage and a disadvantage. Transparency may boost trust by showing patients exactly how their data is being used, but it can also reveal sensitive details and make it harder to keep them private.

- **Consistency:** Distributed networks of nodes are the backbone of blockchain-based healthcare systems, which provide full and accurate data. The reliability and security of the system may be jeopardised if any one of these nodes were to fail, leading to a loss of trust.
- Healthcare providers and patients unfamiliar with blockchain technology may be wary of its potential due to the low adoption rate of blockchain-based solutions. Finally, healthcare systems that use blockchain technology are still in their early stages of deployment.

Ultimately, these issues must be resolved by open and honest communication, thorough education and training, and robust technology solutions if trust in smart and interactive healthcare systems built on the blockchain is to be established. Improving the system's dependability and security, establishing clear regulations and standards, and increasing the technology's use by both patients and medical professionals are all part of this process.

8. FUTURE RESEARCH OPPORTUNITIES TOWARDS USING BLOCKCHAIN IN HEALTHCARE SECTOR

Blockchain technology has several potential applications in healthcare, and there are many interesting areas that might be studied (Yaqoob, Khaled, et al., 2021). Some examples of these possibilities are:

- The creation of reliable privacy and security solutions: As mentioned earlier, healthcare systems that rely on blockchain technology have several challenges when it comes to privacy and security. Research may be conducted to provide fresh and innovative ways to tackle these challenges and guarantee the safety and confidentiality of patient data.
- Looking into standardisation and interoperability: To ensure easy communication and cooperation across healthcare systems, it is crucial to adopt interoperability. It is feasible to conduct studies that look at the potential applications of blockchain technology in developing interoperability solutions and standardising protocols for data exchange.

- Conducting medical research with blockchain technology One possible use of blockchain technology is the safe and transparent management of data used in medical research. Research into the potential uses of blockchain technology to improve research outcomes and facilitate the creation of new medical discoveries is within reach.

- Healthcare supply networks could benefit from blockchain technology's capacity to increase transparency and traceability. Building blockchain-based supply chain management solutions could be the key to achieving this goal. Research may be conducted to examine the potential applications of blockchain technology in ensuring the security and efficacy of healthcare products and tools.

- Increasing patient agency and participation: By granting people more say over their own health records, blockchain technology may increase patient agency and participation. Studying how blockchain-based solutions might be customised to meet patients' needs and improve their healthcare experience overall is a viable area of study to pursue.

- In order to boost innovation in the healthcare industry, protect patient privacy, and enhance patient outcomes, there are a plethora of fascinating research topics that may be explored. Finally, there is a plethora of opportunities to investigate the many possible applications of blockchain technology in healthcare.

9. RESEARCH STATEMENTS FOR USING BLOCKCHAIN IN HEALTHCARE SECTOR

The following are some research claims on the use of blockchain technology in healthcare, as stated in the studies conducted by Tandon, Anushree, et al. in 2020 and Khezr, Seyednima in 2019:

- The goal of this research is to find out how well blockchain-based solutions protect patients' personal information and electronic health records (EHRs).

   The potential applications of blockchain technology in healthcare supply chain management are the focus of this research. Equally important is the examination of the pros and cons of blockchain-based solution implementation.

- Looking at how medical research may benefit from blockchain-based solutions, with an eye on improving data sharing, transparency, and collaboration amongst the parties involved.

- Looking at how blockchain technology can empower patients to have a say in their healthcare records and promote self-management by making it easier for them to access and manage their own information.

- Building a blockchain-based infrastructure to run clinical trials in a secure and transparent manner; this might increase efficiency, decrease costs, and increase patient safety.

- To improve healthcare in developing countries with inadequate infrastructure and resources, researchers are looking at the potential use of blockchain technology.

- Looking at blockchain-based technologies that might help healthcare systems work together more effectively and make it easier for different companies to share patient data.

- Principles for data security, informed consent, and governance should be part of any framework for the appropriate and ethical application of blockchain technology to healthcare.

- Looking into the pros and cons of introducing blockchain-based solutions, as well as the likelihood that blockchain technology may improve the efficiency and accuracy of healthcare payment and billing systems.

So, ultimately, by exploring and making use of blockchain-based solutions to improve medication adherence and decrease medication errors through transparent and secure recording of medicine intake, etc.

10. POTENTIALS FOR BLOCKCHAIN IN NEAR FUTURE

The impending development of several intriguing blockchain-related applications bodes well for the technology's ability to transform a wide range of industries. In this piece, we'll look at a few ways blockchain technology may be used in several industries, including healthcare. The 2020 publication by Poonam Chahal and Amit Kumar Tyagi Amit Kumar Tyagi and G. Rekha were married in 2020. P Released in 2022 by S. Kumari and P. Muthulakshmi Amit Kumar Tyagi, Vinuthna, and Shamila were married in 2023. Tyagi (A.K.) and Madhav (A.V.S.) 2022 The publishing by D. Goyal and A.K. Tyagi in 2020; The 2019 publication by Amit Kumar Tyagi and Rekha G. Tyagi In 2019, the results were published by Amit Kumar Tyagi, V. Krishna Reddy, and Gillala Rekha. "Sai, G.H., Tripathi, K., and Tyagi, A.K. 20,23" was published in 2019 by Shruti Kute, Amit Kumar Tyagi, and Rohit Sahoo. Studies conducted in 2020 by Gudeti, Mishra, and colleagues 21, include Tyagi, Meenu, and others S.S. Kute, Aswathy S.U. 2022, and A.K. Tyagi, in that order According to Nair M.M., Tyagi A.K., and Sravanthi K. 2021, the following subjects can be investigated in the future:

- Digital Identity: Secure and verifiable digital identities may be created with the help of blockchain technology. A variety of activities, like as voting, gaining access to financial services, and data storage, may make use of these identities.
- Supply Chain Management: By integrating blockchain technology into supply chains, we can ensure that all items are legitimate and of high quality. This is achieved through end-to-end transparency and traceability.
- Blockchain technology offers a more efficient and safe way to register and transfer ownership of real estate, which might lead to the elimination of intermediaries like lawyers and title firms in the real estate industry.
- Decentralised Finance (DeFi): Anyone with an internet connection may use blockchain technology to build open, transparent, and accessible decentralised financial systems.
- The healthcare industry has the potential to use blockchain technology to create open-source, secure systems for patient data management, medication usage tracking, and product authenticity verification.
- In the energy sector, blockchain technology has the potential to create decentralised energy grids, which would improve the efficiency of renewable energy and other energy sources' distribution and storage.
- One potential use of blockchain technology in gaming is the creation of decentralised gaming ecosystems where players may own and trade virtual goods and currency.

- Using blockchain technology in the school industry will make credit transfers and job applications easier for students. The adoption of blockchain technology has the potential to provide transparent and secure systems for the recording and validation of academic qualifications.

As a conclusion, blockchain technology has many potential applications, and many exciting new applications will likely appear in the near future as the technology evolves and develops more.

11. CONCLUSION AND FUTURE WORK

By improving patient outcomes, strengthening data security and privacy, and enabling more efficient and cost-effective healthcare delivery, intelligent and interactive healthcare systems built on blockchain technology might radically alter the healthcare industry. Healthcare practitioners can create secure and transparent systems for patient data management, medication consumption tracking, and medical supply and equipment validity verification using the immutability and tamper-proof properties of blockchain technology. In the long run, this may benefit patients' health by increasing their safety and allowing healthcare providers to work together more effectively. The use of smart and interactive technologies like wearables, the internet of things (IoT), and artificial intelligence (AI) can also pave the way for proactive and personalised healthcare. Because of this, medical professionals can improve patient outcomes by responding quickly to issues. Nevertheless, there are a lot of challenges that must be overcome. These include issues related to data protection, meeting regulatory standards, and ensuring that different healthcare systems are interoperable and standardised.

Ultimately, Intelligent and Interactive Healthcare Systems built on the Blockchain might completely transform the healthcare industry. However, for this revolutionary potential to materialise, a great deal of stakeholder collaboration and innovation is required. As blockchain technology has the ability to shake up several non-financial sectors, it bodes well for the technology's future. Healthcare organisations may reduce the risk of data breaches and ensure patient privacy by securely storing and disseminating medical records using blockchain technology. Applying blockchain technology allows this to be achieved. With blockchain's ability to provide transparency and traceability, supply chain management may enhance item monitoring and decrease the chance of fraudulent conduct. To facilitate the exchange of renewable energy, blockchain technology may be able to aid the energy sector in creating decentralised energy markets. Scalability, interoperability, and legal concerns are just a few of the ongoing challenges to blockchain adoption.

The current state of the blockchain infrastructure is not scalable because of its restricted capacity, which limits the amount of transactions that can be processed. Interoperability issues stem from the fact that different blockchain systems do not adhere to any kind of standards. Information communication between networks is made more difficult by the absence of standards. Regulators are worried about blockchain technology since there aren't now clear rules and standards for its usage. Ambiguity and potential legal risks result from this murkiness. To rub salt in the wound, blockchain technology is highly promising and is expected to experience significant growth in the next years. With the constant development of new blockchain platforms and use cases, blockchain technology is poised to revolutionise several sectors while opening up exciting new possibilities for growth and innovation.

Due to its ability to enable a wide range of non-banking businesses, the technology behind blockchain has great promise for the future. Healthcare organisations may reduce the risk of data breaches and ensure patient privacy by securely storing and disseminating medical records using blockchain technology. Applying blockchain technology allows this to be achieved. Because blockchain technology allows for more accurate monitoring of goods and decreases the chance of fraudulent conduct, it can improve supply chain management by making information more transparent and easier to trace. The development of decentralised energy markets, made possible by blockchain technology, may revolutionise the energy industry by allowing for the efficient trading of renewable energy sources. Nevertheless, a lot of challenges still need to be resolved before blockchain technology can be extensively used. Concerns about regulation, interoperability, and scalability are among these hurdles.

REFERENCES

Abou-Nassar, E. M., Iliyasu, A. M., El-Kafrawy, P. M., Song, O.-Y., Kashif Bashir, A., & Abd El-Latif, A. A. (2020). DITrust chain: Towards blockchain-based trust models for sustainable healthcare IoT systems. *IEEE Access : Practical Innovations, Open Solutions*, 8, 111223–111238. doi:10.1109/ACCESS.2020.2999468

Al-Marridi, A. Z., Mohamed, A., & Erbad, A. (2021). Reinforcement learning approaches for efficient and secure blockchain-powered smart health systems. *Computer Networks*, *197*, 108279. doi:10.1016/j.comnet.2021.108279

Ali, A., Pasha, M. F., Fang, O. H., Khan, R., Almaiah, M. A., & Al Hwaitat, A. K. (2022). Big Data Based Smart Blockchain for Information Retrieval in Privacy-Preserving Healthcare System. In *Big Data Intelligence for Smart Applications* (pp. 279–296). Springer International Publishing. doi:10.1007/978-3-030-87954-9_13

Tyagi, A. (2020). Challenges of Applying Deep Learning in Real-World Applications. Challenges and Applications for Implementing Machine Learning in Computer Vision. IGI Global. doi:10.4018/978-1-7998-0182-5.ch004

Chen, M., Malook, T., Rehman, A. U., Muhammad, Y., Alshehri, M. D., Akbar, A., Bilal, M., & Khan, M. A. (2021). Blockchain-Enabled healthcare system for detection of diabetes. *Journal of Information Security and Applications*, *58*, 102771. doi:10.1016/j.jisa.2021.102771

Dasaklis, T. K., Casino, F., & Patsakis, C. ().Blockchain meets smart health: Towards next generation healthcare services. In *2018 9th International conference on information, intelligence, systems and applications (IISA)*, pp. 1-8. IEEE. 10.1109/IISA.2018.8633601

Gudeti, B., Mishra, S., Malik, S., Fernandez, T. F., Tyagi, A. K., & Kumari, S. (2020). *A Novel Approach to Predict Chronic Kidney Disease using Machine Learning Algorithms*. 2020 4th International Conference on Electronics, Communication and Aerospace Technology (ICECA), Coimbatore. 10.1109/ICECA49313.2020.9297392

Hathaliya, J., Sharma, P., Tanwar, S., & Gupta, R. (2019). Blockchain-based remote patient monitoring in healthcare 4.0. In *2019 IEEE 9th international conference on advanced computing (IACC)*, (pp. 87-91). IEEE. 10.1109/IACC48062.2019.8971593

Tyagi, A. (2021). Healthcare Solutions for Smart Era: An Useful Explanation from User's Perspective. Recent Trends in Blockchain for Information Systems Security and Privacy. CRC Press.

Khatoon, A. (2020). A blockchain-based smart contract system for healthcare management. *Electronics (Basel)*, *9*(1), 94. doi:10.3390/electronics9010094

Khezr, S., Moniruzzaman, M., Yassine, A., & Benlamri, R. (2019). Blockchain technology in healthcare: A comprehensive review and directions for future research. *Applied Sciences (Basel, Switzerland)*, *9*(9), 1736. doi:10.3390/app9091736

Khubrani, M. M. (2021). A framework for blockchain-based smart health system. [TURCOMAT]. *Turkish Journal of Computer and Mathematics Education*, *12*(9), 2609–2614.

Kumar, T., Ramani, V., Ahmad, I., Braeken, A., Harjula, E., & Ylianttila, M. (2018). Blockchain utilization in healthcare: Key requirements and challenges. In *2018 IEEE 20th International conference on e-health networking, applications and services (Healthcom)*. IEEE. 10.1109/HealthCom.2018.8531136

Kumari, S., & Muthulakshmi, P. (2022). Transformative Effects of Big Data on Advanced Data Analytics: Open Issues and Critical Challenges. *Journal of Computational Science*, *18*(6), 463–479. doi:10.3844/jcssp.2022.463.479

Kute, S. (2021). Building a Smart Healthcare System Using Internet of Things and Machine Learning. Big Data Management in Sensing: Applications in AI and IoT. River Publishers.

Kute, S. S., Tyagi, A. K., & Aswathy, S. U. (2022). Industry 4.0 Challenges in e-Healthcare Applications and Emerging Technologies. In A. K. Tyagi, A. Abraham, & A. Kaklauskas (Eds.), *Intelligent Interactive Multimedia Systems for e-Healthcare Applications*. Springer. doi:10.1007/978-981-16-6542-4_14

Kute, S. S., Tyagi, A. K., & Aswathy, S. U. (2022). Security, Privacy and Trust Issues in Internet of Things and Machine Learning Based e-Healthcare. In A. K. Tyagi, A. Abraham, & A. Kaklauskas (Eds.), *Intelligent Interactive Multimedia Systems for e-Healthcare Applications*. Springer. doi:10.1007/978-981-16-6542-4_15

Le, H. T., Lam, N. T. T., Vo, H. K., Luong, H. H., Khoi, N. H. T., & Anh, T. D. (2022). Patient-chain: patient-centered healthcare system a blockchain-based technology in dealing with emergencies. In *Parallel and Distributed Computing, Applications and Technologies: 22nd International Conference, PDCAT 2021*. Cham: Springer International Publishing. 10.1007/978-3-030-96772-7_54

Madhav, A. V. S., & Tyagi, A. K. (2022). The World with Future Technologies (Post-COVID-19): Open Issues, Challenges, and the Road Ahead. In A. K. Tyagi, A. Abraham, & A. Kaklauskas (Eds.), *Intelligent Interactive Multimedia Systems for e-Healthcare Applications*. Springer. doi:10.1007/978-981-16-6542-4_22

Nair, M. M., Kumari, S., Tyagi, A. K., & Sravanthi, K. (2021). Deep Learning for Medical Image Recognition: Open Issues and a Way to Forward. In: Goyal D., Gupta A.K., Piuri V., Ganzha M., Paprzycki M. (eds) *Proceedings of the Second International Conference on Information Management and Machine Intelligence. Lecture Notes in Networks and Systems*. Springer, Singapore. 10.1007/978-981-15-9689-6_38

Prabadevi, B. (2021). Toward blockchain for edge-of-things: A new paradigm, opportunities, and future directions. *IEEE Internet of Things Magazine, 4*(2), 102–108. doi:10.1109/IOTM.0001.2000191

Quasim, M. T., Algarni, F., Abd Elhamid Radwan, A., & Goram Mufareh, M. A. (2020). A blockchain based secured healthcare framework. In *2020 International Conference on Computational Performance Evaluation (ComPE)*, (pp. 386-391). IEEE. 10.1109/ComPE49325.2020.9200024

Ramani, V., Kumar, T., Bracken, A., Liyanage, M., & Ylianttila, M. (2018). Secure and efficient data accessibility in blockchain based healthcare systems. In *2018 IEEE Global Communications Conference (GLOBECOM)*. IEEE. 10.1109/GLOCOM.2018.8647221

Sai, G. H., Tripathi, K., & Tyagi, A. K. (2023). Internet of Things-Based e-Health Care: Key Challenges and Recommended Solutions for Future. In: Singh, P.K., Wierzchoń, S.T., Tanwar, S., Rodrigues, J.J.P.C., Ganzha, M. (eds) *Proceedings of Third International Conference on Computing, Communications, and Cyber-Security. Lecture Notes in Networks and Systems*. Springer, Singapore. 10.1007/978-981-19-1142-2_37

Shamila, M., & Vinuthna, K. (2023). Genomic privacy: performance analysis, open issues, and future research directions. Amit Kumar Tyagi, Ajith Abraham (eds.) Data Science for Genomics. Academic Press. doi:10.1016/B978-0-323-98352-5.00015-X

Sharma, A., Tomar, R., Chilamkurti, N., & Kim, B.-G. (2020). Blockchain based smart contracts for internet of medical things in e-healthcare. *Electronics (Basel), 9*(10), 1609. doi:10.3390/electronics9101609

Sharma, P., Moparthi, N. R., Namasudra, S., Shanmuganathan, V., & Hsu, C.-H. (2022). Blockchain-based IoT architecture to secure healthcare system using identity-based encryption. *Expert Systems: International Journal of Knowledge Engineering and Neural Networks, 39*(10), e12915. doi:10.1111/exsy.12915

Singh, S., Sharma, S. K., Mehrotra, P., Bhatt, P., & Kaurav, M. (2022). Blockchain technology for efficient data management in healthcare system: Opportunity, challenges and future perspectives. *Materials Today: Proceedings, 62*, 5042–5046. doi:10.1016/j.matpr.2022.04.998

Soltanisehat, L., Alizadeh, R., Hao, H., & Choo, K.-K. R. (2020). Technical, temporal, and spatial research challenges and opportunities in blockchain-based healthcare: A systematic literature review. *IEEE Transactions on Engineering Management*.

Son, H. X., Le, T. H., Nga, T. T. Q., Hung, N. D. H., Duong-Trung, N., & Luong, H. H. (2021). *Toward a blockchain-based technology in dealing with emergencies in patient-centered healthcare systems*. In Mobile, Secure, and Programmable Networking: 6th International Conference, MSPN 2020, Paris. 10.1007/978-3-030-67550-9_4

Tandon, A., Dhir, A., Islam, A. K. M. N., & Mäntymäki, M. (2020). Blockchain in healthcare: A systematic literature review, synthesizing framework and future research agenda. *Computers in Industry, 122*, 103290. doi:10.1016/j.compind.2020.103290

Tripathi, G., Ahad, M. A., & Paiva, S. (2020). S2HS-A blockchain based approach for smart healthcare system. In Healthcare, 8. Elsevier. doi:10.1016/j.hjdsi.2019.100391

Tyagi, A. (2020). Artificial Intelligence and Machine Learning Algorithms. Challenges and Applications for Implementing Machine Learning in Computer Vision. IGI Global. doi:10.4018/978-1-7998-0182-5.ch008

Tyagi, A. K., & Goyal, D. (2020). A Survey of Privacy Leakage and Security Vulnerabilities in the Internet of Things. 2020 5th International Conference on Communication and Electronics Systems (ICCES). IEEE. 10.1109/ICCES48766.2020.9137886

Tyagi, A.. (2022). Using Multimedia Systems, Tools, and Technologies for Smart Healthcare Services. IGI Global., doi:10.4018/978-1-6684-5741-2

Wu, G., Wang, S., Ning, Z., & Zhu, B. (2021). Privacy-preserved electronic medical record exchanging and sharing: A blockchain-based smart healthcare system. *IEEE Journal of Biomedical and Health Informatics*, *26*(5), 1917–1927. doi:10.1109/JBHI.2021.3123643 PMID:34714757

Xu, J., Xue, K., Li, S., Tian, H., Hong, J., Hong, P., & Yu, N. (2019). Healthchain: A blockchain-based privacy preserving scheme for large-scale health data. *IEEE Internet of Things Journal*, *6*(5), 8770–8781. doi:10.1109/JIOT.2019.2923525

Yaqoob, I., Salah, K., Jayaraman, R., & Al-Hammadi, Y. (2021). Blockchain for healthcare data management: Opportunities, challenges, and future recommendations. *Neural Computing & Applications*, 1–16.

Chapter 8
Impact of Machine Learning and Deep Learning Techniques in Autism

Megha Bhushan

ⓘ https://orcid.org/0000-0003-4309-875X

DIT University, India

Maanas Singal

DIT University, India

Arun Negi

Deliotte USI, India

ABSTRACT

Autism spectrum disorder (ASD) is a behavioural and developmental illness caused by brain abnormalities. Individuals with ASD have difficulty with limited or repeated acts, as well as social communication and participation. Additionally, people with ASD may learn, move, or pay attention in various ways. It should be remembered that some individuals without ASD may also experience some of these symptoms. However, these traits may render life very difficult for those with ASD. Since the trend of machine learning (ML) and deep learning (DL) techniques has been on an onset in every domain, the same is being actively utilized for diagnosis and treatment of this aliment. This chapter provides an in-depth insight into the efforts of researchers on diverse crowd for development and implementation of ML/DL models to assist the ailing individual along with their families and health caregivers. It provides the review of existing works in diverse directions in focus with ASD like prediction, segregation, correlation, etc. between parameters which would help the medical professionals.

DOI: 10.4018/979-8-3693-2359-5.ch008

1. INTRODUCTION

Social communication and common behaviour is hampered in many neurologically ailing individuals by the complicated neurodevelopmental disease known as Autism Spectrum Disorder (ASD). The diagnosis of ASD currently places a significant emphasis on qualitative behavioural assessment. Factors like carer report bias and professionals' lack experience identifying ASD may have a detrimental impact on the diagnostic accuracy. Based on a new meta-analysis of data from 35 countries, the mean age of ASD diagnosis was 60.48 months, and when accounting exclusively for children under the age of 10, it was 43.18 months (van't Hof et al., 2021). The prognosis of the affected youngsters is further impacted by the postponed action that results from the delayed diagnosis (Dawson et al., 2012). Both the extent and the intensity of its symptoms are quite variable. Common signs include difficulty communicating, particularly in social situations, obsessional hobbies, and repeated mannerisms. A thorough examination is needed to detect ASD. This also comprises a thorough evaluation and a range of tests conducted by child psychologists and other licenced experts. Autism Diagnostic Observation Schedule Revised (ADOS-R) and Autism Diagnostic Interview Revised (ADI-R) are two common techniques for diagnosing autism (Duda et al., 2014). Low diagnosis and treatment rates in healthcare institutions are another barrier to rapid ASD detection and therapy. In the United States, just 1% of people with ASD are now identified by primary care HCPs (Monteiro et al., 2019; Rhoades et al., 2007). The American Academy of Paediatrics (AAP) advises clinicians knowledgeable with the Diagnostic and Statistical Manual of Mental Disorders, Fifth Edition (DSM-5) criteria to diagnose ASD or refer patients to a specialist for additional evaluation after a failed ASD screen in primary care (Hyman et al., 2020).

Even with these statistics, 60% of children who fail screenings are neither detected in general care nor directed to a specialist (Monteiro et al., 2019). Primary care diagnosis is frequently hampered by a lack of perceived self-efficacy in making the diagnosis, low confidence in using ASD diagnostic tools due to a lack of specialist training and/or time to administer, and a lack of time to properly review results with carers and discuss treatment recommendations (Fenikilé et al., 2015; Self et al., 2015). Additionally, traditional screening tools used in healthcare contexts may overlook a significant number of instances of ASD. For instance, 61% (278/454) of the kids who received a diagnosis of ASD in a cohort of more than 20,000 kids with outcome data failed a standard screener (Guthrie et al., 2019). Several works have tried to identify and classify ASD using different machine learning approaches. The researchers in (Thabtah & Peebles, 2020) suggested using Rules-Machine Learning (RML) to evaluate the ASD features and discovered that RML improves the performance of classifiers. Similar to how the authors in (Satu et al., 2019) used tree-based classifiers to highlight individual important characteristics of typically developing and autistic children in Bangladesh. In (Abbas et al., 2018), feature encoding approaches were used to address the issues of scarcity, sparsity, and data imbalance. ADI-R and ADOS ML methodologies were merged into a single evaluation. A further work that was published in (Thabtah et al., 2018) offered a CI approach called Variable Analysis (VA), which employed Support Vector Machine (SVM), Decision Tree (DT), and Logistic Reggression (LR) for reliable ASD diagnoses and prognoses (Hossain et al., 2019; Howlader et al., 2018; Thabtah, 2017, 2019); and demonstrated feature-to-feature and feature-to-class associations.

Recent developments in Social Cognitive Neuroscience (SCN) have provided new insights into how people evaluate and describe their ideas, attitudes, and actions (Arya et al., 2022). The branch of study known as SCN investigates biological mechanisms and related cognitive-based elements (Nosek et al., 2011), and it has shown that interpersonal relationships rely on implicit psychophysiological systems that are not controlled consciously (Lieberman, 2010). Implicit assessments frequently evaluate unconscious, automatic biological functions that result from the internal processing of external environmental cues (Arya et al., 2021).

These indicators are a viable substitute for explicit assessments, which cannot independently capture inferred brain functions. Several technologies have improved heathcare (Pathan et al., 2020; V. J. Singh et al., 2015), however; proper implementation of the novel methods requires extensive pre-planning for smooth transition to the said methods. Thus, more recent research has combined biomarkers with conventional evaluation methods in order to address explicit measure inadequacies in the ASD diagnosis (LeDoux & Pine, 2016). Electro-Dermal Activity (EDA) (Alcañiz Raya et al., 2020; Nikula, 1991); Functional Near-Infrared Spectroscopy (fNIRS), Electroencephalography (EEG) (Knyazev et al., 2004), Functional Magnetic Resonance Imaging (fMRI), Heart Rate Variability (HRT) (Nickel & Nachreiner, 2003), and eye tracking currently the most effective biomarkers for studying unconscious processes. While fMRI studies showed that ASD is associated with hyperactivity in brain activation and changes in the cingulate posterior cortex and parts of the insula, EEG study demonstrated that ASD people display more left hemisphere activity in social circumstances (Di Martino et al., 2014). The screening and categorization of body movements which constitute a major part of behavioural biosigns such as facial expressions, limb coordination, eye movement, etc. was also made possible by newly developed technical instruments, such as cameras and/or sensors (M. L. Alcañiz et al., 2019).

Another important improvement is Virtual Reality (VR), an immersive computer-generated experience that lets people experience virtual and unreal worlds. VR makes experienced events and users' emotions more ecologically valid, showing promise for psychological training, evaluation, and treatment (Holloway et al., 1992). In general, Head-Mounted Displays (HMDs) are the most significant, accessible, and cost-effective VR products (S. Parsons et al., 2004).

A semi-immersive room concoited as the Cave-Automatic Virtual Environment (CAVE), equipped, and installed with upto 6 rear-casted surfaces, has been recommended as an alternative VR device that is more suited to the target persons (ASD youngsters) (Bowman et al., 2002; T. D. Parsons, 2011; T. D. Parsons et al., 2009; Pastorelli & Herrmann, 2013).With its semi-immersive design, CAVE eliminates the possibility of users getting "cyber-sick," which is discomfort brought on by sensory-motor discord and cognitive dissonance in a virtual environment. Additionally, the CAVE system can circumvent the severe limitations of HMDs, which are not only inappropriate for children with tiny heads but can also increase their cognitive and sensory contests (Guazzaroni, 2018; Wallace et al., 2010).

There were no appreciable differences between children with ASD and Typically Developing Controls (TD) in previous studies on the viability, safety, and learning capabilities of CAVE environments in ASD children, and improvements in a number of tasks (such as sidewalks and crossings) (Lorenzo et al., 2019). Immersion, interaction, and a sense of presence in the environment are the three core features that all VR systems, independent of technology or brand, share (Biocca et al., 2001; Cipresso et al., 2018; Skalski & Tamborini, 2007; Slater, 2009). A system's ability to isolate a user from reality is known as immersion (Cummings & Bailenson, 2016). The combined use of these research and technology paves the door for more reliable systems to be used by people with ASD, as well as by their families and medical professionals.

2. LITERATURE REVIEW

This chapter presents a review of 32 primary research works collected from various reputed international journals and conferences by renowned publishers including IEEE, Nature, Springer, Wiley and MDPI. Table 1 depicts a detailed summary of these studies.

AdaBoost: Adaptive Boosting; ADT: Abstract Data Type; ANN: Artificial Neural Network; ARIA: Adaptive Robotic Intervention Architecture; ASD: Autism Spectrum Disorder; BA: Bat Algorithm; CART: Classification And Regression Trees; CNN: Convolutional Neural Network; CT: Classification Tree; DBSCAN: Density-Based Spatial Clustering of Applications with Noise; DL: Deep Learning; DNN: Deep Neural Network; DT: Decision Tree; ENS: Ensemble; ET: Extra Trees; FDA: Fisher's Discriminant Analysis; FNN: Fuzzy Neural Network; FPA: Flower Pollination Algorithm; FT: Feature Transformation; GBM: Gradient Boosting Machine; GBT: Gradient Boosted Trees; GWO: Grey Wolf Optimizer; KNN: k-Nearest Neighbors; LDA: Linear Discriminant Analysis; LOSO: Leave-One-Subject-Out; LR: Logistic Regression; LSTM: Long Short-Term Memory; MDA: Multiple Discriminant Analysis; ML: Machine Learning; MLP: Multi-Layer Perceptron; MT: Metric Learning; NB: Naive Bayes; NN: Neural Network; PART: Partial Decision Trees; PDA: Principal Component Discriminant Analysis; PRISM: Prism Decision Tree Algorithm; RCNN: Region-based Convolutional Neural Network; RF: Random Forest; RIDOR: Rule Induction Based On Differential Orderings; RIPPER: Repeated Incremental Pruning to Produce Error Reduction; RML: Rule-Machine Learning; RNN: Recurrent Neural Network; SSD: Single Shot Detector; SVM: Support Vector Machine; TCDM: Tree-structured Clustering with Dynamic Models; TF: TensorFlow; XGBoost: eXtreme Gradient Boosting; YOLO: You Only Look Once; FC: Functional Connectivity; TD: Typically Developing; ADHD: Attention Deficit Hyperactivity Disorder; VFGM: Virulence Factor-related Gut Microbiota; OSHU: Oregon Health and Science University, GE: Gene Expression; BASC: Behavior Assessment System for Children; LFA: Low-Functioning Autism; AUROC: Area Under the Receiver Operating Characteristic

3. OPEN CHALLENGES

The reviewed literature spans across multiple domains including applications with regard to diagnosis, prediction, treatment, segregation, and isolation of the individuals suffering from ASD. The prediction or diagnosis of the neurological condition has been implemented via the use of ML and DL techniques in broadly four spectrums using (i) gene-cluster analysis, (ii) hybrid MRI data, (iii) body movement patterns/speech, and (iv) standard diagnostic questionnaires.

The studies conducted in (Alsuliman & Al-Baity, 2022; M. Wang et al., 2021) use ML and DL techniques for predicting the ASD using human genome data analysis. The studies involve identification and isolation of gene clusters that show correlation with the onset of ASD in infants before and after birth. The open challenges in this area are theoretically oriented as the study of genetics at an advanced level along with super-specialized studies is required before this technique is thoroughly understood to be applied into practice. The studies conducted for autism screening using this domain mainly relies on the isolation of specific gene-clusters whose results are then cross-verified with clinical symptoms. Thus, a lot of independent and collaborating studies are required before this interdisciplinary sub-domain is perfected to be utilized in common practice.

Table 1. Summary of existing studies

Article	Year	Summary	Techniques Used	Advantages	Disadvantages	Precision/Accuracy
(Mastrovito et al., 2018)	2018	To find diagnostically distinct and relevant traits for each condition (autism and schizophrenia) and effectively utilise them to categorise an independent cohort of participants. It greatly aided in the identification of common and divergent connection variations in the default mode network, in addition to in the salience and motor networks.	Linear-SVM	Similar social cognition deficiencies related to ASD and SZ may be connected to alterations in connection within the DMN and salience network's higher order association cortex. It might be utilised to differentiate ASD and SZ individuals.	Finding the appropriate combination of characteristics to maximise diagnostic capacity is a significant problem in discovering diagnostic biomarkers from resting state functional connectivity.	The ASD verification data set yielded 83% accuracy, whereas the SZ verification data set yielded 80% accuracy.
(Omar et al., 2019)	2019	Autism may now be diagnosed at an early stage because of advances in AI and ML. A model for prediction based on ML techniques was presented, as well as a mobile app was created for predicting ASD in people of any age.	LR, SVM, NB, RF, and CART	The results demonstrated superior performance when compared to other known approaches to screen for autism. The model is capable of predicting autism features for multiple age groups.	On an actual dataset, the findings revealed mediocre accuracy performance (77% to 85%). This was primarily caused by the real dataset having inadequate samples or data.	Accurately predict autism in children, adolescents, and adults with 92.26%, 93.78%, and 97.10%, correspondingly.
(C. Wang et al., 2019)	2019	A ML framework was presented to identify autistic patients from the normal populace. It used "rs-fMRI" for collecting data to implement the framework for increasing classification accuracy on the whole ABIDE dataset.	SVM-RFE, and Auto-encoder NN	The suggested solution is entirely data-driven and requires no prior knowledge, making it a little simpler to work with. The first FC characteristics in this study originated from entire brain areas instead of local regions like the default mode network, which aids broad generalization of results.	Even though the sample was drawn from the entire ABIDE dataset, the identification outcome using solely DL was unsatisfactory since the sample was tiny in comparison to the number of FC characteristics.	Correctly identified autism with a 93.59% accuracy with a sensitivity of 92.52%, and specificity clocking at 94.56%.
(Akter et al., 2019)	2019	The study collected early stage diagnosed ASD data samples from several phases of life (toddler, child, adolescents, and adults). It used multiple feature transformation algorithms to compress the data. Following that, several classification approaches were used to evaluate performance.	Adaboost, FDA, C5.0, LDA, MDA, PDA, SVM, and CART	It collected early detection ASD datasets from several phases of life (toddler, child, adolescent, and adult) and analysed the results using a variety of different classifiers to examine the key aspects of ASD, which provided some extremely valuable insights.	Some of the classifiers did not consistently give excellent findings because, while having excellent precision, they produced biased results for the datasets they were used in since there was not enough ASD data to properly address these issues.	Accuracy of 97.20% was achieved for children using AdaBoost. Similarly 93.89% accuracy was achieved for adolescents using GLMBoost, and 93.86% accuracy for adults using AdaBoost.
(Raj & Masood, 2020)	2020	A study was carried out on three publicly available, non-clinical ASD datasets, with multiple ML algorithms for ASD Diagnosis in candidate data being used. For adults, children, and adolescents, datasets 1, 2, and 3 yielded excellent accuracies.	NB, SVM, LR, NN, CNN, and KNN	When compared to existing studies, the CNN classifier outperformed SVM in terms of incorporating all of its feature properties after managing missing values.	The optimal accuracy number appears only when the omitted values had been successfully effectively resolved using some standard process.	Accuracies attained using CNN are 99.53%, 98.30%, and 96.88% for adults, kids, and teenagers, respectively.

continues on following page

Table 1. Continued

Article	Year	Summary	Techniques Used	Advantages	Disadvantages	Precision/Accuracy
(Lai et al., 2020)	2020	For the purpose of screening methods for kids with ASD utilising ML and DL techniques, 46 ASD participants were chosen from 3 special needs schools, while 24 normal controls were chosen from the community.	ResNet-50, CNN, ARIA, Glmnet, and SVM	According to cup and disc associated metrics, the study has shown that retinal images may be used to build an objective risk category for ASD based on a variety of retinal and nerve fiber-related features.	Data collection for screening may be challenging in backward or orthodox communities where ASD along with other neuro-logical diseases that are considered taboo in society.	The classification model's sensitivity and specificity were 95.7% (95% CI 76.0%, 99.8%) and 91.3% (95% CI 70.5%, 98.5%), correspondingly.
(Thabtah & Peebles, 2020)	2020	A ML approach dubbed R-ML was deveoped, which not only detects autistic features in cases and controls but also provides users with knowledge bases (or rules) that domain experts may use to explain the rationale for the classification.	RIPPER, RIDOR, NNGE, Bagging, CART, RML, PRISM, AdaBoost, and C4.5	It not only improves the sensitivity, specificity, and predicted accuracy of the ASD screening procedure, but it also provides automatic categorization as well as comprehensive rule sets for physicians, carers, patients as well as their families, and teachers.	The scoring systems were built during the evaluation stage based on handcrafted guidelines and hence are susceptible to criticism for being subjective.	Adult=6 through RML, Adolescent=12 via AdaBoost, and Children=6 via RML were the lowest error rates.
(Peral et al., 2020)	2020	An architecture centred on data integration and analytics was created, to enable the distributed processing of the input information for Early ASD screening. Furthermore, it made possible to identify significant characteristics as well as hidden relationships between parameters.	DT, RF, Bayes, Adaboost, PART, ANN, SVM, and AttSelClass	It identified many critical characteristics for the diagnosis of ASD, as well as demonstrated correlations between different factors through a battery of tests.	Since datasets were not always acquired according to the same standards, changes in the parameters for the same might provide a range of outcomes. The models may encounter a bottleneck in this area, notwithstanding their value in order to maintain consistency and streamline data integration.	AttSelClass obtained the highest overall complete accuracy possible (97%) with DT baseline estimation at 92%.
(Alcaniz Raya et al., 2020)	2020	In the experimental study, 25 children with normal neurodevelopment and 24 children with ASD participated in a multidimensional VR experience while having their body movements tracked by a depth sensor camera as auditory, visual, and scent stimuli were presented.	SVM-RFE, LOSO, C-SVM, and LIBSVM	The variations between groups, as well as a diverse collection of trained ML models incorporating body characteristics and stimulus conditions, were used to assess the discriminability of ASD and TD youngsters using body movement, which aided in establishing a link between stimuli-based movement and ASD.	Limited to small participant sample sizes for each group. Usage of higher sample sets could make it possible to validate the ML technique and test the model.	The accuracy of the models that included the head and trunk joints was 82.98%, and it stayed the same for the model that used the foot joints.

continues on following page

121

Table 1. Continued

Article	Year	Summary	Techniques Used	Advantages	Disadvantages	Precision/Accuracy
(Yassin et al., 2020)	2020	Developed and compared classifiers that can distinguish between individuals with schizophrenia, ASD, and TD based on their MRI scans. It identify the most crucial categories of brain features influencing the categorization; and assess the classifiers' uniformity with the degree of clinical severity.	LR, SVM, RF, AdaBoost, DT, and KNN	The results advances our knowledge of the most effective categorization strategies among individuals with ASD, schizophrenia as well as TD as well as the most significant clusters of brain features that affect categorization	The ASD individuals considered in this study were only men. The mere fact that none of the ASD participants, several of the UHR and FEP participants, or all of the schizophrenia patients had taken medication might also have affected the results.	The classifiers' accuracy rates for the subcortical volume feature group were SVM (80%), AdaBoost (75%), KNN (85%), RF (75%), and LR (75%).
(Vabalas et al., 2020)	2020	Employed an imitation task with altered movement style to see if kinematic and eye movement activity variables might predict autism diagnosis. With kinematic data, the generated models attained a categorization accuracy of 73% and with eye movement data, a categorization accuracy of 70%.	t-test, SVM-RFE, ReliefF, and mRMR	It used layered validation and feature selection aiming at selection stability to overcome overfitting and consistent feature selection difficulties. It demonstrated that even small-sample studies may generate statistically meaningful predictions that generalize to unseen data.	Complex implementation of the suggested task. Also, there is a need for extensive data pre-processing.	ReliefF (76%) had the highest combined data accuracy, and SVM-RFE (66%) had the lowest performance.
(Leblanc et al., 2020)	2020	The study looked at the effect of missing value and feature imputation approaches on two previously reported autism detection classifiers that had been refined on standard-of-care equipment scoresheets and tested on evaluations of 140 kids YouTube videos.	ADT and LR	The experimental investigation demonstrates that by employing algorithmic-driven substitute queries to take the place of missing data and dynamically personalising feature imputation approaches to the YouTube video under consideration, UAR for both LR9 and ADTree7 may be increased.	The possibility of overfitting in the broad and adaptive feature substitution techniques that were incorporated into the pipeline is one of the primary issues. There is a greater chance of performance degradation for unusual rating vectors as well as rating kinds that are greatly dissimilar from the training set.	LR9 achieved 98.9% sensitivity and 89.4% specificity in subsequent independent studies, whereas ADTree7 attained, at worst, 89.9% sensitivity and 79.7% specificity.
(M. Wang et al., 2021)	2021	VFGM genes and IgA levels were utilised to identify ASD using ML. Studies on the sequencing of metagenome data from people with ASD (n = 43) and TD (n = 31) were carried out for over the genes in the virulence component repository.	RF	Use of ML approaches segregated ASD using levels of IgA levels and VFGM genes.	The sexes of ASD and TD children were not properly matched since the male-to-female ratio in ASD children reached 4:1 or higher, reflecting the ASD frequency in the general community.	The AUC for three new GBS genes was 0.833 (95% CI:0.74 0.33) whereas AUC for four non-GBS VF genes in the SRP182132 study was 0.929 (95% CI:0.87 0.24).

continues on following page

Table 1. Continued

Article	Year	Summary	Techniques Used	Advantages	Disadvantages	Precision/Accuracy
(Tartarisco et al., 2021)	2021	To enhance classification of autism screening and diagnosis tools, ML is being actively used in behavioural science. Similarly, in the study, ML was used to assess the precision and dependability of the Q-CHAT in differentiating younger individuals with autism from their counterparts using five different algorithms.	KNN, NB, RF, SVM, and LR.	The data from the findings verified the Q-CHAT's excellent performance and multicultural validity, and also supports the use of ML to build shorter, quicker versions of the tool while keeping its high accuracy in classification.	Before using the screener in clinical practice, despite the encouraging results, there are a few prerequisites that must be met, such as figuring out how characteristics are assessed (in what contexts, using what mediums and by which clinicians).	The findings have shown an average accuracy of about 90%, with SVM leading the pack with a 95% accuracy rate.
(Zhao et al., 2021)	2021	The potential of employing head movement characteristics to identify people with ASD was studied. Ten yes/ no questions were given to children with ASD and TD, and they were instructed to respond by nodding or shaking their heads. The range of head rotation and the amount of rotations per minute were measured and analyzed.	SVM, LDA, DT, RF, and ENS	The findings demonstrated that social movement of the head contained kinematic data that might be used to detect ASD.	Previous research indicates that the lower usage of head nodding/shaking in ASD patients may be detected exclusively in unintended settings. This shows that the research's task was inadequate to identify a difference in the frequency of head nodding or shaking between those with ASD and those with TD.	With just three features, SVM produced the greatest accuracy (81%) of any algorithm.
(Eslami et al., 2021)	2021	A DL model ASD-DiagNet was presented that has consistently good accuracy for distinguishing ASD brain imaging results from neuro-typical scans. It also included the first merging of classic ML and DL algorithms, allowing the researchers to extract ASD indicators from MRI records.	MLP, ASD-DiagNet, Auto-ASD-Network, and DL	The method based on ML and DL algorithms, will aid in quantifying existing psychiatric diagnoses and will improve the precision of diagnosis, prognosis, and therapy of difficult-to-assess mental diseases such as ADHD and ASD.	For appropriate implementation and suitable data pre-processing, the suggested integrated method necessitates a specific level of technical skill or understanding.	The OHSU dataset yielded the highest accuracy (82%) when utilising ASD-DiagNet.
(Liang et al., 2021)	2021	To obtain slow-changing biassed self-stimulatory behaviour characteristics, the study used temporal coherency between consecutive frames as free supervision and defined a global discriminative margin. To describe the suggested model, the Layer-wise Relevance Propagation (LRP) approach was used.	TCDN, KNN, SVM, LDA, FT, MT, and CT	The study revealed that acquiring knowledge from unlabeled films can improve visual comprehension in the area of self-stimulatory behavioural studies that relied on the collected set of experimental data.	It is restricted to tiny data collection, which prevented it from being generalised to data on a national or even broader scale on an international or worldwide scale.	The suggested TCDN model produced an accuracy of 98.3% that was substantially optimised.

continues on following page

123

Table 1. Continued

Article	Year	Summary	Techniques Used	Advantages	Disadvantages	Precision/Accuracy
(Sharif & Khan, 2022)	2022	An ML-based system was developed for automated identification of ASD utilising characteristics collected from test individuals' corpus callosum and intracranial brain volume. The framework not only achieved high recognition accuracy, but it significantly decreased the level of sophistication of the training ML model.	LDA, SVM, RF, MLP, and KNN	In the context of ASD screening, the study's investigation illustrated the prospective advantages of ML. The experiment also demonstrated how ML algorithms may be utilised with structural MRI data to recognise individuals with ASD automatically.	Predictions utilising the suggested framework need a significant amount of data pre-processing, in addition to the fact that accuracy is only 60%.	For LDA, SVM, RF, MLP, and KNN, the framework obtained average accuracy of 56.21%, 51.34%, 54.61%, 56.26%, and 52.16%, respectively.
(Alsuliman & Al-Baity, 2022)	2022	Different optimised methods were compared for selecting features using bio-inspired algorithms over various kinds of data to select a model with greater precision. Enhanced the classification process of ASD using a comparison of 16 diverse optimised ML models.	GWOSVM, GWO-NB, GWO-KNN, FPA-KNN, GWO-DT, FPA-NB, FPA-SVM, FPA-DT, BA-NB, BA-SVM, BA-KNN, BA-DT, ABC-NB, ABC-DT, ABV-KNN, and ABC-SVM	The suggested models have shown promising efficacy in terms of ASD prediction accuracy, particularly when the GE dataset was used. As a result, the study's findings imply a broad possibility for acceptance into ordinary practice.	Various ML algorithms were employed for ASD identification; however, a few of them are unduly laborious and susceptible to error by humans, and therefore by the time the disease is discovered, the patient may already be in a difficult-to-manage stage of ASD.	When tested separately, GWO-SVM, using GE and PBC data sets, had the best accuracy (99.34%, and 99.66% respectively).
(M. Alcañiz et al., 2022)	2022	Differentiated between autistic and normally developing children by employing visual attention behaviours as a measure of sensitivity to and retrieval of socially significant information in a virtual world using an eye-tracking paradigm.	SVM, RF, NB, XGBoost, and KNN	Through eye-tracking paradigms, analysed virtual social and nonsocial visual perception and comprehension in TD toddlers in contrast to those with autism as an indicator of sensitivity to, and extraction of, socially significant information, allowing for a rapid diagnosis.	Due to the small sample size, the large number of characteristics, and the models' lack of application to an isolated sample becomes the limitation.	Complete dataset using SVM with 9 features (accuracy = 0.86 +/- 0.1), compared to complete dataset using KNN with 7 significant features (accuracy = 0.77 +/- 0.06).
(Elshoky et al., 2022)	2022	A model was developed to recognise autism from face photos utilising several classical, DL, and AutoML approaches. The findings clearly suggest that AutoML is a cutting-edge way for implementing ML techniques while utilising time as a resource.	DNN, Transfer Learning, CNN, AutoML, DT, RF, GBM, SVM, LR and KNN	Greater ML model performance may be obtained with optimizations and hyperparameters utilizing AutoML, saving the effort and time necessary for feature engineering.	Although AutoML attained the highest level of accuracy, it still has the same model interpretability issue as DL "Black-Box" models.	VGG-16 offered the best efficiency, having test accuracy of 89% at 10 Epoch along-with ET clocking at 72.64% in 4.25 seconds.

continues on following page

Table 1. Continued

Article	Year	Summary	Techniques Used	Advantages	Disadvantages	Precision/Accuracy
(Yang et al., 2022)	2022	A thorough and useful evaluation of ASD classification based on data from the ABIDE repository by using traditional ML and DL algorithms is provided. In order to discriminate between individuals with ASD and those with TD, the study looked at several brain networks and evaluated their functional connectivity.	LR, LSVM, KSVM, and DNN	BASC has the highest predictive value for ASD categorization, whereas the correlation metric is a particularly stable option amongst the models studied.	Through experimental research, it may be inferred that classical ML had already produced the best results possible and that there were no practical limits to how much more could be done to boost its accuracy, sensitivity, and specificity.	The functional atlas BASC444 and RBF kernel SVM, along with the correlation measure, were used to generate the experimental findings. The accuracy was 69.43% and the equivalent specificity was 73.61%.
(H. Wang et al., 2022)	2022	A novel and dynamic ASD diagnostic tool was created which allowed parents and healthcare providers to act on early concerns. To fulfil these objectives, a few-shot learning system which integrates a Siamese network along with a Wide and Deep network to acquire both linear and non-linear connections from tiny ASD datasets was devised.	ASDPred, SNN, WDM, KNN, and ANN	A diagnostic tool "ASDPred" integrated within a web-based system was developed to enable ASD diagnosis using the defined model, thereby accomplishing the stated purpose.	Complex initial design and deployment of the platform for customised adoption by individual users or corporations.	Using ASDPred, the best outcome was obtained with an F1-score of 0.97 and a specificity of 0.98.
(Kim et al., 2022)	2022	ML classifiers were used to analyse features from T1-weighted MRI and DTI data from 58 children with ASD (ages 3-6 years) and 48 TDC. The experimental findings show that the proposed ML-based MRI processing system could distinguish low-functioning ASD kids in preschool from TDCs.	SVM, LR, RF, AdaBoost, and MLP	When T1w MRI and DTI data were integrated, classification accuracy improved, as predicted. The experimental findings highlight the possible benefits of multidimensional scanning for identifying LFA pre-schoolers.	As far as the authors are aware, this was the first research to use ML approaches to separate kids with LFA from age-matched TDCs using both T1w and DTI characteristics, which results in an absence of reference for comparability.	RF classifier produced the best performance numbers, with 88.8% accuracy and 93.0% sensitivity.
(Wawer & Chojnicka, 2022)	2022	DNNs were used for diagnosing ASD from textual utterances, especially narrations provided by people with ASD. This was accomplished by a thorough analysis of two text encoders, ELMo and USE, as well as three categorization methods.	XGBoost, SVM, and DenseNN	The negative predictive values, specificities, positive predictive values, sensitivities, and values of the ELMo and USE text encoders were all very promising. The findings show that page-level embeddings are highly beneficial for representing utterances in the ADOS-2 picture book assignment.	The main drawback was the relatively small number of participants, large age range, and imperfect matching of participants' IQ scores. Because of this, the study was unable to separate the participants into subcategories according to age, sex, or IQ level.	Using ELMo with SVM on a single embedding vector, the maximum sensitivity was attained (0.76), along with a specificity of 0.60.

continues on following page

Table 1. Continued

Article	Year	Summary	Techniques Used	Advantages	Disadvantages	Precision/Accuracy
(Esqueda-Elizondo et al., 2022)	2022	Attention is a cognitive function that allows us to respond to relevant inputs in a timely manner. The study proposed a mechanism for measuring attention on a 13-year-old kid with ASD using EEG data. The EEG data were collected using an Epoc+ Brain-Computer Interface (BCI) while constructing different learning exercises on the Emotiv Pro platform.	NB, SGD, DT, SVM-RBF, KNN, MLPNN, RF, and ET	It provided quantitative information regarding the efficiency of ML models when an ASD user undertakes didactic/learning activities, the latter with the goal of supporting the teacher's or therapist's view.	A limited scope of generalisation because it was a case study on a single participant who generated all of the processing data for the suggested model's implementation.	Best performance was provided by the MLP-NN, which had an AUC of 0.9299.
(Mellema et al., 2022)	2022	Evaluated and compared the effectiveness of 12 most prominent and powerful ML models. With the help of 15 different arrangements of fMRI and sMRI characteristics, each of the evaluated model was trained and optimised separately. The models discovered repeatable potential biomarkers for the detection of ASD as well as new cerebellar biomarkers.	NB, RF, ERT, AdaBoost, GB, SVM, LassoR, RidgeR, Dense-FNN, LSTM-RNN, and BrainNet CNN	It identified and quantified consensus neuroimaging properties that were reproducible across processing methodologies, models, and a large number of reasonably large datasets. In the neuroimage processing community, improved repeatability and trust in experimental outcomes is critical.	The work has the opportunity to be improved upon even if it considerably improves the fabrication of ML tools for automated accurate ASD diagnosis. The IMPAC dataset only comprises binary diagnoses, which means that the model depends on the input dataset.	The DFNN and LSTM algorithms performed well, with highest AUROC of 80.4% and 79.0%, respectively.
(Wolff et al., 2022)	2022	The main objective of the research was to determine for the event for which of the components of the clinical diagnostic tests for ASD (ADI-R, ADOS) would most successfully separate across four groups of individuals assigned to specialised ASD clinics.	SVM	Detecting ASD in those with suspected signs of the illness, including those with concurrent ADHD, is doable with much fewer items than the original ADOS/2 and ADI-R algorithms while maintaining reasonably good diagnostic accuracy.	It suggested ASD and ADHD are distinct mental health problems, both seem to be closely associated. In fact, evidence reveals that ASD and ADHD diagnoses commonly co-occur. A significant restriction is a lack of theoretical understanding in this sector.	The ASD ADOS/2 total cut-offs were satisfactory by 76% of the group with ASD and 68% of the group with ASD and ADHD.
(Betts et al., 2023)	2023	A unique approach was offered to the problem of ASD identification by merging ML with infant and maternal health administrative information to build a model for predicting autistic disorder in the population as a whole.	LR with elastic net regularization and GBTs	Combining ML with routinely gathered administrative data, with greater refinement and higher accuracy than the suggested technique, might play an essential part in the early identification of autistic problems.	Since earlier attempts to predict autism have typically relied on at-risk samples (rather than the general population) that were purposefully recruited and resource-intensive measurements, it is challenging to compare the performance of the proposed model with that of earlier attempts.	For Verification AUC-ROC, the metrics were GBT=0.73 (0.70, 0.76) and ENR-LR=0.73 (0.70, 0.76).

continues on following page

Table 1. Continued

Article	Year	Summary	Techniques Used	Advantages	Disadvantages	Precision/Accuracy
(Di Giovanni et al., 2023)	2023	An advanced ML approach was proposed based on the analysis of clusters on genotypical/phenotypical embedding spaces to uncover biological processes. It may function as pathophysiological substrates for ASD. This was employed for assessment based on the VariCarta database.	UMAP, HDBSCAN Clustering, Agglomerative Clustering, DBSCAN, and K-Means	The VariCarta database was utilised to identify genetic categories of individuals with ASD. A ML technique that utilized a clustering analysis on an amended embedding space was used. The results produced several clusters of ASD-associated genes and retrieved the set of related genes from each cluster.	The main drawback is the lack of data on a sample of persons without ASD in VariCarta, which prevented the same research from being done on them. Due to this constraint, it is impossible to differentiate among "de novo" mutations versus those that were present in the biological parents' genomes.	The experimental findings suggest that two gene clusters—Clusters 2 and 7—have a higher clinical significance than the other nine recovered gene clusters.
(Voinsky et al., 2023)	2023	The absence of solid biomarkers makes ASD diagnosis a time-consuming process. A variety of ML-generated models based on information about RNA gene expression were offered by the study as prospective ASD diagnostic tools.	ET, and RF	The presented ML-generated tools might be seen as a proof-of-concept inquiry and a starting point for future research on transcriptomics-based diagnosis of ASD.	The main weaknesses are its limited sample size and a possibility for model overfitting because there are no separate validation cohorts.	The RF classifier produced the maximum accuracy for predictors #3 and #5 (accuracy = 82.178%).
(A. Singh et al., 2023)	2023	The study revealed a low-cost, socially built robot named 'Tinku,' which was created to help teach special needs youngsters. It is low-cost yet feature-rich, with capabilities such as offline voice processing and computer vision enabling nonverbal communication, conveying emotions in a humanistic manner, and so on.	Tiny-YOLO, TF-lite, Faster-RCNN, and SSD	The robotic framework for assisting clinical trials for ASD rehabilitation was effectively evaluated in the experimental investigation. As a result, the objective problem of high costs associated with establishing advanced configurations such as a robotic device for widespread use was overcome.	The suggested model may be improved by putting it to the test on various test situations and conducting comprehensive clinical trials. This strategy will be more reliable to utilise in the case of ASD due to the psychological component of testing.	While Tiny-YOLO's metrics were 23% at 0.7, TF-Lite (SSD Mobilenet) provided a mAP of 82% at 2.5 FPS detection speed.

The research works such as the approach presented in (Eslami et al., 2021; Sharif & Khan, 2022) take a standard DL or a hybrid ML-DL augmented approach for diagnosis or prediction of ASD in any category of individuals on various types of processed MRI data. The said approaches work by extraction of relevant data from the imaging data by utilizing image processing techniques using a purely DL or a hybrid ML-DL approach. The researchers have a broad scope of interest in this sub-domain even though the accuracy scores of the experimental studies are borderline. Thus, the primary target of the ML/DL researchers should be to optimize the data processing algorithms for better predictability.

The approach undertaken by researchers for the same objective like in studies conducted in (Alcaniz Raya et al., 2020; Vabalas et al., 2020) augments the concept of VR in the mix. The motion sensitive depth sensing cameras track the orientation of the individual to generate image data that is further refined by DL algorithms and is then fed into ML algorithms for classification results. This type of research work draws a comprehensive comparison between the body movements of a TDC and that of an individual suffering from ASD. The classification accuracy scores in studies utilizing this particular approach show optimistic results with high metrics. A similar approach is followed in the study where the text utterance in response to prompt or external stimuli is analysed through ML algorithms (Alcaniz Raya et al., 2020) for a through comparison which is then used for classification between TDC and ASD individuals. This particular study can be used for the treatment purposes as well with chat-bot or virtual personal assistant-like approach.

The most commonly used method of diagnosing the ASD is utilized in studies as in (Tartarisco et al., 2021; H. Wang et al., 2022). The questionnaires are provided to the individuals for screening purposes which can not only be used for classification between TDC and ASD, but can also gauge the severity of the symptoms which aid in sub-categorization. The application of ML algorithms on this standard test for diagnosis of autism can also be used to segregate those suffering from schizophrenia rather than autism. The reason for the requirement of the said contrast is because the many symptoms of either the diseases or conditions are not unique and overlap each other in many cases. Thus, for proper intervention and treatment; the researchers in their future endeavours should work on the details for finer contrast studies for effective categorization.

Other than the predicting or diagnosis studies, the works like the one conducted in (A. Singh et al., 2023) employs the ML/DL frameworks for creating a personal assistant type of bot which can have either virtual or physical presence or both. These types of studies have the intervention and treatment objective as their target which may be suited for helping the individual himself or the family members and care-givers for that matter. Since a chat-bot may help like a personal assistant or a nanny for younger individuals, a physically present robotic construct is more ideal for older individuals. Thus, the open challenge in this particular scenario is the development of a unique product, construct, or application that is compatible for use by individuals of all ages and severities of ASD.

Lastly, the research conducted in studies like (Yang et al., 2022; Yassin et al., 2020) present the co-joint presence of multiple disorders that may latch themselves on individuals suffering for some categories of ASD. The most common types of these "side-symptoms" include OCD, ADHD, etc. which require separate interventional treatments as they might have a degrading effect on the individuals' health. The concurrent ailments might make it difficult for an individual to undergo a particular set of treatments which then requires appropriate measures for the same. This domain required the researchers to fine tune the contrasting techniques along with identification of isolated symptoms for easy identification and categorization.

In summary, the open challenges of the reviewed studies reveal a diverse domain of various tasks that are required to be performed for fine-tuning of the ML/DL framework that is being utilized in the said study. The broadest open challenge of all, along-with being the toughest one is the integration of multiple models and approaches for diverse objectives to perform in a unison, i.e., the creation of a unified framework. The said framework should be a one-stop total all-in-one solution for ASD individuals or their family members and healthcare professionals or care-givers. This would allow the suffering individual to be at ease to the maximum degree of cushion the framework would provide.

4. CONCLUSION AND FUTURE SCOPE

The presented review of the diverse technological domain oriented studies for tackling the challenge of ASD has been analyzed in great detail in this chapter. ASD will remain a very challenging and insightful area or sub-domain of research as it harbors the potential of integration of multiple technological and pure knowledge-based domains. The challenges that come along-with this particular ailment spans across technical, social, economic, and cultural values. This is primarily due to the fact that many cultures consider neuro-ailments and its subject itself as a societal taboo which further degrades the life of those affected. In contrast, not all but many western cultures are a bit more broad-minded in this aspect and hence the balance of research in this particular domain tilts towards the west.

The scope of utilization of ML and DL frameworks with augmentation of few other technologies is an open-ended problem statement which provides a broad horizon for the conduction of research in this domain. The studies reviewed contained a diverse field of interest yet were similar in the objective--prediction or diagnosing of ASD. The research works presented multiple techniques for the same objective along with a few steps further like isolating the common features or parameters from the data.

These studies collectively establish a foundation of correlations between clinical, and socio-specific features or parameters which can help in early diagnosis for effective intervention and treatment. Some of these studies also dived into gene-level identification of such specifics which have a broad scope of improvement using ML/DL implementations for tackling the challenge of autism. Finally, a few of the studies were also conducted for aiding the treatment or helping the affected individuals or the family members and health professionals for a better life quality of those who are already fighting this condition. In summary, the work on the subject of autism or any neurological condition for that matters spans across multiple domains and sub-domains in terms of applications, and usage.

The future scope will be to implement the presented novel or hybrid approach on a larger, and more generalized crowd for further fine-tuning and error-reduction. This issue was almost present in each study as the amount of data samples to be worked upon were very limited. Thus, the researchers can augment or combine multiple studies and collaborate on creating a unified system that can help each individual affected in unison, i.e., a unified system that can diagnose, intervene, and offer treatment to the suffering individual directly or by aiding the health care-givers, professional and family members. Such a work could also be implemented virtually through interactive chat-bots or physically using robotic apparatus or constructs.

REFERENCES

Abbas, H., Garberson, F., Glover, E., & Wall, D. P. (2018). Machine learning approach for early detection of autism by combining questionnaire and home video screening. *Journal of the American Medical Informatics Association : JAMIA*, *25*(8), 1000–1007. doi:10.1093/jamia/ocy039 PMID:29741630

Akter, T., Satu, M. S., Khan, M. I., Ali, M. H., Uddin, S., Lio, P., Quinn, J. M. W., & Moni, M. A. (2019). Machine learning-based models for early stage detection of autism spectrum disorders. *IEEE Access : Practical Innovations, Open Solutions*, *7*, 166509–166527. doi:10.1109/ACCESS.2019.2952609

Alcañiz, M., Chicchi-Giglioli, I. A., Carrasco-Ribelles, L. A., Marín-Morales, J., Minissi, M. E., Teruel-García, G., Sirera, M., & Abad, L. (2022). Eye gaze as a biomarker in the recognition of autism spectrum disorder using virtual reality and machine learning: A proof of concept for diagnosis. *Autism Research*, *15*(1), 131–145. doi:10.1002/aur.2636 PMID:34811930

Alcañiz, M. L., Olmos-Raya, E., & Abad, L. (2019). Uso de entornos virtuales para trastornos del neurodesarrollo: una revisión del estado del arte y agenda futura. *Medicina (Buenos Aires)*, *79*(1), 77–81.

Alcañiz Raya, M., Chicchi Giglioli, I. A., Marín-Morales, J., Higuera-Trujillo, J. L., Olmos, E., Minissi, M. E., Teruel Garcia, G., Sirera, M., & Abad, L. (2020). Application of supervised machine learning for behavioral biomarkers of autism spectrum disorder based on electrodermal activity and virtual reality. *Frontiers in Human Neuroscience*, *14*, 90. doi:10.3389/fnhum.2020.00090 PMID:32317949

Alcaniz Raya, M., Marín-Morales, J., Minissi, M. E., Teruel Garcia, G., Abad, L., & Chicchi Giglioli, I. A. (2020). Machine learning and virtual reality on body movements' behaviors to classify children with autism spectrum disorder. *Journal of Clinical Medicine*, *9*(5), 1260. doi:10.3390/jcm9051260 PMID:32357517

Alsuliman, M., & Al-Baity, H. H. (2022). Efficient Diagnosis of Autism with Optimized Machine Learning Models: An Experimental Analysis on Genetic and Personal Characteristic Datasets. *Applied Sciences (Basel, Switzerland)*, *12*(8), 3812. doi:10.3390/app12083812

Arya, R., Kumar, A., & Bhushan, M. (2021). Affect Recognition using Brain Signals: A Survey. In V. Singh, V. K. Asari, S. Kumar, & R. B. Patel (Eds.), *Computational Methods and Data Engineering* (pp. 529–552). Springer Singapore. doi:10.1007/978-981-15-7907-3_40

Arya, R., Kumar, A., Bhushan, M., & Samant, P. (2022). Big five personality traits prediction using brain signals. [IJFSA]. *International Journal of Fuzzy System Applications*, *11*(2), 1–10. doi:10.4018/IJFSA.296596

Betts, K. S., Chai, K., Kisely, S., & Alati, R. (2023). Development and validation of a machine learning-based tool to predict autism among children. *Autism Research*, *16*(5), 941–952. doi:10.1002/aur.2912 PMID:36899450

Biocca, F., Harms, C., & Gregg, J. (2001). *The networked minds measure of social presence: Pilot test of the factor structure and concurrent validity. 4th Annual International Workshop on Presence*, Philadelphia, PA.

Bowman, D. A., Gabbard, J. L., & Hix, D. (2002). A survey of usability evaluation in virtual environments: Classification and comparison of methods. *Presence (Cambridge, Mass.)*, *11*(4), 404–424. doi:10.1162/105474602760204309

Cipresso, P., Giglioli, I. A. C., Raya, M. A., & Riva, G. (2018). The past, present, and future of virtual and augmented reality research: A network and cluster analysis of the literature. *Frontiers in Psychology*, *9*, 2086. doi:10.3389/fpsyg.2018.02086 PMID:30459681

Cummings, J. J., & Bailenson, J. N. (2016). How immersive is enough? A meta-analysis of the effect of immersive technology on user presence. *Media Psychology*, *19*(2), 272–309. doi:10.1080/1521326 9.2015.1015740

Dawson, G., Jones, E. J. H., Merkle, K., Venema, K., Lowy, R., Faja, S., Kamara, D., Murias, M., Greenson, J., Winter, J., Smith, M., Rogers, S. J., & Webb, S. J. (2012). Early behavioral intervention is associated with normalized brain activity in young children with autism. *Journal of the American Academy of Child and Adolescent Psychiatry*, *51*(11), 1150–1159. doi:10.1016/j.jaac.2012.08.018 PMID:23101741

Di Giovanni, D., Enea, R., Di Micco, V., Benvenuto, A., Curatolo, P., & Emberti Gialloreti, L. (2023). Using Machine Learning to Explore Shared Genetic Pathways and Possible Endophenotypes in Autism Spectrum Disorder. *Genes*, *14*(2), 313. doi:10.3390/genes14020313 PMID:36833240

Di Martino, A., Yan, C.-G., Li, Q., Denio, E., Castellanos, F. X., Alaerts, K., Anderson, J. S., Assaf, M., Bookheimer, S. Y., Dapretto, M., Deen, B., Delmonte, S., Dinstein, I., Ertl-Wagner, B., Fair, D. A., Gallagher, L., Kennedy, D. P., Keown, C. L., Keysers, C., & Milham, M. P. (2014). The autism brain imaging data exchange: Towards a large-scale evaluation of the intrinsic brain architecture in autism. *Molecular Psychiatry*, *19*(6), 659–667. doi:10.1038/mp.2013.78 PMID:23774715

Duda, M., Kosmicki, J. A., & Wall, D. P. (2014). Testing the accuracy of an observation-based classifier for rapid detection of autism risk. *Translational Psychiatry*, *4*(8), e424–e424. doi:10.1038/tp.2014.65 PMID:25116834

Elshoky, B. R. G., Younis, E. M. G., Ali, A. A., & Ibrahim, O. A. S. (2022). Comparing automated and non-automated machine learning for autism spectrum disorders classification using facial images. *ETRI Journal*, *44*(4), 613–623. doi:10.4218/etrij.2021-0097

Eslami, T., Raiker, J. S., & Saeed, F. (2021). Explainable and scalable machine learning algorithms for detection of autism spectrum disorder using fMRI data. In *Neural engineering techniques for autism spectrum disorder* (pp. 39–54). Elsevier. doi:10.1016/B978-0-12-822822-7.00004-1

Esqueda-Elizondo, J. J., Juárez-Ramírez, R., López-Bonilla, O. R., García-Guerrero, E. E., Galindo-Aldana, G. M., Jiménez-Beristáin, L., Serrano-Trujillo, A., Tlelo-Cuautle, E., & Inzunza-González, E. (2022). Attention measurement of an autism spectrum disorder user using EEG signals: A case study. *Mathematical & Computational Applications*, *27*(2), 21. doi:10.3390/mca27020021

Fenikilé, T. S., Ellerbeck, K., Filippi, M. K., & Daley, C. M. (2015). Barriers to autism screening in family medicine practice: A qualitative study. *Primary Health Care Research and Development*, *16*(4), 356–366. doi:10.1017/S1463423614000449 PMID:25367194

Guazzaroni, G. (2018). *Virtual and augmented reality in mental health treatment.* IGI Global.

Guthrie, W., Wallis, K., Bennett, A., Brooks, E., Dudley, J., Gerdes, M., Pandey, J., Levy, S. E., Schultz, R. T., & Miller, J. S. (2019). Accuracy of autism screening in a large pediatric network. *Pediatrics, 144*(4), e20183963. doi:10.1542/peds.2018-3963 PMID:31562252

Holloway, R., Fuchs, H., & Robinett, W. (1992). Virtual-worlds research at the University of North Carolina at Chapel Hill as of February 1992. *Visual Computing: Integrating Computer Graphics with Computer Vision*, 109–128.

Hossain, M. A., Islam, S. M. S., Quinn, J. M. W., Huq, F., & Moni, M. A. (2019). Machine learning and bioinformatics models to identify gene expression patterns of ovarian cancer associated with disease progression and mortality. *Journal of Biomedical Informatics, 100*, 103313. doi:10.1016/j.jbi.2019.103313 PMID:31655274

HowladerK. C.SatuM. S.BaruaA.MoniM. A. (2018). Mining significant features of diabetes mellitus applying decision trees: A case study in bangladesh. BioRxiv, 481994. doi:10.1101/481994

Hyman, S. L., Levy, S. E., Myers, S. M., Kuo, D. Z., Apkon, S., Davidson, L. F., Ellerbeck, K. A., Foster, J. E. A., Noritz, G. H., Leppert, M. O., Saunders, B. S., Stille, C., Yin, L., Weitzman, C. C., Childers, D. O. Jr, Levine, J. M., Peralta-Carcelen, A. M., Poon, J. K., Smith, P. J., & Bridgemohan, C. (2020). Identification, evaluation, and management of children with autism spectrum disorder. *Pediatrics, 145*(1), e20193447. doi:10.1542/peds.2019-3447

Kim, J. I., Bang, S., Yang, J.-J., Kwon, H., Jang, S., Roh, S., Kim, S. H., Kim, M. J., Lee, H. J., & Lee, J.-M. (2022). Classification of preschoolers with low-functioning autism spectrum disorder using multimodal MRI data. *Journal of Autism and Developmental Disorders*, 1–13. PMID:34984638

Knyazev, G. G., Slobodskaya, H. R., & Wilson, G. D. (2004). *Personality and brain oscillations in the developmental perspective.*

Lai, M., Lee, J., Chiu, S., Charm, J., So, W. Y., Yuen, F. P., Kwok, C., Tsoi, J., Lin, Y., & Zee, B. (2020). A machine learning approach for retinal images analysis as an objective screening method for children with autism spectrum disorder. *EClinicalMedicine, 28*, 100588. doi:10.1016/j.eclinm.2020.100588 PMID:33294809

Leblanc, E., Washington, P., Varma, M., Dunlap, K., Penev, Y., Kline, A., & Wall, D. P. (2020). Feature replacement methods enable reliable home video analysis for machine learning detection of autism. *Scientific Reports, 10*(1), 1–11. doi:10.1038/s41598-020-76874-w PMID:33277527

LeDoux, J. E., & Pine, D. S. (2016). Using neuroscience to help understand fear and anxiety: A two-system framework. *The American Journal of Psychiatry, 173*(11), 1083–1093. doi:10.1176/appi.ajp.2016.16030353 PMID:27609244

Liang, S., Sabri, A. Q. M., Alnajjar, F., & Loo, C. K. (2021). Autism spectrum self-stimulatory behaviors classification using explainable temporal coherency deep features and SVM classifier. *IEEE Access : Practical Innovations, Open Solutions, 9*, 34264–34275. doi:10.1109/ACCESS.2021.3061455

Lorenzo, G., Lledó, A., Arráez-Vera, G., & Lorenzo-Lledó, A. (2019). The application of immersive virtual reality for students with ASD: A review between 1990–2017. *Education and Information Technologies, 24*(1), 127–151. doi:10.1007/s10639-018-9766-7

Mastrovito, D., Hanson, C., & Hanson, S. J. (2018). Differences in atypical resting-state effective connectivity distinguish autism from schizophrenia. *NeuroImage. Clinical*, *18*, 367–376. doi:10.1016/j.nicl.2018.01.014 PMID:29487793

Mellema, C. J., Nguyen, K. P., Treacher, A., & Montillo, A. (2022). Reproducible neuroimaging features for diagnosis of autism spectrum disorder with machine learning. *Scientific Reports*, *12*(1), 3057. doi:10.1038/s41598-022-06459-2 PMID:35197468

Monteiro, S. A., Dempsey, J., Berry, L. N., Voigt, R. G., & Goin-Kochel, R. P. (2019). Screening and referral practices for autism spectrum disorder in primary pediatric care. *Pediatrics*, *144*(4), e20183326. doi:10.1542/peds.2018-3326 PMID:31515298

Nickel, P., & Nachreiner, F. (2003). Sensitivity and diagnosticity of the 0.1-Hz component of heart rate variability as an indicator of mental workload. *Human Factors*, *45*(4), 575–590. doi:10.1518/hfes.45.4.575.27094 PMID:15055455

Nikula, R. (1991). Psychological correlates of nonspecific skin conductance responses. *Psychophysiology*, *28*(1), 86–90. doi:10.1111/j.1469-8986.1991.tb03392.x PMID:1886966

Nosek, B. A., Hawkins, C. B., & Frazier, R. S. (2011). Implicit social cognition: From measures to mechanisms. *Trends in Cognitive Sciences*, *15*(4), 152–159. doi:10.1016/j.tics.2011.01.005 PMID:21376657

Omar, K. S., Mondal, P., Khan, N. S., Rizvi, M. R. K., & Islam, M. N. (2019). A machine learning approach to predict autism spectrum disorder. *2019 International Conference on Electrical, Computer and Communication Engineering (ECCE)*, (pp. 1–6). IEEE. 10.1109/ECACE.2019.8679454

Parsons, S., Mitchell, P., & Leonard, A. (2004). The use and understanding of virtual environments by adolescents with autistic spectrum disorders. *Journal of Autism and Developmental Disorders*, *34*(4), 449–466. doi:10.1023/B:JADD.0000037421.98517.8d PMID:15449520

Parsons, T. D. (2011). Neuropsychological assessment using virtual environments: enhanced assessment technology for improved ecological validity. *Advanced Computational Intelligence Paradigms in Healthcare 6. Virtual Reality in Psychotherapy, Rehabilitation, and Assessment*, 271–289.

Parsons, T. D., Rizzo, A. A., Rogers, S., & York, P. (2009). Virtual reality in paediatric rehabilitation: A review. *Developmental Neurorehabilitation*, *12*(4), 224–238. doi:10.1080/17518420902991719 PMID:19842822

Pastorelli, E., & Herrmann, H. (2013). A small-scale, low-budget semi-immersive virtual environment for scientific visualization and research. *Procedia Computer Science*, *25*, 14–22. doi:10.1016/j.procs.2013.11.003

Pathan, S., Bhushan, M., & Bai, A. (2020). A study on health care using data mining techniques. *Journal of Critical Reviews*, *7*(19), 7877–7890.

Peral, J., Gil, D., Rotbei, S., Amador, S., Guerrero, M., & Moradi, H. (2020). A machine learning and integration based architecture for cognitive disorder detection used for early autism screening. *Electronics (Basel)*, *9*(3), 516. doi:10.3390/electronics9030516

Raj, S., & Masood, S. (2020). Analysis and detection of autism spectrum disorder using machine learning techniques. *Procedia Computer Science*, *167*, 994–1004. doi:10.1016/j.procs.2020.03.399

Rhoades, R. A., Scarpa, A., & Salley, B. (2007). The importance of physician knowledge of autism spectrum disorder: Results of a parent survey. *BMC Pediatrics*, *7*(1), 1–10. doi:10.1186/1471-2431-7-37 PMID:18021459

Satu, M. S., Sathi, F. F., Arifen, M. S., Ali, M. H., & Moni, M. A. (2019). Early detection of autism by extracting features: a case study in Bangladesh. *2019 International Conference on Robotics, Electrical and Signal Processing Techniques (ICREST)*, (pp. 400–405). IEEE. 10.1109/ICREST.2019.8644357

Self, T. L., Parham, D. F., & Rajagopalan, J. (2015). Autism spectrum disorder early screening practices: A survey of physicians. *Communication Disorders Quarterly*, *36*(4), 195–207. doi:10.1177/1525740114560060

Sharif, H., & Khan, R. A. (2022). A novel machine learning based framework for detection of autism spectrum disorder (ASD). *Applied Artificial Intelligence*, *36*(1), 2004655. doi:10.1080/08839514.2021.2004655

Singh, A., Raj, K., Kumar, T., Verma, S., & Roy, A. M. (2023). Deep learning-based cost-effective and responsive robot for autism treatment. *Drones (Basel)*, *7*(2), 81. doi:10.3390/drones7020081

Singh, V. J., Bhushan, M., Kumar, V., & Bansal, K. L. (2015). Optimization of segment size assuring application perceived QoS in healthcare. *Proceedings of the World Congress on Engineering, 1*, (pp. 1–3). IEEE.

Skalski, P., & Tamborini, R. (2007). The role of social presence in interactive agent-based persuasion. *Media Psychology*, *10*(3), 385–413. doi:10.1080/15213260701533102

Slater, M. (2009). Place illusion and plausibility can lead to realistic behaviour in immersive virtual environments. *Philosophical Transactions of the Royal Society of London. Series B, Biological Sciences*, *364*(1535), 3549–3557. doi:10.1098/rstb.2009.0138 PMID:19884149

Tartarisco, G., Cicceri, G., Di Pietro, D., Leonardi, E., Aiello, S., Marino, F., Chiarotti, F., Gagliano, A., Arduino, G. M., Apicella, F., Muratori, F., Bruneo, D., Allison, C., Cohen, S. B., Vagni, D., Pioggia, G., & Ruta, L. (2021). Use of machine learning to investigate the quantitative checklist for autism in toddlers (Q-CHAT) towards early autism screening. *Diagnostics (Basel)*, *11*(3), 574. doi:10.3390/diagnostics11030574 PMID:33810146

Thabtah, F. (2017). Autism spectrum disorder screening: machine learning adaptation and DSM-5 fulfillment. *Proceedings of the 1st International Conference on Medical and Health Informatics 2017*, (pp. 1–6). IEEE. 10.1145/3107514.3107515

Thabtah, F. (2019). Machine learning in autistic spectrum disorder behavioral research: A review and ways forward. *Informatics for Health & Social Care*, *44*(3), 278–297. doi:10.1080/17538157.2017.1399132 PMID:29436887

Thabtah, F., Kamalov, F., & Rajab, K. (2018). A new computational intelligence approach to detect autistic features for autism screening. *International Journal of Medical Informatics*, *117*, 112–124. doi:10.1016/j.ijmedinf.2018.06.009 PMID:30032959

Thabtah, F., & Peebles, D. (2020). A new machine learning model based on induction of rules for autism detection. *Health Informatics Journal, 26*(1), 264–286. doi:10.1177/1460458218824711 PMID:30693818

Vabalas, A., Gowen, E., Poliakoff, E., & Casson, A. J. (2020). Applying machine learning to kinematic and eye movement features of a movement imitation task to predict autism diagnosis. *Scientific Reports, 10*(1), 1–13. doi:10.1038/s41598-020-65384-4 PMID:32433501

van't Hof, M., Tisseur, C., van Berckelear-Onnes, I., van Nieuwenhuyzen, A., Daniels, A. M., Deen, M., Hoek, H. W., & Ester, W. A. (2021). Age at autism spectrum disorder diagnosis: A systematic review and meta-analysis from 2012 to 2019. *Autism, 25*(4), 862–873. doi:10.1177/1362361320971107 PMID:33213190

Voinsky, I., Fridland, O. Y., Aran, A., Frye, R. E., & Gurwitz, D. (2023). Machine Learning-Based Blood RNA Signature for Diagnosis of Autism Spectrum Disorder. *International Journal of Molecular Sciences, 24*(3), 2082. doi:10.3390/ijms24032082 PMID:36768401

Wallace, S., Parsons, S., Westbury, A., White, K., White, K., & Bailey, A. (2010). Sense of presence and atypical social judgments in immersive virtual environments: Responses of adolescents with Autism Spectrum Disorders. *Autism, 14*(3), 199–213. doi:10.1177/1362361310363283 PMID:20484000

Wang, C., Xiao, Z., Wang, B., & Wu, J. (2019). Identification of autism based on SVM-RFE and stacked sparse auto-encoder. *IEEE Access : Practical Innovations, Open Solutions, 7*, 118030–118036. doi:10.1109/ACCESS.2019.2936639

Wang, H., Chi, L., & Zhao, Z. (2022). ASDPred: An End-to-End Autism Screening Framework Using Few-Shot Learning. *Proceedings of the 31st ACM International Conference on Information & Knowledge Management*, (pp. 5004–5008). ACM. 10.1145/3511808.3557210

Wang, M., Doenyas, C., Wan, J., Zeng, S., Cai, C., Zhou, J., Liu, Y., Yin, Z., & Zhou, W. (2021). Virulence factor-related gut microbiota genes and immunoglobulin A levels as novel markers for machine learning-based classification of autism spectrum disorder. *Computational and Structural Biotechnology Journal, 19*, 545–554. doi:10.1016/j.csbj.2020.12.012 PMID:33510860

Wawer, A., & Chojnicka, I. (2022). Detecting autism from picture book narratives using deep neural utterance embeddings. *International Journal of Language & Communication Disorders, 57*(5), 948–962. doi:10.1111/1460-6984.12731 PMID:35555933

Wolff, N., Kohls, G., Mack, J. T., Vahid, A., Elster, E. M., Stroth, S., Poustka, L., Kuepper, C., Roepke, S., Kamp-Becker, I., & Roessner, V. (2022). A data driven machine learning approach to differentiate between autism spectrum disorder and attention-deficit/hyperactivity disorder based on the best-practice diagnostic instruments for autism. *Scientific Reports, 12*(1), 18744. doi:10.1038/s41598-022-21719-x PMID:36335178

Yang, X., Zhang, N., & Schrader, P. (2022). A study of brain networks for autism spectrum disorder classification using resting-state functional connectivity. *Machine Learning with Applications, 8*, 100290. doi:10.1016/j.mlwa.2022.100290

Yassin, W., Nakatani, H., Zhu, Y., Kojima, M., Owada, K., Kuwabara, H., Gonoi, W., Aoki, Y., Takao, H., Natsubori, T., Iwashiro, N., Kasai, K., Kano, Y., Abe, O., Yamasue, H., & Koike, S. (2020). Machine-learning classification using neuroimaging data in schizophrenia, autism, ultra-high risk and first-episode psychosis. *Translational Psychiatry*, *10*(1), 278. doi:10.1038/s41398-020-00965-5 PMID:32801298

Zhao, Z., Zhu, Z., Zhang, X., Tang, H., Xing, J., Hu, X., Lu, J., & Qu, X. (2021). Identifying autism with head movement features by implementing machine learning algorithms. *Journal of Autism and Developmental Disorders*, 1–12. PMID:34250557

KEY TERMS AND DEFINITIONS

ADOS-R: A standardised evaluation instrument that aids in the diagnosis of autism spectrum disorders (ASD) in both children and adults is the Autism Diagnostic Observation Schedule-Revised (ADOS-R).

Autism: The neurological and developmental illness known as autism spectrum disorder (ASD) has an impact on a person's ability to engage with others, communicate, and learn.

Dense NN: A common layer in neural networks is the dense layer, which is highly interconnected, meaning that each neuron in the layer receives input from every neuron in the layer below it.

fNIRS: It is a non-intrusive optical brain observing approach that estimates cortical hemodynamic function in accordance with neural activity using near-infrared light.

Gradient Boosting: It is a ML method used in regression and classification applications. It provides an ensemble of weak models for predictions, often decision trees, as a prediction model.

Linear Discriminant Analysis: It is a generalisation of Fisher's linear discriminant, which is a method used in statistics and other fields to find the linear combination of characteristics that describes or distinguishes multiple categories based on a given parameter.

Long Short Term Memory: It is a type of ANN that is used in artificial intelligence as well as deep learning. Unlike traditional feedforward neural networks, LSTM includes feedback connections.

Multi-Layer Perceptron: It is a type of feedforward ANN that is fully linked. Various feedforward ANNs are referred to as MLPs, but the word is also used to refer more specifically to networks made up of multiple layers of perceptrons.

Social Cognitive Neuroscience: It is a new multidisciplinary area of study that investigates the biological mechanisms that guide social cognition.

Temporal Coherence: It is defined as the mean correlation in the magnitude of a wave and itself, skipped by T (the time period of the wave's oscillation) for any combination of certain points.

Typically Developing Control: The individuals that do not fall into the category of any severe neurological disorder ailment are generally referred as TDCs.

Virtual Reality: It is an innovation that generates an artificially-generated setting with realistic-looking scenes and objects, giving the user the impression that they are immersed in the environment around them.

Chapter 9
Web–Based Application for Physical to Digital ECG Signal Analysis for Cardiac Dysfunctions

Hariharan S.
SASTRA University (Deemed), India

Hemalatha Karnan
SASTRA University (Deemed), India

Uma Maheshwari D.
SASTRA University (Deemed), India

ABSTRACT

Electrocardiogram (ECG) acts as a symptomatic tool that routinely analyzes the functions of the heart. Till recently, most ECG records were kept on thermal paper. The evaluation of ECG charts needs considerable training and can be time-consuming and daunting process. The evaluation of ECG charts needs considerable training and can be time-consuming and daunting process. We can perform diagnosis and analysis with automation by digitizing the paper ECG. We can perform diagnosis and analysis with automation by digitizing the paper ECG. The main goal of this chapter is physical to-digital fusion of ECG signal and implement machine learning algorithm. This can be achieved by extracting the P, QRS, and T waves in ECG signals to demonstrate the heart's electrical activity using various techniques. The web-based application can make use of a machine-learning algorithm that analyzes and diagnoses cardiac disorders and normal conditions by uploading the ECG image. Thereby it reduces the time-consuming and daunting process for the analysis of ECG reports.

DOI: 10.4018/979-8-3693-2359-5.ch009

1. INTRODUCTION

According to the World Health Organization, cardiovascular disease is the primary factor of death. This has persisted as the major cause of death for the last 20 years. This paper emphasizes more on Signal and image processing of ECG image reports. By digitizing ECG records, the need for prolonged manual influence can be eliminated. Digitization provides the analysis and the diagnosis with less computational efficiency. The study developed and validated an algorithm for the digitization of ECG paper images. The algorithm showed a high degree of accuracy in identifying and extracting relevant ECG features such as waveforms, intervals, and segments. The algorithm was also able to produce digital ECG tracings that were comparable to those generated by standard ECG machines. The study used a dataset of 1,000 ECG paper images to develop and validate the algorithm. The images were digitized using a high-resolution scanner, and the algorithm was developed using a combination of image processing and machine learning techniques. The algorithm was trained and tested using the dataset and the performance is evaluated. One of the main limitations of the study is that it only evaluated the algorithm performance on a single dataset. Further studies are needed to evaluate the algorithm's performance on a larger and more diverse dataset. Additionally, the study did not compare the algorithm's performance to other existing methods for ECG digitization, which could provide insights into the strengths and weaknesses of the proposed approach (Randazzo et al., 2022). The study used a deep learning approach to develop a fully-automated paper ECG digitization algorithm. The algorithm was developed and trained using a large dataset of over 10,000 ECG paper images. The algorithm used a convolutional neural network (CNN) to automatically detect and extract relevant ECG features such as waveforms, intervals, and segments. The algorithm was analyzed using an individual test set of ECG paper images. The proposed algorithm achieved high accuracy in digitising ECG paper images. The algorithm provides high sensitivity and specificity in detecting various ECG abnormalities, including left bundle branch block, ST depression, and ST elevation. The algorithm has the potential to be used in clinical settings to improve ECG analysis and diagnosis. The study only evaluated the proposed algorithm's performance on a single dataset, which was relatively small. Further studies are needed to evaluate the algorithm's performance on larger and more diverse datasets. The study did not provide a detailed analysis of false positives and false negatives, which could help identify areas for further improvement. The study did not compare the proposed algorithm to other existing methods for ECG digitization, which could provide insights into the strengths and weaknesses of the proposed approach (Wu et al., 2022). The study used a deep learning approach to digitize ECG paper records and diagnose abnormal ECG signals. The dataset comprised 1000 ECG paper records, which were scanned and pre-processed to remove noise and improve image quality. The paper used a convolutional neural network (CNN) to identify ECG features such as QRS complexes, P waves, and T waves. The study also used a recurrent neural network (RNN) to classify the ECG signals as normal or abnormal. The proposed algorithm achieved high accuracy in digitizing ECG paper records. The RNN-based classification model also achieved high accuracy, with an overall accuracy of 95.6% in classifying ECG signals as normal or abnormal. The study demonstrated that the proposed technique has the ability to enhance the efficiency of ECG diagnosis. The main limitation of the study is that it only evaluated the algorithm's performance on a single dataset. Further studies are needed to evaluate the algorithm's performance on a larger and more diverse dataset. Additionally, the study did not compare the proposed approach to other existing methods for ECG diagnosis, which could provide insights into the strengths and weaknesses of the proposed approach. Finally, the study did not provide a detailed analysis of false positives and false negatives, which could help identify areas for further improvement (Mishra et al., 2021). The proposed paper-based ECG records use image processing techniques. The paper used a flatbed scanner to acquire the ECG paper records and developed a MATLAB-based program to pre-process and enhance the images. The program used techniques such as image thresholding and edge detection to identify the ECG waveforms and extract relevant features such as QRS complexes, P waves, and T waves. The extracted features were then validated against the original ECG records to ensure accuracy. The proposed method achieved high accuracy in digitizing ECG paper records. The method also has high sensitivity and specificity in detecting various ECG abnormalities, including ST elevation, ST depression, and arrhythmias. The paper suggests that their approach has the potential to be integrated with machine learning algorithms to improve ECG diagnosis. Algorithm performance and the results presented in the paper may be specific to the dataset used for evaluation. The effectiveness of the algorithm might vary when applied to different types of ECG paper records or datasets from diverse populations. The paper may not provide information about the computational requirements or complexity of the proposed algorithm. It could be beneficial to understand the resources needed for implementing the algorithm in real-world applications (Baydoun et al., 2019). The study proposed a method for digitizing ECG traces and classifying them into different categories using machine learning algorithms. The authors used a scanner to acquire the ECG traces and developed a MATLAB-based program to preprocess and enhance the images. The program used techniques such as image thresholding and morphological operations to extract relevant features such as QRS complexes, P waves, and T waves. The features that were extracted were deployed to train an SVM classifier and to classify the ECG traces into different categories such as ventricular hypertrophy, normal, right bundle branch block, left bundle branch block. The proposed method achieved high accuracy in digitizing ECG traces. The SVM classifier also achieved high accuracy in classifying ECG traces into different categories, with an accuracy of 94.2%. The analysis demonstrated that the suggested method has the potential to enhance the efficiency of ECG diagnosis. The overall efficiency is enhanced by the advanced work progress. This involves developing a fuzzy-based expert system that assists in the diagnosis and generating automatic diagnosis reports as well (Angelovirgin & Sangeetha, 2017). The study proposed a method for digitizing ECG graphs and detecting heart disease using machine learning algorithms. The authors used a scanner to acquire the ECG graphs and developed a MATLAB-based program to preprocess and extract features from the images. The program used techniques such as image thresholding, filtering, and edge detection to extract relevant features such as QRS complexes, P waves, and T waves. The features that were extracted were then deployed to train a backpropagation neural network (BPNN) classifier to detect heart disease. The presented method is precise in digitizing ECG graphs, with an average accuracy of 99.2% in detecting QRS complexes, 97.5% in detecting P waves, and 98.1% in detecting T waves. The BPNN classifier also highly precise in detecting heart disease, with an overall accuracy of 95.7%. The analysis demonstrated that the presented approach has the potential to enhance the efficiency of ECG diagnosis. By augmenting the size of the sample utilized in BPNN the capacity to identify the cardiac arrhythmia is increased. This can be enhanced by expanding the range of detection features (Aruselvi, 2020). The paper proposes a modified DenseNet model for arrhythmia detection and visualization using Grad-CAM. Two hypotheses about Grad-CAM were established and an experiment was conducted to achieve high-performance deep learning models with comprehensible visualization. The training was repeated to determine the optimal parameters in each model structure, and the test set was evaluated using the parameters that exhibited the best performance in the validation set. The DenseNet used in this study consisted of two modules, Conv Block and Transition Block, with hyperparameters including Growth rate, Window size, and Reduction. The proposed method achieved a classification performance of 0.98 accuracy, with clear visualization of the response area using Grad-CAM. The experiments demonstrated that all models in the study were better at classifying ECGs than AlexNet, with high performance and comparable visualization. The paper acknowledges that although the developed model enables better visualization than the comparative model, it does not guarantee complete visualization of all data. Further research is needed to provide meaningful visualizations of all data and to create a quantitative evaluation criterion for the visualization of the model's judgment basis (Kim et al., 2022). The paper proposes an automatic method for classifying Aortic valvular stenosis (AS) using ECG images by training CNNs (Convolutional neural networks) with annotated diagnoses from medical doctors who observe echocardiograms. One-beat ECG images for 12-leads and 4-leads are generated from ECGs and used to train the CNNs. The Grad-CAM technique is applied to the trained CNNs to detect feature areas in the early time range of the one-beat ECG image. The trained CNN for the 4-lead achieves classification performance close to expert medical doctors' diagnoses, by limiting the time range of the ECG image to the feature area detected by Grad-CAM. The classification results for 4-lead ECG images are better than those for one-beat ECG images. The paper highlights the need for an automatic system for diagnosing AS using ECG due to the shortage of medical doctors and the high cost of echocardiography in rural areas. The paper also emphasizes the lack of clarity in how deep learning networks interpret inputs and output judgments, and the need to verify the appropriateness of network judgments from a medical point of view. The study focuses on AS, which is one of the most serious valvular diseases, and aims to output echocardiography based on diagnosis by inputting only ECG of an unknown patient to the trained network (Hata et al., 2020). The study developed DenseNet and CNN models for the classification of healthy subjects and patients with ten classes of myocardial infarction (MI) based on the location of myocardial involvement. ECG signals from the Physikalisch-Technische Bundesanstalt (PTB) database were pre-processed, and the ECG beats were extracted using an R peak detection algorithm. The beats were then fed to the DenseNet and CNN models separately. An enhanced class activation mapping (CAM) technique called Grad-CAM was applied to the outputs of both models to visualize the specific ECG leads and portions of ECG waves that were most influential for the predictive decisions made by the models. Both DenseNet and CNN models attained high classification accuracies of more than 95%. DenseNet was preferred for the classification task due to its low computational complexity and higher classification accuracy compared to the CNN model. Lead V4 was the most activated lead in both the DenseNet and CNN models. The study established the different leads and parts of the signal that get activated for each class, providing some level of explainability for the classification decisions of deep models. The dataset used in the study was imbalanced, and a public database was used instead of authentic hospital data. The study is the first to map the classification decision of deep models to specific ECG leads and locations, providing some level of explainability that clinicians can relate. The study contributes significantly to the medical field by providing visible explainability of the inner workings of the models, which may help garner clinical acceptance and potential implementation for ECG triage of MI diagnosis in hospitals and remote out-of-hospital settings (Jahmunah et al., 2022).

2. METHODOLOGY

This paper uses 4 categories for image classification for our ECG images. It includes normal, myocardial infarction, abnormal heartbeat, and history of myocardial infarction. All the ECG images from the Mendeley dataset (Aruselvi, 2020). The scheme of workflow is shown in the Fig. 1. It includes the crucial step which consists of Data preparation and Preprocessing. The steps involved are converting all ECG images to grayscale and resizing images per requirements. Divide the images into 12 sections for each image extracting 12 lead values (1-12). Remove gridlines from each lead image and convert them to a binary image. The next steps include Data feature Extraction and Data Engineering which consists of tracing and extracting only the necessary signal from images and using the contour technique. The image is converted to a one-dimensional signal. After that, MinMaxScaler is used to scale the image. For each lead, (1-12) signal in all ECG images, save the 1D signal values in an a.csv file. In a single CSV file, combine all 12 lead values with the target label added. We tested various algorithms and then utilized the ensemble technique to stack algorithms to enhance performance because it was a classification problem. We tested various algorithms and then utilized the ensemble technique to stack algorithms to enhance performance because it was a classification problem.

Figure 1. Scheme of workflow

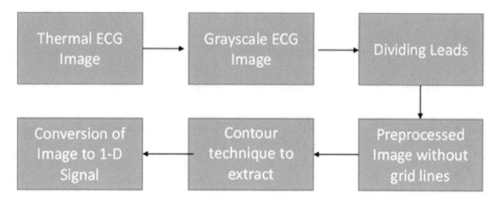

3. RESULTS AND DISCUSSION

3.1. Image and Signal Processing

The thermal paper ECG image which needs to be converted into a one-dimensional signal is loaded as the input. In this paper, we have used four sets of ECG images namely Normal ECG, Myocardial Infarction, abnormal heartbeat, and history of myocardial infarction. The required ECG is loaded and it follows the algorithm which is used to convert into the signals and analyse the condition of the beneficiary according to the features extracted and machine learning is used to analyse the report with the training and testing processes. The RGB thermal paper ECG image which is uploaded as input is show in the Fig. 2. The next step of the algorithm includes the conversion of the RGB image to the grayscale of the input ECG image. This reduces the complexity of the data and allows for easier analysis and processing. The resulting grayscale image can be easily converted into a one-dimensional signal for further analysis.

The process involves resizing of the thermal paper ECG image according to the requirements. The ECG image is divided into 13 sections for each image extracting 13 lead values (1-13). Further processing can be easily done using the divided lead images. So, the division of the ECG images is an important process in the quantization of the ECG image to signal. The division of the different leads of the thermal paper ECG is shown in Figure 3.

Figure 2. Input thermal paper ECG image

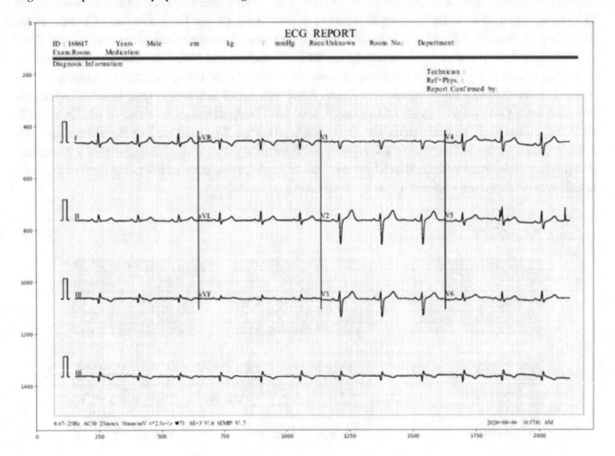

In order to further process the leads each lead undertakes a series of transformations. This process includes the removal of grid lines which is depicted in Fig. 4, the conversion of grayscale, applying the Gaussian filtering and the thresholding used for the conversion of the image to binary format.

The contouring technique involves image processing to extract and represent the boundaries or shapes of objects. The process involves a combination of image preprocessing and signal processing techniques. Through the contour technique the transformed image is traced, and isolated, and the signals are extracted. The resulting output representing the 2D signal is stored in CSV format. Figure 5 depicts the relevant information extracted from the thermal paper ECG that is used for the conversion of the signal.

Based on the observation the X axis represents the high and the low points and the Y axis captures the curve or the shape depicted in the Fig. 6. In our analysis the high and low points are concentrated and thus the X axis is saved independently as the normalized and scaled 1D signal in CSV file.

Using the transpose operation the 1D rows were transformed into the columns. With the availability of both the 1D and 2D CSV files which is depicted in Fig. 7. Once we extract the 1D values from the ECG image, it is merged as a single CSV file for the analysis. The dimensionality reduction is also performed and further applies various machine learning algorithms.

Figure 3. Different leads of the ECG

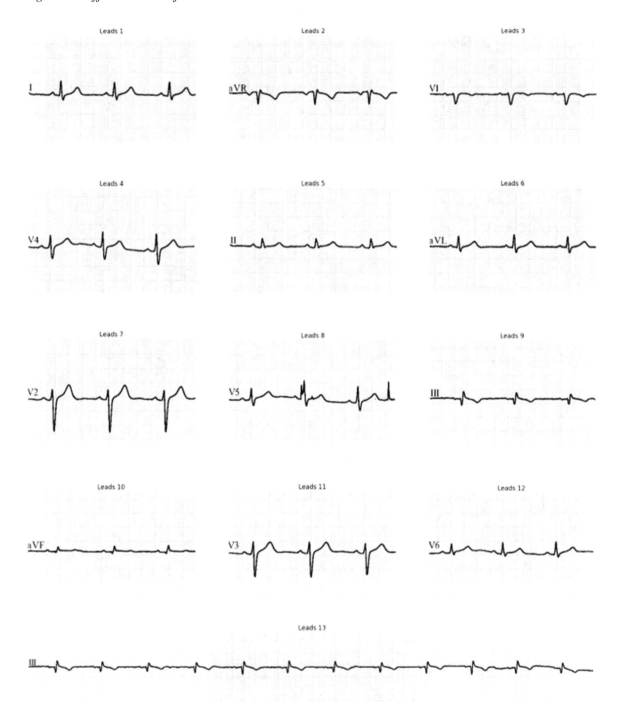

Figure 4. Pre-processed image without gridlines

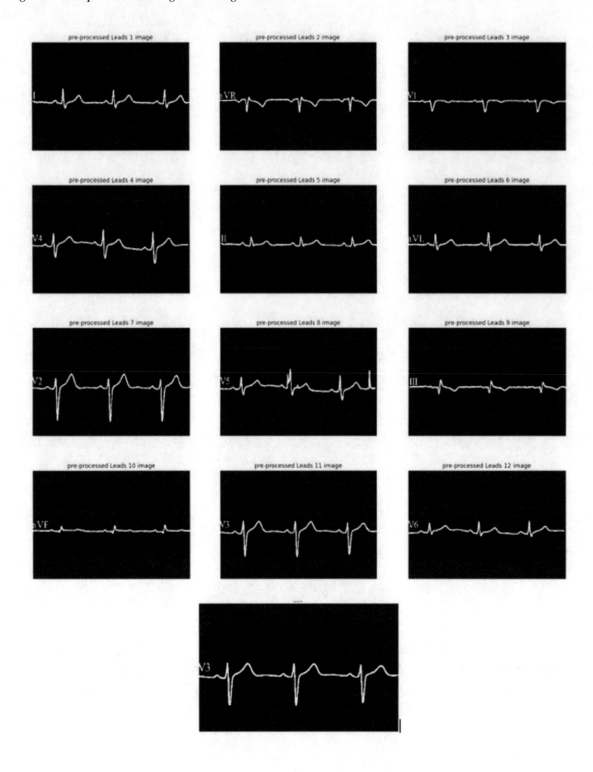

Figure 5. Contour images

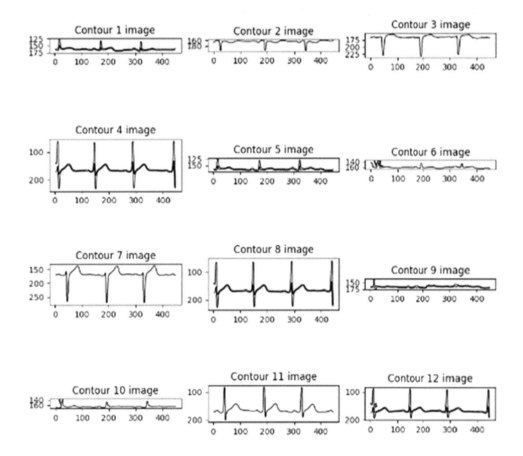

The Grad-CAM (Gradient-weighted Class Activation Mapping) is a technique used for visualizing and interpreting the decisions made by a neural network, particularly in the context of image classification tasks. It helps to understand which regions of the input image are contributing the most to the model's prediction. Grad-CAM is generally applied to convolutional neural networks (CNNs), which are commonly used for image-related tasks. The goal of Grad-CAM is to generate a heatmap that highlights the important regions of an input image that contribute to a specific class prediction made by the network. During the forward pass, gradients are computed with respect to the final convolutional layer's output. These gradients represent how much each element in the output feature map contributes to the overall prediction. Global Average Pooling is applied to the gradients, which results in a set of weights for each feature map. This step is important for obtaining a class-discriminative localization map. The original feature maps are then linearly combined using the obtained weights, creating a weighted sum that represents the importance of each feature map for the target class. The result is passed through a ReLU activation to eliminate negative values. The final heatmap is upsampled to the original input image size, providing a spatial localization of important regions. The Grad-CAM heatmap visually indicates which regions of the input image were most crucial for the network to make a certain prediction. The ECG signals are converted into images or spectrograms that can be fed into a CNN. Each class could represent a specific type of cardiac condition. Train a CNN on the ECG data for classification tasks. After training, Grad-CAM can be applied to visualize which parts of the ECG signals contributed the most to the model's decision for a particular class. Clinicians and researchers can use the Grad-CAM visualizations to gain insights into the neural network's decision-making process. For example, they can identify specific patterns or regions in the ECG signal that are indicative of certain cardiac conditions. The normal one-dimensional ECG of four conditions is compared with the Grad Cam Visualisation in the Figure 8

Figure 6. Normalised 2D signal

	X	Y
0	0.739819	0.000000
1	0.737127	0.010660
2	0.720877	0.018884
3	0.699773	0.025480
4	0.696124	0.032170
...	...	...
250	0.710078	0.974109
251	0.692782	0.980873
252	0.705865	0.987214
253	0.727418	0.993963
254	0.747485	1.000000

Figure 7. Normalised 1D signal

	0	1	2	3	4	5	6	7	8	9	...	245	246	247	248	249	:
X	0.739819	0.737127	0.720877	0.699773	0.696124	0.719836	0.738314	0.76047	0.772462	0.766114	...	0.747437	0.741823	0.73248	0.729167	0.72661	0.710(

Figure 8. Normal and grad cam visualisation of normal, MI, PMI, HB

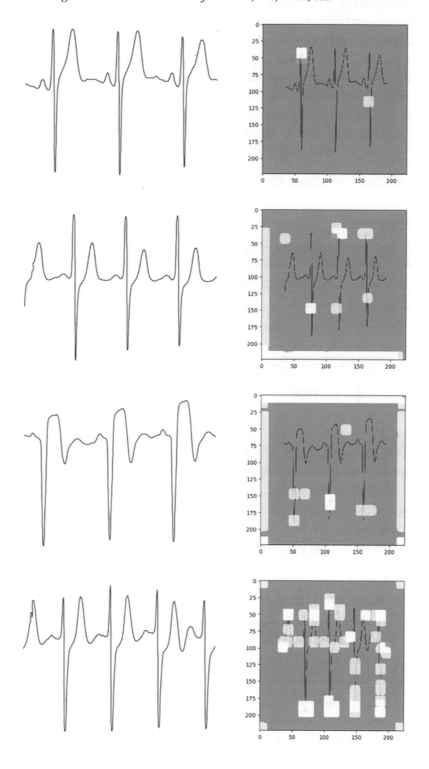

3.2. Machine Learning Algorithms

Several researchers have utilized various data mining techniques to identify and predict the heart anomalies such as Neural networks, KNN, and Decision tree classifiers. ECG images pertaining to four categories such as normal, myocardial infarction, abnormal heartbeat and the history of myocardial infarction. Post-dimensionality reduction of KNN involves applying dimensionality reduction techniques on the feature space before utilizing the KNN algorithm to leverage the benefits of reduced dimensionality and enhance the model's performance. The K- Nearest Neighbors (KNN) algorithm is a supervised machine learning technique capable of addressing both the classification and regression predictive tasks. The classification report of the KNN algorithm can be observed in Table 1.

Table 1. Performance metrics of KNN

Parameters	Precision	Recall	F1 Score	Support
0	1.00	1.00	1.00	51
1	0.98	1.00	0.99	50
2	1.00	1.00	1.00	52
3	1.00	0.97	0.98	33
Accuracy			0.99	186
Macro avg	1.00	0.99	0.99	186
Weighted avg	0.99	0.99	0.99	186

Post-dimensionality reduction of logistic regression involves applying dimensionality reduction techniques on the feature space before training the logistic regression model. This can help mitigate challenges associated with high-dimensional data and improve the model's performance in terms of predictive accuracy and interpretability. Logistic regression is a statistical approach utilized for analyzing a dataset with one or more independent variables that influence the outcome. It is employed for modeling the binary classification problems. The classification report of Logistic Regression can be found in Table 2.

Table 2. Performance metrics of logistic regression

Parameters	Precision	Recall	F1 Score	Support
0	1.00	0.96	0.98	51
1	0.96	0.98	0.97	50
2	1.00	1.00	1.00	52
3	0.97	1.00	0.99	33
Accuracy			0.98	186
Macro avg	0.98	0.99	0.98	186
Weighted avg	0.98	0.98	0.98	186

Post-dimensionality reduction of SVM involves applying dimensionality reduction techniques on the feature space before training the SVM model. This can help mitigate the challenges of high-dimensional data and improve the performance and efficiency of the SVM algorithm. Support vector machines (SVMs) are adaptable supervised machine learning algorithms widely employed for classification and regression tasks. SVM exhibit distinctive implementation approaches compared to other machine learning algorithms. The classification report can be found in the Table. 3

Table 3. Performance metrics of SVM

Parameters	Precision	Recall	F1 Score	Support
0	0.58	1.00	0.74	51
1	1.0	1.00	1.00	50
2	1.00	0.61	0.76	52
3	1.00	0.68	0.81	33
Accuracy			0.82	186
Macro avg	0.90	0.82	0.83	186
Weighted avg	0.90	0.82	0.83	186

The application of the KNN algorithm directly on the original feature space without any prior reduction of the number of features. When using KNN without dimensionality reduction, the algorithm considers all the available features in the dataset to compute distances and determine the nearest neighbors. This means that each feature contributes equally to the calculation of distances, and no specific feature selection or dimensionality reduction techniques are applied. The classification report of KNN is shown in Table 4.

When using logistic regression without dimensionality reduction, the algorithm considers all the available features in the dataset to estimate the coefficients that define the association of the features and the target variable. Each feature is assigned a weight or coefficient that indicates its contribution to the prediction. Without dimensionality reduction, all the features are treated equally, and no specific feature selection or dimensionality reduction techniques are applied. The classification report of Logistic Regression is shown in Table 5.

Table 4. Performance metrics of KNN with reduction

Parameters	Precision	Recall	F1 Score	Support
0	1.00	1.00	1.00	51
1	1.00	1.00	1.00	50
2	1.00	1.00	1.00	52
3	1.00	1.00	1.00	33
Accuracy			1.00	186
Macro avg	1.00	1.00	1.00	186
Weighted avg	1.00	1.00	1.00	186

Table 5. Performance metrics of logistic regression with reduction

Parameters	Precision	Recall	F1 Score	Support
0	1.00	1.00	1.00	51
1	1.00	0.98	0.99	50
2	1.00	1.00	1.00	52
3	0.97	1.00	0.99	33
Accuracy			0.99	186
Macro avg	0.99	0.99	0.99	186
Weighted avg	0.99	0.99	0.99	186

When using SVM without dimensionality reduction, the algorithm considers all the available features in the dataset to find the optimal hyperplane. Each feature contributes equally to the determination of the hyperplane and the classification/regression process. Without dimensionality reduction, the SVM algorithm calculates the distances between data points in the original feature space to define the support vectors and determine the decision boundaries. The SVM model learns the relationships between the features and the target variable based on the provided data without explicitly reducing the number of features. The classification report of SVM is shown in Table. 6.

Table 6. Performance metrics of SVM with reduction

Parameters	Precision	Recall	F1 Score	Support
0	0.77	0.92	0.84	51
1	1.00	1.00	1.00	50
2	0.90	0.90	0.90	52
3	0.97	0.70	0.81	33
Accuracy			0.90	186
Macro avg	0.91	0.88	0.89	186
Weighted avg	0.91	0.90	0.90	186

XGBoost, or Extreme Gradient Boosting, is an ensemble learning algorithm that combines the predictions of multiple weak decision tree models to make accurate predictions. Without dimensionality reduction, XGBoost considers all the available features in the dataset during the construction of decision trees and the learning process. Each feature contributes to the overall prediction, and the algorithm determines the importance of each feature based on its relevance to the target variable. XGBoost a powerful implementation of gradient-boosted decision trees is specially engineered for exceptional speed, performance, and dominance in machine learning. The classification report of XG Boost is shown in Table 7.

Ensemble learning involves training multiple models on the same dataset in machine learning and their predictions are aggregated to produce a consolidated final prediction. Each individual model in the ensemble is often referred to as a base model or weak learner. Without dimensionality reduction, an ensemble can consist of various types of models, such as decision trees, random forests, gradient-boosting machines, or neural networks. Each base model in the ensemble may utilize all the available features in the original feature space to make predictions. In Voting-based Ensemble classification, a combination of three Machine learning models k-nearest neighbors (KNN), Support Vector Machine (SVM), and Random Forest Classifier is employed. The models are stacked and their predictions are combined through voting to determine the model that achieves the highest accuracy. Hyperparameters tuning is conducted using GridSearchCV to optimize the performance of the results.. Based on the voting, the classification report is printed as shown below in Table. 8. Once the model is acceptable, we will pickle the model for future use and prediction.

Table 7. Performance metrics of XG boost with reduction

Parameters	Precision	Recall	F1 Score	Support
0	1.00	1.00	1.00	51
1	1.00	1.00	1.00	50
2	1.00	1.00	1.00	52
3	1.00	1.00	1.00	33
Accuracy			1.00	186
Macro avg	1.00	1.00	1.00	186
Weighted avg	1.00	1.00	1.00	186

Table 8. Performance metrics of ensemble with reduction

Parameters	F	Recall	F1 Score	Support
0	0.95	0.95	0.95	51
1	1.00	1.00	1.00	50
2	0.86	0.90	0.88	52
3	0.86	0.79	0.83	33
Accuracy			0.92	186
Macro avg	0.92	0.91	0.91	186
Weighted avg	0.92	0.92	0.92	186

To begin with, the user uploads the ECG images through our web app. Subsequently, a series of image conversion techniques, including RGB to grayscale conversion, denoising, gaussian filtering, thresholding, and contouring are employed to extract signals devoid of grid lines. The signal is then subjected to dimensionality reduction and the essential waves are isolated through segmentation. These extracted waves are then inputted into our pre-trained model for analysis. Upon completion of the analysis, the results are relayed back to the user based on their finding.

The analysis outcomes are displayed in Figure 9.

Figure 9. Analysis report of thermal paper ECG

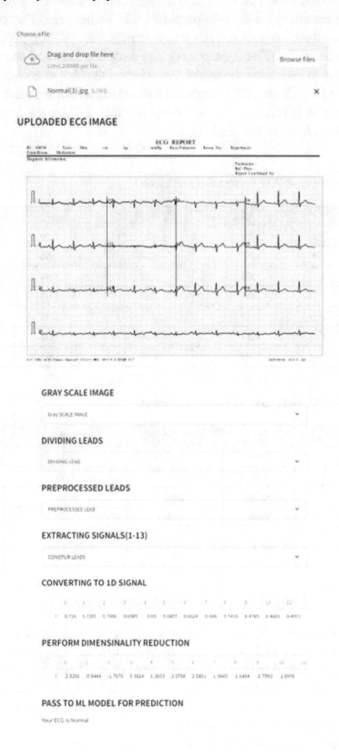

4. CONCLUSION

The digital quantization of thermal paper ECG is obtained using signal and image processing techniques. The analysis result can be done quickly with more accuracy. Thereby it helps the beneficiary to look after their health report immediately. This paper considers the four different conditions namely normal, abnormal, myocardial infarction, and history of myocardial infarction. Patients with normal and abnormal conditions can be identified by the machine learning algorithm. The machine learning algorithm is carried out with and without dimensionality reduction and the classification report for the different algorithm are obtained. The KNN and XG Boost algorithm with the dimensionality reduction is more accurate with an accuracy of 100%. This paper can also be extended by training and testing the other different conditions of cardiovascular diseases. Different machine learning algorithms can also be implemented with low computational time and power. Hence the prediction or analysis of the ECG can be done quickly with a higher rate of accuracy.

REFERENCES

Angelovirgin, G., & Sangeetha, M. (2017). Conversion of ecg graph into digital format and detecting the disease. *Mathematics, A. Ijpam.Eu, 116*, 465–471.

Aruselvi, K. (2020). Digitization of ECG Trace and Classification. *International Journal of Emerging Technologies and Innovative Research.* www.jetir.org

Baydoun, M., Safatly, L., Abou Hassan, O. K., Ghaziri, H., El Hajj, A., & Isma'eel, H. (2019, November 7). High Precision Digitization of Paper-Based ECG Records: A Step Toward Machine Learning. *IEEE Journal of Translational Engineering in Health and Medicine, 7*, 1900808. doi:10.1109/JTEHM.2019.2949784 PMID:32166049

Hata, E., Seo, C., Nakayama, M., Iwasaki, K., Ohkawauchi, T., & Ohya, J. (2020). Classification of Aortic Stenosis Using ECG by Deep Learning and its Analysis Using Grad-CAM. *Proc. Annu. Int. Conf. IEEE Eng. Med. Biol. Soc.* IEEE. 10.1109/EMBC44109.2020.9175151

Jahmunah, V., Ng, E. Y. K., Tan, R. S., Oh, S. L., & Acharya, U. R. (2022). Explainable detection of myocardial infarction using deep learning models with Grad-CAM technique on ECG signals. *Computers in Biology and Medicine, 146*, 105550. doi:10.1016/j.compbiomed.2022.105550 PMID:35533457

Kim, J. K., Jung, S., Park, J., & Han, S. W. (2022). Arrhythmia detection model using modified DenseNet for comprehensible Grad-CAM visualization. *Biomedical Signal Processing and Control, 73*, 103408. doi:10.1016/j.bspc.2021.103408

Mishra, S., Khatwani, G., Patil, R., Sapariya, D., Shah, V., Parmar, D., Dinesh, S., Daphal, P., & Mehendale, N. (2021). ECG Paper Record Digitization and Diagnosis Using Deep Learning. *Journal of Medical and Biological Engineering, 41*(4), 422–432. doi:10.1007/s40846-021-00632-0 PMID:34149335

Randazzo, V., Puleo, E., Paviglianiti, A., Vallan, A., & Pasero, E. (2022). Development and Validation of an Algorithm for the Digitization of ECG Paper Images. *Sensors (Basel)*, *22*(19), 7138. doi:10.3390/s22197138 PMID:36236237

Wu, H., Patel, K. H. K., Li, X., Zhang, B., Galazis, C., Bajaj, N., Sau, A., Shi, X., Sun, L., Tao, Y., Al-Qaysi, H., Tarusan, L., Yasmin, N., Grewal, N., Kapoor, G., Waks, J. W., Kramer, D. B., Peters, N. S., & Ng, F. S. (2022). A fully-automated paper ECG digitisation algorithm using deep learning. *Scientific Reports*, *12*(1), 20963. doi:10.1038/s41598-022-25284-1 PMID:36471089

Chapter 10
Real–Time Symptomatic Disease Predictor Using Multi–Layer Perceptron

Pancham Singh

 https://orcid.org/0009-0005-0435-7941

Ajay Kumar Garg Engineering College, Ghaziabad, India

Mrignainy Kansal

 https://orcid.org/0009-0005-2610-040X

Ajay Kumar Garg Engineering College, Ghaziabad, India

Ayush Pratap Singh

Ajay Kumar Garg Engineering College, Ghaziabad, India

Ayushi Verma

Ajay Kumar Garg Engineering College, Ghaziabad, India

Snigdha Tyagi

Ajay Kumar Garg Engineering College, Ghaziabad, India

Aditya Vikram Singh

Ajay Kumar Garg Engineering College, Ghaziabad, India

ABSTRACT

Early disease diagnosis is crucial for effective treatment, but current healthcare methods have limitations. Supervised machine learning algorithms, particularly deep learning networks, have proven effective in developing medical diagnostics and real-time applications for detecting high-risk diseases. This paper evaluates five algorithms: Multilayer perceptron (MLP), random forest, decision tree, Naive Bayes, and K-Nearest neighbours (KNN) for predicting diseases based on user-entered symptoms. MLP outperformed other algorithms, achieving an accuracy of 97.2%, which is 4-5% higher than existing disease prediction models. Notably, existing techniques account for only 94% accuracy on average. Highlighting the potential of MLP in early disease diagnosis, this paper concludes by summarizing its goals, challenges, and outcomes.

DOI: 10.4018/979-8-3693-2359-5.ch010

1. INTRODUCTION

Algorithms for artificial intelligence (AI) and machine learning (ML) make it easier to create systems with tools that mimic human abilities like the capacity for logic, reason, and generalisation based on data from prior experiences. The proposed system is built on a machine learning model, which is a system of computer programming used to process data Fields(Sawhney et al., 2023). The expansion of technology has made everything crueller and more varied. In today's digital age, medical professionals will do anything to save lives. It is not practical for doctors to be on call constantly. However, we can always use this forecasting system to increase productivity when using modern techniques. Data in the form of the patient's symptoms, age, and gender can be sent to the ML model for additional processing. AI-based systems typically train on pre-processed datasets that can be used to obtain the desired results. Data science is a methodology and statistical combination that can be computed to analyse data to discover trends and forecast the future. Python is known to be one of the most efficient programming languages that can yield adequate results due to its dynamic nature which makes it feasible to operate.

These methods can aid in forming smart processes that can benefit the current healthcare sector by making it inexpensive, more effective, and equitable (Dangare & Apte, 2012). The doctor can use data collected from numerous facilities and patients to forecast treatment strategies that are superior to conventional practices and improve all facets of the healthcare industry. We can boost the economy and ensure the general welfare of society by utilising such methods in the healthcare sector. This system would help identify and examine the patient's symptoms in various body parts, and then careful analysis could be carried out to determine the necessary results (Mariappan et al., 2022). Providing a suitable and organised medical assessment of the ill is a crucial step in the treatment process. This system is very helpful for patients to track their health through self-analysis and management in addition to helping doctors during routine check-ups. Documenting all of the patient's data from the start of treatment, such as a thorough list of the patient's symptoms, lab results, and X-ray reports, can help to more accurately predict a disease (Devarapalli et al., 2012). In the healthcare industry, AI and MI algorithms have assisted in achieving success by automating routine diagnostic and therapeutic procedures and coming to conclusions about strategies that can also help medical professionals carry out a variety of tasks that cannot yet be automated. Using machine learning techniques makes it easier to identify people with more common diseases, which is also useful for classifying these diseases. Diseases are difficult to predict because similar types of symptoms can result in various outcomes.

As a result, the proposed system uses the data set and a deep learning algorithm to predict disease and then provides a disease prognosis based on the symptoms that the user has added. Early-stage detection of any chronic diseases can also benefit the diagnosis during the initial stages to bypass substantial concerns in the future. The disease prediction system can be useful for an entire range of individuals irrespective of their age group.

2. LITERATURE REVIEW

A literature review for symptomatic disease prediction in healthcare is an in-depth examination of existing research, studies, and publications that explore various methods, models, and technologies used to predict diseases based on symptoms. This type of literature review plays a crucial role in understanding the current state of knowledge, advancements, and gaps in the field of disease prediction and diagnosis. We have taken literature review of some papers on disease prediction are given below:

1. (Meghriche et al., 2008) provided a model to predict multiple diseases using widely popular techniques like Decision Tree and Random Forest while introducing a new technique known as LightGBM. While all three algorithms attained high accuracy scores for the side effect prediction only 95 could be scrutinized out of a total of 132 to prevent the model from overfitting.

2. (Di Noia et al., 2013) used data mining techniques to come up with a disease prediction model. The proposed model uses the power of different Artificial Intelligence calculations like Choice Tree, Irregular Timberland, Guileless Bayes Classifier calculations, and Innocent Bayes along with normal language processing to obtain accurate and precise outcomes. Tokenization is used for text preparation, additionally mixed with exception calculations to test the similarity of and back.

3. (Bilandi et al., 2021) came up with a model that uses X-ray and CT images to predict COVID-19 using CNN with an accuracy of 94% Although the proposed model has high accuracy for COVID-19 prediction it does not represent a production-ready solution, especially with a smaller count of images.

4. (Chen, 2021) suggested a model for disease prediction using CNN over Big Data. This model was able to handle frequent incompleteness in the healthcare data. The findings also include that the sample size chosen was less which affected the accuracy score.

5. (Rajamhoana et al., 2018) proposed a system for heart disease prediction KNN, Decision Tree, SVM and Linear Regression which achieved good accuracy. This model was based on biological parameters like heart rate, blood pressure, cholesterol etc. which had to be provided as input by the user. For these parameters, users have to depend on external entities. This makes the model dependent on external entities as a result failing to reduce cost.

6. (Lu et al., 2002) proposed a heart disease prediction model that uses the concept of a neural network in its multimodal prediction algorithm and uses real-time data from hospital records. The proposed model has increased computational cost.

7. (Edeh et al., 2022) explained streamlines ML for the prediction of chronic diseases. It achieves an accuracy score of 94.8% using a Decision tree map, Naive Bayes and Random Forest using both structured and unstructured data. It runs at a regular speed which is quicker than other existing unimodal prediction algorithms.

8. (Do et al., 2017) proposed a diabetes prediction system. The data preparation is done using K-Means Clustering and classification is performed using a Decision tree, thus attaining a high accuracy score of 98.7% with high sensitivity. It uses the Pima Indians Diabetes (PID) dataset which comprises 768 instances under 8 numerical attributes. Out of 768, 198 samples are removed as noise in the dataset during data preparation and only 570 samples are taken as input data which makes it unclear whether this system provides the same high accuracy scores for a larger dataset or not.

9. (da Silva et al., 2021) suggested a model for similar disease prediction. For Breast cancer detection this model provides 98.57% accurate results using the AdaBoost classifier. As for Heart disease and Diabetes prediction, they produce significantly less accurate results using Logistic Regression (87.1% accuracy) and SVM (85.71 accuracy) respectively. The proposed model also has high-improvement scopes for feature selection, pre-processing and model fitting.

10. (Sailaja et al., 2021) proposed a Skin Cancer prediction model. The model uses SVM and KNN classifiers where SVM performs producing an accuracy of 97.8% compared to KNN's accuracy of

86.25%. The model uses 2017's ISIC dataset with 1000 instances. The AUC recorded for textural features was 0.94.

3. MULTILAYER PERCEPTRON (MLP)

This project utilised the Multilayer Perceptron (MLP) technique found in the Deep Learning Algorithm. The Multilayer Perceptron (MLP) is a distributed parallel processing structure with numerous processing nodes. They are linked together by connections, which are one-way signalling channels. Input, output, and hidden layers make up a multilayer perceptron (MLP). Multiple nodes, which can be represented by circles, can be found in these layers (Kansal, Singh, Srivastava, et al., 2023). The data flow from one node to another is depicted by the lines joining the nodes. Signals are sent to the input layer using a few external nodes. The weighted connecting channels are used to transfer the output from the input layer to the hidden layer. It performs calculations and transmits the results to the output layer using hidden layers and weighted connections. After the last computation, the output layer generates the outcome. Every node other than the input nodes functions as a processing element, neuron, or activation function with a minimum threshold. MLP trains networks using a supervised learning technique known as back propagation in which the information pursues only a forward path that starts from the input nodes, through the hidden nodes, and concludes at the output nodes. Error calculation is performed in the opposite direction. The major applications of MLP are pattern classification, recognition, prediction, and approximation in Figure 1. MLP is nothing but a modification made in the standard linear perceptron that can distinguish linearly inseparable data.

Figure 1. Multilayer perceptron neural network model

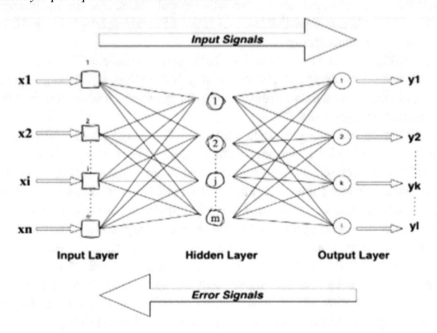

The network's output is compared to the desired output, and if there is a discrepancy between the two, the network weights are adjusted backwards and recalculated to maintain the network's performance. The proposed network model can be learned through this process. (Qteat & Awad, 2021). This is known as training the network. After we are done with training the network, tests are run on a new dataset where no target output has been provided to the network. The generalized and step-by-step working of Multilayer Perceptron (MLP) can be summarized as

1. At first, the input is provided to the input layer through some external nodes for processing and the predicted output is produced.
2. This output thus produced is subtracted from the actual output to calculate the final error value.
3. A back propagation algorithm is then used by the network to adjust the weights.
4. To adjust the weights, work backwards through the network, starting with the weights between the output layer node and the last hidden layer node.
5. The forward process starts once the back propagation is finished.
6. This process is performed in repetition so that the error between the predicted output and the actual output is minimized.

4. METHODOLOGY

We have used data from the University of Columbia following their study done at New York-Presbyterian Hospital which consists of 150 prevalent diseases along with their symptoms (Javaid et al., 2023). It is converted into a CSV file. The training dataset contains a total of 4920 rows and 133 columns whereas the testing dataset contains 41 rows and 133 columns. The dataset is made up of binary 0 and 1. The following steps have been taken into account for our proposed system:

- Firstly, we will be collecting the dataset of disease and possible symptoms of an unhealthy body.
- Then we will collect the information so that we can associate the symptoms with possible diseases to obtain disease information.
- Then treating the patient's symptoms as input, we will process them with the aid of machine learning algorithms (Multilayer Perceptron).
- Then we will predict the disease that is possible for the acquired symptoms.
- The system will show the most possible diseases and provide the user with remedies and cures.

The detailed flow chart of the methodology is given below in Figure 2: Before taking any algorithm into account in our project we performed a comparative analysis between different algorithms. We have successfully developed such a system to predict multiple diseases based on symptoms using five different machine-learning algorithms (Kansal, Singh, Shukla, et al., 2023). A model regarding ML has played a significant role in creating accuracy and determining results with the aid of training data. On average, we achieved an accuracy of about 94%, proving that MLP is the most accurate of all five algorithms.

1. Collect Symptom's data Set: Data collection involves gathering a comprehensive dataset that includes a wide range of symptoms and the diseases they correspond to. This data can be collected from medical records, health databases, and other credible sources. It's important to ensure that the data covers a diverse population to improve the model's generalizability.

2. Search for disease-Associated to the Symptoms: A wide range of diseases is associated with various symptoms, covering everything from common conditions like constipation and coughs to more severe illnesses such as diabetes, heart disease, and different types of cancer.

3. Match disease related to the Symptoms: To match diseases to specific symptoms accurately, it's crucial to analyze the symptoms in detail and refer to medical resources or databases that catalog diseases based on their symptoms. Without knowing the specific symptoms you're interested in, it's challenging to provide a direct match. For comprehensive matching, consider using online symptom checkers or consulting healthcare professionals for precise diagnosis and information.

4. Take input from user as Symptoms: "Take input from user as symptoms" refers to the process of collecting or receiving information from a person (the user) about their physical or mental health conditions that are indicative of a disease, disorder, or illness. This process is a fundamental part of medical consultations, health assessments, and diagnostic procedures.

5. Apply ML Models: Applying machine learning (ML) models for real-time symptomatic disease prediction involves a series of steps to design, train, and deploy models that can analyze symptoms and other relevant data to predict diseases. This process can significantly enhance healthcare delivery by providing rapid, data-driven insights for early diagnosis and treatment. Here's an overview of how to apply ML models for this purpose are Data Collection and Preparation, Feature Selection, Model Selection and Training, Deployment for Real-Time Prediction, Continuous Monitoring and Updating.

6. Generate output as possible disease: Generating output as a possible disease using machine learning (ML) models involves analyzing input data, typically symptoms provided by users or patients, to predict the most likely disease or condition. This process leverages historical health data, patterns, and relationships discovered through ML algorithms to make informed predictions.

4.1 Multilayer Perceptron

Multilayer Perceptron, a class of artificial neural networks, maps input to the desired output. MLP consists of multiple layers with unidirectional directed graphs. Except for the input nodes, each node has its activation threshold. The hidden layer's activation unit is calculated as layer's activation unit is calculated as

$$z_1^{(h)} = a_0^{(in)} w_{0,1}^{(h)} + a_1^{(in)} w_{1,1}^{(h)} + \dots + a_m^{(in)} w_{m,1}^{(h)}$$

$$a_1^{(h)} = \phi\left(z_1^{(h)}\right)$$

Figure 2. Methodology

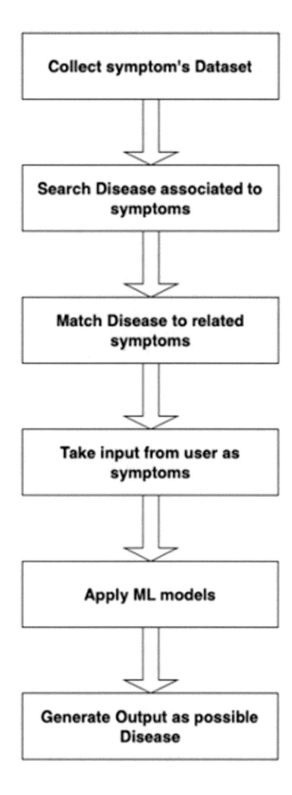

The ith value of the input layer is represented by a(in), weight coefficient is represented by w. By applying an activation function φ on the z value one can obtain the activation unit. The activation function can be calculated as

$$\phi(z) = \frac{1}{1 + e^{-z}}$$

The results of the Multilayer Perceptron implementation outdone other algorithms and were accurate up to ~97%.

4.2 Decision Tree

Decision trees can be thought of as a very powerful and adaptable classification method. Decision trees can be used for image classification and pattern recognition. As a result of its high adaptability, it is used to categorise extremely complex problems (Rahman et al., 2021). The issue with higher dimensions can also be solved by it. In addition, Herbold claimed that the decision tree algorithm is regarded as a flowchart similar to a tree structure. It has an internal mode that shows the results and the decision rule's branches. It divides nodes into sub-branches to get to the result using an if-else structure. Other algorithms may be used by Decision Tree to divide a node into sub-nodes. Several of these algorithms include

ID3 → (extension of *D3*)
C4.5 → (successor of *ID3*)
CART → (Classification and Regression Tree)

To choose the best possible attributes as a root node or branch node one can use either the Information Gain or Gini Index method-

Information Gain = Entropy-[(Weighted Average)*Entropy]
Gini Index = 1-sum of the squared probabilities of each class

The results of the Decision Tree implementation were accurate up to ~95%.

4.3 Random Forest

The Random Forest Algorithm is a supervised learning algorithm that can be applied to both classification and regression. This random forest algorithm is helpful for both classification and regression problems (Fan et al., 2016). Additionally, it can work with categorical and continuous variables. Starting with each chosen random data sample from the dataset, a decision tree is built. After that, votes are cast on each compiled result. Following the idea of bagging or bootstrap aggregating is a random forest. If bagged repeatedly, a random sample will be chosen and the training set will be replaced to fit the trees to this sample for a training set X1, X2,... Xn with responses as Y1, Y2,... Yn. Predictions for the unseen sample can be made by majority vote or by averaging predictions across all distinct regression trees:

$$f = \frac{1}{B} \sum_{b=1}^{B} f_b(x')$$

Here B is the number of times the bagging has happened, x′ is unseen samples and fb is the regression tree. The results of the Random Forest implementation were accurate up to ~93%.

4.4 Naive Bayes

A Naive Bayes algorithm is a collection of algorithms built on the Naive Bayes theorem. The idea that each prediction pair is independent of the other is one that they frequently adhere to (Wang et al., 2020). It is also assumed that traits make independent and equal contributions to prediction. In the proposed system, we used a simple Bayesian algorithm to get about ~93% accurate predictions.

It is a conditional probability-based $y = \underset{k \in \{1,\ldots,K\}}{\arg\max} \, p(C_k) \prod_{i=1}^{n} p(x_i|C_k)$ model which attaches

probability to each possible outcome [23]. The Bayes Theorem governs the Naive Bayes as

$$p(C_k|x) = \frac{p(C_k)p(x|C_k)}{p(x)}, \rightarrow\rightarrow posterior = \frac{prior \times likelihood}{evidence}$$

K is the possible outcomes; x is the problem instance that has to be classified and Ck is the class. A classifier can be obtained using this known as the Bayes Classifier.

4.5 K-Nearest Neighbour

K-Nearest Neighbour, also known as KNN, is a kind of supervised learning algorithm. This is a fundamental algorithm that is frequently used in pattern searching and data mining processes to find data patterns that link input to results, enhancing pattern recognition with each subsequent iteration (Abdul-Kareem et al., 2002). In the words of Tjahjadi and Ramli, this method can be used based on a neighbour's majority vote. Also, the k-neighbour is given a weight of age. One can start the classification by selecting the K number of neighbours. Then find the Euclidean Distance of K number of neighbours as

$$Euclidean \, distance \, between \, A_1 \, and \, B_2 = \sqrt{(X_2 - X_1)^2 + (Y_2 - Y_1)^2}$$

Take the K-nearest neighbour after that, according to Euclidean distance. Count how many data points of each type there are in each of these k neighbours. Choose the class with the most neighbours to receive new data points. With up to 92% accuracy, we classified the disease dataset using the K Nearest Neighbour method.

5. RESULT

We attempted to highlight the most well-liked machine learning techniques in this study. This essay discusses the strategy, current difficulties, and a comparison of the current and suggested systems, as shown in Table 1. A list of diseases from the dataset serves as the system's output. Multilayer perceptron (MLP) achieved the highest accurate prediction in the proposed system, which is 97%. According to a comparison of popular techniques, Multilayer Perceptron can produce results that are at least 5-6% more accurate than other prediction models in Figure 3.

Table 1. Model evaluation metrics (by comparison between different ML techniques

Algorithm	Accuracy
Multilayer Perceptron	97.2273
Decision Tree	95.1219
Random Forest	93.1433
Naive Bayes	93.0227
K Nearest Neighbor	92.3418

In Figure 4, KNN provided approximately 92% accurate predictions, Naive bias provided approximately 93%, Random Forest provided approximately 93% and Decision Tree provided approximately 95% accurate Prediction.

Figure 3. Bar graph comparison for accuracy of algorithms

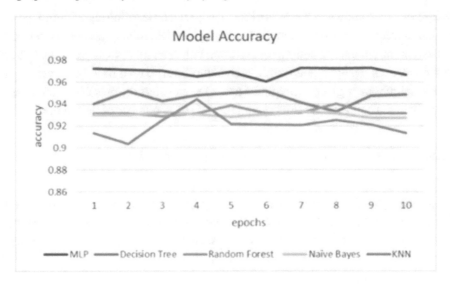

Provides an accurate comparison between the existing technologies and MLP model when implemented on the Columbia University Disease Dataset based on Presbyterian Hospital admitted during 2004.

Figure 4. Linear comparison for accuracy of algorithms

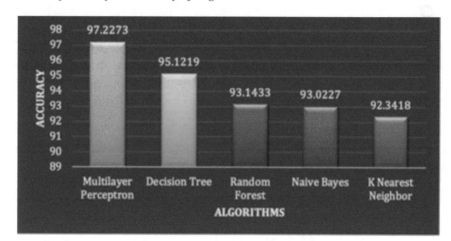

6. DISCUSSION

In this paper we have used data from the University of Columbia the following study done at New York-Presbyterian Hospital which consists of 150 prevalent diseases along with their symptoms (Javaid et al., 2023). The training dataset contains a total of 4920 rows and 133 columns whereas the testing dataset contains 41 rows and 133 columns. The dataset is made up of binary 0 and 1. In this paper Multilayer perceptron (MLP) achieved the highest accuracy in the proposed system, which is 97%. According to a comparison of popular techniques, Multilayer Perceptron can produce results that are 5-6% more accurate than other prediction models like KNN provided approximately 92%, Naive bias provided approximately 93%, Random Forest provided approximately 93%, and Decision Tree provided approximately 95% accuracy. So it's clear that the accuracy of Multilayer perceptron is on the same data set is higher than others existing algorithms.

7. CONCLUSION AND FUTURE WORK

A cutting-edge disease prediction system has been developed using the multilayer perceptron. Compared to other methods currently in use, this strategy has been shown to produce results that are more precise and significant. Our system helps users identify potential diseases by carefully analysing symptoms. The algorithms Multilayer Perceptron, Random Forest, Decision Tree, Naive Bayes, and K-Nearest Neighbour were used to build the model that is being presented. Our future work will involve conducting a thorough investigation into neural networks to gather and store real-time data for users everywhere using cloud computing. Data imbalance is one of the main issues with this system's accuracy. When creating a classification model, the final model will be biased if one class receives significantly more data than the other classes. We also intend to add extra features, like online doctor consultations. These consultations will be based on the user's understanding of symptoms, as it is not uncommon for individuals to misinterpret symptoms, resulting in inaccurate disease predictions and improper treatment.

REFERENCES

Abdul-Kareem, S., Baba, S., Zubairi, Y. Z., Prasad, U., Ibrahim, M., & Wahid, A. (2002). Prognostic systems for NPC: A comparison of the multi layer perceptron model and the recurrent model. *Proceedings of the 9th International Conference on Neural Information Processing, 2002*. IEEE. 10.1109/ICONIP.2002.1202176

Bilandi, N., Verma, H. K., & Dhir, R. (2021). An intelligent and energy-efficient wireless body area network to control coronavirus outbreak. *Arabian Journal for Science and Engineering*, *46*(9), 1–20. doi:10.1007/s13369-021-05411-2 PMID:33680703

Chen, D. (2021). Analysis of machine learning methods for COVID-19 detection using serum Raman spectroscopy. *Applied Artificial Intelligence*, *35*(14), 1147–1168. doi:10.1080/08839514.2021.1975379

da Silva, C. C., de Lima, C. L., da Silva, A. C. G., Silva, E. L., Marques, G. S., de Araújo, L. J. B., Albuquerque, L. A. Junior, de Souza, S. B. J., de Santana, M. A., & Gomes, J. C. (2021). Covid-19 dynamic monitoring and real-time spatio-temporal forecasting. *Frontiers in Public Health*, *9*, 641253. doi:10.3389/fpubh.2021.641253 PMID:33898377

Dangare, C., & Apte, S. (2012). A data mining approach for prediction of heart disease using neural networks. [IJCET]. *International Journal of Computer Engineering and Technology*, *3*(3).

Devarapalli, D., Apparao, A., Narasinga Rao, M. R., Kumar, A., & Sridhar, G. R. (2012). A Multi-layer perceptron (MLP) neural network based diagnosis of diabetes using brain derived neurotrophic factor (BDNF) levels. *Int. J. Adv. Comput*, *35*(12), 2051–0845.

Di Noia, T., Ostuni, V. C., Pesce, F., Binetti, G., Naso, D., Schena, F. P., & Di Sciascio, E. (2013). An end stage kidney disease predictor based on an artificial neural networks ensemble. *Expert Systems with Applications*, *40*(11), 4438–4445. doi:10.1016/j.eswa.2013.01.046

Do, Q., Son, T. C., & Chaudri, J. (2017). Classification of asthma severity and medication using TensorFlow and multilevel databases. *Procedia Computer Science*, *113*, 344–351. doi:10.1016/j.procs.2017.08.343

Edeh, M. O., Dalal, S., Dhaou, I. B., Agubosim, C. C., Umoke, C. C., Richard-Nnabu, N. E., & Dahiya, N. (2022). Artificial intelligence-based ensemble learning model for prediction of hepatitis C disease. *Frontiers in Public Health*, *10*, 892371. doi:10.3389/fpubh.2022.892371 PMID:35570979

Fan, X., Wang, L., & Li, S. (2016). Predicting chaotic coal prices using a multi-layer perceptron network model. *Resources Policy*, *50*, 86–92. doi:10.1016/j.resourpol.2016.08.009

Javaid, M., Sarfraz, M. S., Aftab, M. U., Zaman, Q., Rauf, H. T., & Alnowibet, K. A. (2023). WebGIS-Based Real-Time Surveillance and Response System for Vector-Borne Infectious Diseases. *International Journal of Environmental Research and Public Health*, *20*(4), 3740. doi:10.3390/ijerph20043740 PMID:36834443

Kansal, M., Singh, P., Shukla, S., & Srivastava, S. (2023). A Comparative Study of Machine Learning Models for House Price Prediction and Analysis in Smart Cities. In F. Ortiz-Rodríguez, S. Tiwari, P. Usoro Usip, & R. Palma (Eds.), Electronic Governance with Emerging Technologies (pp. 168–184). Springer Nature Switzerland. doi:10.1007/978-3-031-43940-7_14

Kansal, M., Singh, P., Srivastava, M., & Chaurasia, P. (2023). Empowering Agriculture With Conversational AI: An Application for Farmer Advisory and Communication. In Convergence of Cloud Computing, AI, and Agricultural Science (pp. 210–227). IGI Global. doi:10.4018/979-8-3693-0200-2.ch011

Lu, W. Z., Fan, H. Y., Leung, A. Y. T., & Wong, J. C. K. (2002). Analysis of pollutant levels in central Hong Kong applying neural network method with particle swarm optimization. *Environmental Monitoring and Assessment*, *79*(3), 217–230. doi:10.1023/A:1020274409612 PMID:12392160

Mariappan, M. B., Devi, K., Venkataraman, Y., & Fosso Wamba, S. (2022). A large-scale real-world comparative study using pre-COVID lockdown and post-COVID lockdown data on predicting shipment times of therapeutics in e-pharmacy supply chains. *International Journal of Physical Distribution & Logistics Management*, *52*(7), 512–537. doi:10.1108/IJPDLM-05-2021-0192

Meghriche, S., Boulemden, M., & Draa, A. (2008). Agreement between multi-layer perceptron and a compound neural network on ECG diagnosis of aatrioventricular blocks. *WSEAS Trans. Biol. Biomed*, *5*(1), 12–22.

Qteat, H., & Awad, M. (2021). Using Hybrid Model of Particle Swarm Optimization and Multi-Layer Perceptron Neural Networks for Classification of Diabetes. *International Journal of Intelligent Engineering & Systems*, *14*(3), 11–22. doi:10.22266/ijies2021.0630.02

Rahman, M. M., Islam, M. M., Manik, M. M. H., Islam, M. R., & Al-Rakhami, M. S. (2021). Machine learning approaches for tackling novel coronavirus (COVID-19) pandemic. *SN Computer Science*, *2*(5), 1–10. doi:10.1007/s42979-021-00774-7 PMID:34308367

Rajamhoana, S. P., Devi, C. A., Umamaheswari, K., Kiruba, R., Karunya, K., & Deepika, R. (2018). Analysis of neural networks based heart disease prediction system. *2018 11th International Conference on Human System Interaction (HSI)*, (pp. 233–239). IEEE.

Sailaja, N. V., Yelamarthi, M., Chandana, Y. H., Karadi, P., & Yedla, S. (2021). Early detection of sepsis on clinical data using multi-layer perceptron. Machine Learning Technologies and Applications. *Proceedings of ICACECS, 2020*, 223–233.

Sawhney, R., Malik, A., Sharma, S., & Narayan, V. (2023). A comparative assessment of artificial intelligence models used for early prediction and evaluation of chronic kidney disease. *Decision Analytics Journal*, *6*, 100169. doi:10.1016/j.dajour.2023.100169

Wang, R. Y., Guo, T. Q., Li, L. G., Jiao, J. Y., & Wang, L. Y. (2020). Predictions of COVID-19 infection severity based on co-associations between the SNPs of co-morbid diseases and COVID-19 through machine learning of genetic data. *2020 IEEE 8th International Conference on Computer Science and Network Technology (ICCSNT)*, (pp. 92–96).

Chapter 11
Mental Health Monitoring in the Digital Age:
A Comprehensive Analysis

Mrignainy Kansal
https://orcid.org/0009-0005-2610-040X
Ajay Kumar Garg Engineering College, Ghaziabad, India

Pancham Singh
https://orcid.org/0009-0005-0435-7941
Ajay Kumar Garg Engineering College, Ghaziabad, India

Prashant Srivastava
Ajay Kumar Garg Engineering College, Ghaziabad, India

Radhika Singhal
Ajay Kumar Garg Engineering College, Ghaziabad, India

Nishant Deep
Ajay Kumar Garg Engineering College, Ghaziabad, India

Arpit Singh
Ajay Kumar Garg Engineering College, Ghaziabad, India

ABSTRACT

Social media has become a significant factor in the development of mental diseases, with the potential to significantly impact people's lives. This study explores the use of computational approaches and deep learning models to identify linguistic indicators suggestive of mental diseases such as depression, anorexia, and self-harm. The study also highlights the complex relationship between emotions and the underlying causes of mental diseases, emphasizing the need for understanding emotional triggers. The research demonstrates the effectiveness of machine learning models in detecting anxiety and depression on websites like Twitter, Facebook, and Reddit, particularly during the COVID-19 pandemic. The study highlights the potential of data mining techniques for automating the diagnosis of Social Network Mental Disorders among social media users, aiming to improve lives and address the rising incidence of mental illnesses in society.

DOI: 10.4018/979-8-3693-2359-5.ch011

1. INTRODUCTION

Mental illness is a health disorder which affects an individual's opinions, feelings, and behaviours. Presently, mental diseases are one of the most significant aspects of the public medical condition and this continues to be a major cause of disability and poor health around the world. Depression, Anxiety disorder, eating disorder, Addiction behaviours, ASD, and other psychoses are some of the most frequent mental illnesses. According to the report of WHO, one-eighth of people suffer from one or more mental illnesses, which places a significant financial burden on the government's authorities. Additionally, the COVID-19 pandemic has increased the suffering of people as well as the authorities (Kim et al., 2020). The judgment that is associated with mental illness and lack of knowledge about mental health assessments prevent most affected people with mental illnesses from receiving effectual treatment and diagnosis, even though treatments and efficacious preventive measures are available. This leads to early identification of mental illness which helps in the treatment of the condition as well as preventing it from getting worse. Due to exponential growth in recent years of social platform users, it has set off a key basis of data. The usage of social media platforms like x(Twitter), LinkedIn, Instagram, and Facebook to express views as well as sentiments is growing progressively popular, particularly among young people. This leads to the growth of study interest in detecting mental illness through analysis of textual content generated by users in their social media posts. Nowadays, social media sites like X(Twitter), Facebook, Instagram, and Reddit, offer opportunities for communication with a wide range of people. Social networks also have negative aspects that can be harmful to society as well as an individual. Depression as well as suicide are mental illnesses that can be treated, and the risk of suicide can be reduced. Suicide is a deliberate act that ends a person's life.

In this study, with the centre on three detailed illnesses anorexia, depression, and self-harm we make several contributions to the research on the automatic finding of mental illnesses at different levels. To this end, we investigate the use of machine learning techniques to detect mental illnesses from writing data on social media platforms and compare them with different designs, including ranked attention transformers and networks. We develop models as shown in Figure 1 for the automated calculation of illnesses using social media platform data and concurrently measure their efficiency. We finally move beyond the static approach and suggest this, to fully comprehend the signs and symptoms of mental illnesses, we should adopt a dynamical perspective that considers how symptoms change over time, particularly how emotions change in connection to cognitive styles.

Recent advances in natural language processing (NLP) have made it possible to perform tasks like analyzing emotions, identifying rumours, and screening for mental health on social media data more easily. The increasing fascination with investigating novel techniques for the detection of mental disorders is explained by developments in natural language processing technologies and deep learning models (Tariq et al., 2019). For instance, frameworks for deep learning enable models to autonomously acquire features, eliminating the necessity for laborious feature engineering, and replacing feature Methods rooted in engineering, like CNN and RNN. Additionally, When utilized with datasets related to mental healthcare, PLMs like BERT, RoBERTa, and Mental BERT have demonstrated competitive performance in detecting mental illnesses, showcasing their potential value.

Figure 1. Architecture design

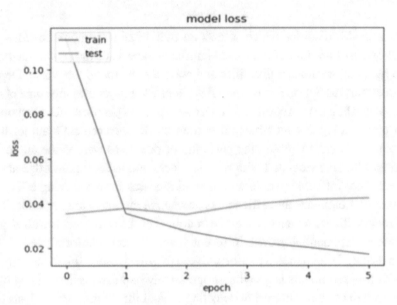

Since feelings play a significant role in human nature and have the power to influence how people behave and feel, many academic disciplines, including psychology and behavioural science, have made significant advances in our understanding of them. Researchers have discovered a link between feelings and mental illnesses like depression. The main reason is Individuals experiencing clinical depression may find it challenging to control their emotions, which leads to less emotional complexity. Therefore, from a psychological standpoint, knowledge of emotions can help with mental illness diagnosis.

Psychologists have investigated how social media emotions may affect mental health. According to several studies, people with mental illnesses express different emotions in their online posts than people without mental illnesses do (Zeberga et al., 2022). Social media service-related posts like Suicidal posts are connected to the user's mental state, with negative feelings appearing remarkably more frequently as compared to positive feelings, according to a study on the finding of suicidal feelings in posts on social media platforms. These studies highlight the often combination or integration of feelings into medical applications to support the detection of mental illness. This article is the starting analysis of textual feelings information combination for mental illness detection, as far as we are aware. To better understand the importance of feelings information in establishing mental illness as well as the role of feelings combination strategies in aiding this identification, this thorough survey.

Numerous depressing posts circulate on social media, necessitating an automatic identification system to save human lives. There are three Reddit posts, two of which have yellow backgrounds to indicate suicidal content, and one of which has a green background to indicate depressive content. The user expresses explicit thoughts of suicide in the first post, which expresses conflicting emotions (Karmegam et al., 2020). The user mentions having suicidal thoughts in the back of his mind in the third post. In the second post, the user discusses their struggle with bipolar disorder as well as his feelings of depression and anxiety. The second post's user may experience severe depression in the future; as a result, this user requires medical therapy.

2. RESEARCH QUESTION

Q1: How may social media users' language detection in the early detection of mental illnesses?
   Q2: How well do Machine Learning algorithms recognize the symptoms of mental disorders?

3. LITERATURE REVIEW

A literature review for the project on "Mental Illness Detection using Machine Learning" is essential to understand the existing research, methodologies, and technologies related to mental health diagnosis and machine learning applications. Here is a brief literature review covering some relevant areas:

1. **Machine Learning in Mental Health Diagnosis:** In the paper "Machine Learning for Mental Health in social media: Bibliometric Study "Numerous studies have explored the application of machine learning algorithms in mental health diagnosis (Losada et al., 2018). highlights the growth in this area and various techniques used for sentiment analysis and mental health prediction based on social media data.
2. **Textual Data Analysis:** In the paper "Detecting Depression with Social Media" Textual data from social media platforms, online forums, and electronic health records have been extensively used for mental health assessment (Kim et al., 2021) demonstrates the feasibility of identifying individuals with depression based on language patterns in their social media posts.
3. **Physiological Data and Wearable Sensors:** In the paper "A Preliminary Study" Utilizing physiological data from wearable sensors has gained attention in mental health research. "Wearable Sensors for Mood Recognition in Bipolar Disorder (Guntuku et al., 2017a) explores the use of wearable technology to monitor mood and detect episodes in bipolar disorder patients.
4. **Feature Engineering and Data Pre-processing:** In the paper "Feature Engineering for Machine Learning: Principles and Techniques for Data Scientists" Feature engineering plays a vital role in extracting meaningful information from diverse data sources (Guidi et al., 2016) and provides insights into best practices in feature selection and engineering.
5. **Machine learning models:** In the paper "Deep Learning for Mental Health Prediction from Social Media Text" Various machine learning models have been applied to mental health prediction tasks. For instance, (Zheng & Casari, 2018) discusses the use of deep learning techniques for mental health prediction based on social media text.
6. **User interface and deployment:** In the paper Research on "Designing User Interfaces for an Artificial Intelligence-Based Application for Mental Health Monitoring" User-friendly interfaces and deployment strategies are crucial for the practical application of mental health detection systems (Ameer et al., 2022) and address the usability aspects of such systems.
7. **Ethical and Privacy Considerations:** In the paper "Ethical Issues in Predictive Mental Health Algorithms" Ensuring privacy and ethical use of data is paramount in mental health applications (Bharti et al., 2020) discusses ethical challenges and considerations when developing AI-based mental health tools.

8. **Real-world application:** In the paper " condition. By conducting a comprehensive literature review, you can build upon existing knowledge and a methodology to design and implement an effective mental illness detection system using machine learning, considering the unique aspects of your project and data sources. Additionally, this review will help you identify gaps in the current research that your project can address. Machine Learning for Early Prediction of Alzheimer's Diagnosis and Progression" Case studies and real-world applications of machine learning in mental health diagnosis provide valuable insights. (Loch et al., 2022) is an example of applying machine learning to detect Alzheimer's disease, a type of mental health.

4. RELATED WORK

Many studies in the field tend to rely on quantifiable assessments and predictive models established through machine learning algorithms as a common approach, while a smaller proportion of research ventures into more innovative territory by employing deep learning techniques like various Convolutional Neural Network (CNN) or Recurrent Neural Network (RNN) models, as well as word embeddings. Notably, prior research consistently highlights the significance of linguistic features, such as LIWC categories, emotional expressions, and pronoun usage, in the context of detecting mental disorders from social media posts (D'Alfonso, 2020). To the best of our knowledge, our study takes a novel approach by utilizing a deep neural architecture that incorporates a diverse range of linguistic variables to model the indicators of mental disorders within the content of social media posts. Recent advances in the field have seen an increasing interest in applying deep learning techniques to classify mental disorders, often leveraging word order as a critical feature. The models we have selected for this endeavour stand out for their exceptional performance and understanding, largely attributed to their utilization of hierarchical structures, helpfulness, and the incorporation of various linguistic features.

Figure 2. Research challenges

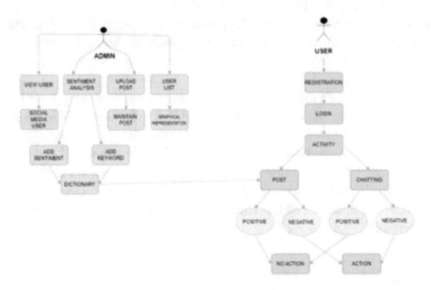

While previous research has acknowledged the implication of feelings in modelling psychological disorders, limited studies spread beyond basic measurable analysis. Through three different investigations focused on identifying depression, anorexia, and self-abuse as shown in Figure 2, we introduce a substitute approach that prioritises a comprehensive exploration of feelings to represent psychological health circumstances through linguistic analysis (Gkotsis et al., 2017). In our emotional model, we move our focus towards tracing the progress of emotions over time in conjunction with cognitive styles and, the presentation of distinct correlation shapes specific to many mental illnesses.

In the quest to recognize mental health conditions, there has been a rising interest in the concept of feeling fusion. We have accurately examined different literature databases to conduct a widespread analysis of published works exploring the application of feeling fusion approaches in mental illness detection (Liu et al., 2022). Feelings, intricate states of feeling ambitious by neurophysiological changes, exert a deep influence on frequent facets of individual existence. Given the extensive use of natural language to convey feelings, the field of NLP, i.e., Natural Language Processing has become progressively capitalized in the study of human emotional expression, which is a vital module in most real-world applications, mainly in the domain of feeling detection.

As sentiment exhibits a close link with feeling, it comes within the view of our article. Sentiment entails a psychological stance or thought influenced by feelings. An important module of NPL techniques, sentiment analysis, finds wide-ranging applications in the field like social media platforms, author identification, consumer reaction, rumour analysis, and health IP (Guntuku et al., 2017a). These sentiment analysis structures can classify social media comments into positive, neutral, or negative, sentiment classifications, or scale the strength of sentiment depending on the specific circumstance.

Scarce research endeavours have integrated multiple language-based variables into their prototypes for measuring the hypothetical emergence of psychological health issues. An earlier study searching the early identification of self-abuse leanings proposed a classified neural network comprising LSTM, i.e., Long Short-Term Memory and CNN, i.e., Convolutional Neural Network layers (Guntuku et al., 2017b). This network was trained on social media comments, merging content elements, sensitive cues, and technical features. Few investigations concurrently deliberate multiple psychological health illnesses. Quantitative analyses of previous research on mental illnesses uncover that individual with depression frequently noticeable linguistic changes, including sensitive usage of negative feelings or comment on social media platforms. Other computational studies have figured out specific recurrent subjects among individuals revealing depression, like confessing about health treatments or physical issues like sleeplessness, as well as looks of hopelessness and irritation (Salas-Zárate et al., 2022). However, linking lessons have restrictions in uncovering more subtle links with textual characters and the tendency for psychological illness.

Additionally, most of the computer-based research signifies the symptoms of psychological disorders as static actions, but the development of psychological illness displays as well as the frequency with which they look in social media user-comments is an important indicator of an individual's chance of budding a psychological disease (Ji et al., 2022). We signify one earlier research. The tendency of machine learning and deep learning algorithms to quickly define users who have been analyzed with a condition is tested by handling the stream of chronologically arranged social media comments. However, few suggestions try to classify the input data as a replication of a dynamic process; in its place, comments are provided at the consumer level and are static.

4. METHODOLOGY

Figure 3. Methodology

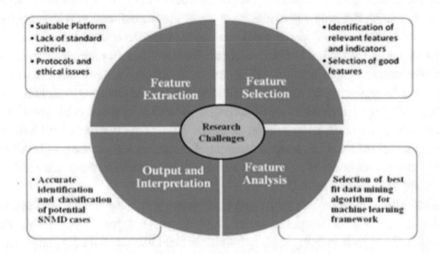

1. **Dataset creation principles**: For the investigation of complicated emotion-cause pair extraction, there is currently no large-scale relation dataset available. The following guidelines should be followed when creating a sizable dataset on emotion-cause relations (Kansal et al., 2023).
2. **Simpleness**: To give more meta-information on the word level, complex sequence tagging systems have been developed; however, these solutions are not replicable for large-scale corpora. The encoders' annotation efforts should be reduced by giving less meta-information because data annotation is expensive.
3. **Extensibility**: There are now several dispersed causal association datasets accessible, and while having many different annotation techniques, they are not incompatible. For the advancement of causality identification, incompatibility is starting to act as a roadblock (Hosseini et al., 2021). The extensible annotation method makes it possible to transform existing datasets into a single format.
4. **Adaptability**: Prior research only included simple causal ties in the datasets and ignored the significance of interaction for complex causal relations because they did not take into account the distinctions between simple causal relations and complex causal relations (Singh et al., 2023). To discover how different spans interact, a lot of intricate causal relationships should be used.
5. **Data collection**: We gathered emotional data from Reddit to discover the emotions and the associated causes of mental illness groups. Phrases are used by those who are experiencing mental health issues. Reddit is made up of a sizable number of online communities specifically, subreddits), where users may exchange user-generated content or leave comments on posts made by others (Crestani et al., 2022). There are a lot of subreddits devoted to mental health issues. The most prevalent mental diseases were selected to enhance the data coverage and utilized as search terms to find the subreddits related to these mental health issues. Following the keyword mapping, many of These keywords' related subreddits were found. Given the vagueness of the terms, we looked at the metaprofile data of subreddits to see if they were linked to mental health issues. Particularly,

all These Reddit threads were divided into two categories (related to and unconnected to mental health concerns), two coders manually subreddits. The agreement of the data that were labelled was measured using the Pearson Correlation (PCCs) (Loch et al., 2022). We learn that The labelled results agree with PCCs =0.92 in all cases. When the original two coders couldn't agree on how to code the subreddits, a third coder one another. If the third coder disagrees with the first two coders, those subreddits are disregarded. Lastly, the Data was gathered from subreddits that are directly related to mental health. We gathered the comments and Using the Pushshift API, you may add metadata, such as user names, timestamps, and community information.

6. **The Annotated data**: We developed the user interface for data annotation and hired three native English speakers. Phrase-level annotation is a requirement for all volunteers. The introduction of several word-level annotation techniques (McClellan et al., 2017). Volunteers must spend a lot of time and effort tagging each word in the training examples.

It is been briefly examined in current computer-based studies on psychological illnesses, models based on neural networks are pretty operative for many NLP applications as shown in Figure 3. However, neural networks are disreputable and hard to understand. Recently, there has been a rise in significance in the speciality of machine learning techniques, predominantly in NLP, which requests to understand neural network judgments (Verma et al., 2022). The psychological situation recognition tool's judgment procedure must be vibrant if it is to help users of social media platforms.

Figure 4. Flow diagram

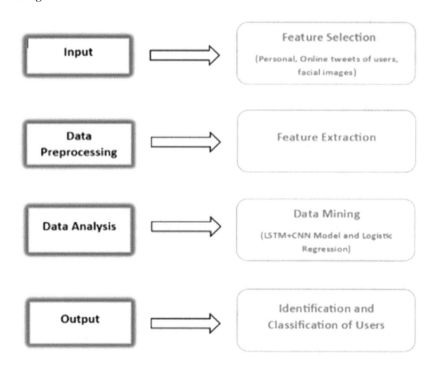

Figure 4 shows the overall classification of the different modules used to detect mental illness on social media platforms. Four categories make up the classification: Datasets, Algorithms, Models, and Features. Several social media platforms, including Instagram, Reddit, and Facebook, X(Twitter) provide instruction datasets (Tao & Fisher, 2022). It is standard to perform some pre-processing on these datasets, such as tokenization, removal of stop words and/or special terms, and normalization.

The next category is Features, which are fragmented into four parts: distributed features, Linguistic Features, Statical Features, and Domain Features. Whereas distributed signs have been broadly used in Deep Learning-related models, the starting three points are typically obtained using NLP techniques. Regarding finding models, there are deep learning-related and outdated machine learning-related approaches. The classification's final category, titled "Algorithm" is divided into three main categories: supervised, semi-supervised and unsupervised learning (Kim et al., 2021). The latter group can be further segmented into fully supervised, semi-supervised, and distantly supervised methods. According to their volume to accomplish greater implementation when qualified using high-grade datasets, many models for the finding of mental illness use supervised learning methods.

5. PROPOSED ALGORITHM

Depression is a common mental health disorder that negatively affects how you feel, the way you think and how you act. It can lead to a variety of emotional and physical problems and can decrease your ability to function at work and home. Social media platforms, such as Twitter, have become popular platforms for people to express their thoughts and feelings (Ameer et al., 2022). This has led to a growing interest in using social media data to detect depression. In this project, we developed and evaluated two models for depression detection in tweets: an LSTM+CNN model and a logistic regression model as shown in Figure 5.

Figure 5. Proposed methodology

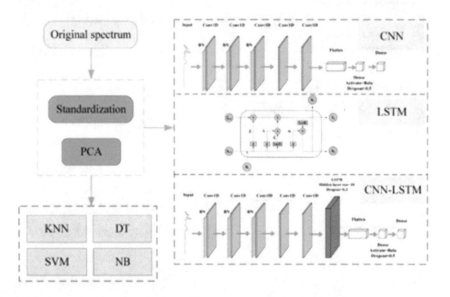

1. **LSTM+CNN Model:** LSTM+CNN models are a type of deep learning model that combines the strengths of two different types of neural networks: Long Short-Term Memory (LSTM) networks and Convolutional Neural Networks (CNNs). LSTM networks are well-suited for tasks such as sentiment analysis and text classification because they can learn long-range dependencies in text (Teague et al., 2022). CNNs are well-suited for tasks such as image classification and feature extraction because they can learn local features from data. In our LSTM+CNN model, the LSTM layer is used to learn long-range dependencies in the tweets, and the CNN layer is used to learn local features from the text. The output of the CNN layer is then fed to a dense layer to produce the final prediction.

2. **Logistic Regression Model:** Logistic regression is a simple but effective machine learning algorithm that can be used for classification tasks. In logistic regression, a linear function is used to predict the probability that a given example belongs to a particular class. In our logistic regression model, we used a variety of features as shown in Figure 6, including the number of words in a tweet (Zhang et al., 2022), the number of hashtags, the number of retweets, and the number of likes, to predict whether or not a tweet is indicative of depression.

Figure 6. Logistic regression

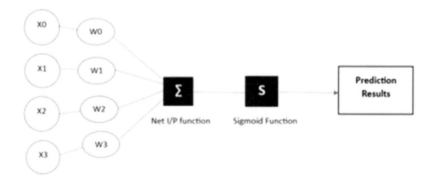

3. **Data:** We used a dataset of 3200 tweets, half of which were labelled as depressive and the other half of which were labelled as non-depressive as shown in Figure 7. The tweets were collected from a variety of sources, including Twitter accounts of people with depression, and Twitter accounts of people who are not depressed.

In the research work, we have conducted two experiments for the evaluation of our model

*   **Experiment 1:** We trained and evaluated our LSTM+CNN model and our logistic regression model on a held-out test set.
    *   **Result**: Our LSTM+CNN model achieved an accuracy of 98.98% on the held-out test set. Our logistic regression model achieved an accuracy of 76.53% on the held-out test set.

- **Experiment 2:** We compared the accuracy of our LSTM+CNN model to the accuracy of our logistic regression model.
  - ○ **Result:** Our LSTM+CNN model outperformed our logistic regression model on the held-out test set by 3.5%.

Figure 7. Data distribution graph

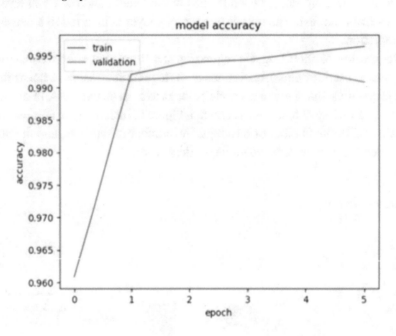

6. RESULTS

In recent years, there has been an increase in interest in using social media to identify mental illnesses. This article offers a thorough analysis of the emotion fusion techniques used for this job, dividing them into deep learning-based and feature engineering-based approaches. The survey's findings show that fusing emotions is a highly successful strategy.

The work targets three distinct diseases (depression, anorexia, and self-harm) and proposes an automated identification of mental disorders based on language cues retrieved from social media. Deep learning algorithms are effective in identifying social media users who run the risk of developing a mental illness (RQ1) as shown in Figure 8. They reflect the messages they publish online with linguistic elements at several levels, including the message's substance, as well as the user's writing style and the emotions conveyed. The study also emphasizes the significance of tracking afflicted people's language from the moment the disease first manifests itself and simulating how linguistic signals change over time (Parry et al., 2022). Although emotions are particularly important for mental health, it makes more sense to treat each emotion independently and link it to certain subjects' cognitive styles as shown by language indicators. Through computer analysis of these multidimensional linguistic variables time, distinguishable patterns that differentiate between users with and without mental disorders (RQ3) were found.

Figure 8. Accuracy graph

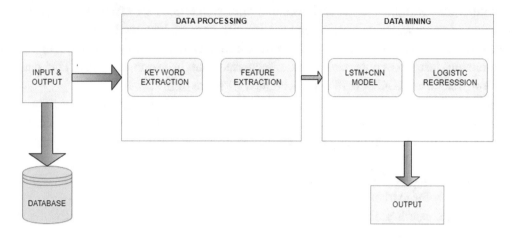

Figure 9. Error graph

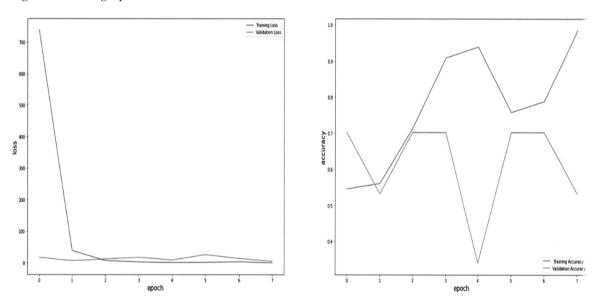

The examination of emotion evolution has shown that understanding linguistic indicators of mental health in more detail requires understanding the time element of mental illness symptoms reflected in language. The creation of a dataset with annotations that are momentarily aware might be a useful area for future study. Our model of emotion evolution through time in connection to several psycho-linguistic categories may be useful for sentiment analysis as well as the broader study of semantic change in language, which goes beyond the field of mental disease identification. To capture the intricate inter-play between many causes and feelings, we developed a large-scale emotion-cause dataset containing complicated emotion-cause instances and presented a contrastive learning-based technique (Shannon et al., 2022). On three datasets, several experiments were run to assess the model's performance. The main findings reveal that N2NCause performs better at extracting complicated emotion-cause pairings as shown in Figure 9. Our suggested remedies may be used to identify emotional distribution triggers among communities with mental health issues and offer suggestions for efficiency. This study on the categorization of material for depression and suicide risk showed how well the suggested framework recognized the possibility of mental illness from Reddit social media postings. Where long Reddit postings predominate, fast Text contextual analysis increased categorisation accuracy. This data's binary classification yielded an AUC of 0.78 and a weighted F1 score of 0.71.

Numerous unpleasant emotions and anxiety-based traits can enhance this research. The multiclass categorization may be added in the future to examine the severity of depression and suicide postings. Another potential area for future study is an automated detection system to pinpoint users who require urgent medical attention. It's fascinating to consider the use of Social Network Mental Disorders Detection Analysis while considering the potential of Natural Language Processing for automated text analysis. It is used occasionally for marketing and in social media trend research. Modern, ready-to-use packages make it simple to create SNMD Analysis programs in Python. By determining in advance whether a person is depressed and even sending them motivating posts based on the severity of their depression, the suggested system would assist suspected individuals in saving their lives.

7. DISCUSSION

Our results show that the LSTM+CNN model is more effective at detecting depression in tweets than the logistic regression model. This is likely because the LSTM+CNN model can learn long-range dependencies in the text, which are important for understanding the sentiment and tone of a tweet. Our results also suggest that social media data can be used to effectively detect depression. This is important because social media data can be collected passively and non-intrusively, which makes it a scalable and cost-effective way to screen for depression.

8. CONCLUSION

In conclusion, "Mental Health Monitoring in Digital Age" is a game-changer in the field of mental health care since it uses a complex combination of logistic regression and LSTM+CNN models. Deep learning and conventional algorithms are integrated to provide sophisticated social media data analysis for the early identification of mental health problems. This creative method offers a scalable and user-friendly solution while simultaneously giving ethical data practices, user privacy, and responsible AI priority. This research work, which combines cutting-edge technology with careful design, not only helps with early intervention but also paves the way for a future in mental health treatment and awareness that is more knowledgeable, compassionate, and helpful.

9. FUTURE WORK

In the future, use a larger and more diverse dataset of depressive tweets and then improve the model accordingly. Explore the use of other features, such as the sentiment of the tweets and the topics that the tweets are about. Also plan to investigate the use of other types of deep learning models, such as transformers. We believe that our work has the potential to help develop new tools for screening for depression and other mental health disorders.

REFERENCES

Ameer, I., Arif, M., Sidorov, G., Gòmez-Adorno, H., & Gelbukh, A. (2022). *Mental Illness Classification on Social Media Texts using Deep Learning and Transfer Learning* (arXiv:2207.01012). arXiv. http://arxiv.org/abs/2207.01012

Bharti, U., Bajaj, D., Batra, H., Lalit, S., Lalit, S., & Gangwani, A. (2020). Medbot: Conversational artificial intelligence powered chatbot for delivering tele-health after covid-19. *2020 5th International Conference on Communication and Electronics Systems (ICCES),* (pp. 870–875). IEEE. https://ieeexplore.ieee.org/abstract/document/9137944/

Crestani, F., Losada, D. E., & Parapar, J. (2022). *Early Detection of Mental Health Disorders by Social Media Monitoring: The First Five Years of the ERisk Project (Vol. 1018).* Springer Nature. https://books.google.com/books?hl=en&lr=&id=03KJEAAAQBAJ&oi=fnd&pg=PR5&dq=Mental+Health+Monitoring+from+social+media+content&ots=imytRcJRhF&sig=66ToTnyQucKr9ulHSUQZA4Po-Hg

D'Alfonso, S. (2020). AI in mental health. *Current Opinion in Psychology, 36,* 112–117. doi:10.1016/j.copsyc.2020.04.005 PMID:32604065

Gkotsis, G., Oellrich, A., Velupillai, S., Liakata, M., Hubbard, T. J., Dobson, R. J., & Dutta, R. (2017). Characterisation of mental health conditions in social media using Informed Deep Learning. *Scientific Reports, 7*(1), 45141. doi:10.1038/srep45141 PMID:28327593

Guidi, A., Lanata, A., Baragli, P., Valenza, G., & Scilingo, E. P. (2016). A wearable system for the evaluation of the human-horse interaction: A preliminary study. *Electronics (Basel), 5*(4), 63. doi:10.3390/electronics5040063

Guntuku, S. C., Yaden, D. B., Kern, M. L., Ungar, L. H., & Eichstaedt, J. C. (2017a). Detecting depression and mental illness on social media: An integrative review. *Current Opinion in Behavioral Sciences, 18,* 43–49. doi:10.1016/j.cobeha.2017.07.005

Guntuku, S. C., Yaden, D. B., Kern, M. L., Ungar, L. H., & Eichstaedt, J. C. (2017b). Detecting depression and mental illness on social media: An integrative review. *Current Opinion in Behavioral Sciences, 18,* 43–49. doi:10.1016/j.cobeha.2017.07.005

Ji, S., Li, X., Huang, Z., & Cambria, E. (2022). Suicidal ideation and mental disorder detection with attentive relation networks. *Neural Computing & Applications, 34*(13), 10309–10319. doi:10.1007/s00521-021-06208-y

Kansal, M., Singh, P., Shukla, S., & Srivastava, S. (2023). A Comparative Study of Machine Learning Models for House Price Prediction and Analysis in Smart Cities. In F. Ortiz-Rodríguez, S. Tiwari, P. Usoro Usip, & R. Palma (Eds.), Electronic Governance with Emerging Technologies (pp. 168–184). Springer Nature Switzerland. doi:10.1007/978-3-031-43940-7_14

Karmegam, D., Ramamoorthy, T., & Mappillairajan, B. (2020). A systematic review of techniques employed for determining mental health using social media in psychological surveillance during disasters. *Disaster Medicine and Public Health Preparedness*, *14*(2), 265–272. doi:10.1017/dmp.2019.40 PMID:31272518

Kim, J., Lee, D., & Park, E. (2021). Machine learning for mental health in social media: Bibliometric study. *Journal of Medical Internet Research*, *23*(3), e24870. doi:10.2196/24870 PMID:33683209

Kim, J., Lee, J., Park, E., & Han, J. (2020). A deep learning model for detecting mental illness from user content on social media. *Scientific Reports*, *10*(1), 11846. doi:10.1038/s41598-020-68764-y PMID:32678250

Liu, D., Feng, X. L., Ahmed, F., Shahid, M., & Guo, J. (2022). Detecting and measuring depression on social media using a machine learning approach: Systematic review. *JMIR Mental Health*, *9*(3), e27244. doi:10.2196/27244 PMID:35230252

Loch, A. A., Lopes-Rocha, A. C., Ara, A., Gondim, J. M., Cecchi, G. A., Corcoran, C. M., Mota, N. B., & Argolo, F. C. (2022). Ethical implications of the use of language analysis technologies for the diagnosis and prediction of psychiatric disorders. *JMIR Mental Health*, *9*(11), e41014. doi:10.2196/41014 PMID:36318266

Losada, D. E., Crestani, F., & Parapar, J. (2018). Overview of eRisk: Early Risk Prediction on the Internet. In P. Bellot, C. Trabelsi, J. Mothe, F. Murtagh, J. Y. Nie, L. Soulier, E. SanJuan, L. Cappellato, & N. Ferro (Eds.), Experimental IR Meets Multilinguality, Multimodality, and Interaction (Vol. 11018, pp. 343–361). Springer International Publishing. doi:10.1007/978-3-319-98932-7_30

McClellan, C., Ali, M. M., Mutter, R., Kroutil, L., & Landwehr, J. (2017). Using social media to monitor mental health discussions- evidence from Twitter. *Journal of the American Medical Informatics Association : JAMIA*, *24*(3), 496–502. doi:10.1093/jamia/ocw133 PMID:27707822

Parry, D. A., Fisher, J. T., Mieczkowski, H., Sewall, C. J., & Davidson, B. I. (2022). Social media and well-being: A methodological perspective. *Current Opinion in Psychology*, *45*, 101285. doi:10.1016/j.copsyc.2021.11.005 PMID:35008029

Salas-Zárate, R., Alor-Hernández, G., Salas-Zárate, M. del P., Paredes-Valverde, M. A., Bustos-López, M., & Sánchez-Cervantes, J. L. (2022). Detecting depression signs on social media: A systematic literature review. *Health Care*, *10*(2), 291. https://www.mdpi.com/2227-9032/10/2/291 PMID:35206905

Shannon, H., Bush, K., Villeneuve, P. J., Hellemans, K. G., & Guimond, S. (2022). Problematic social media use in adolescents and young adults: Systematic review and meta-analysis. *JMIR Mental Health*, *9*(4), e33450. doi:10.2196/33450 PMID:35436240

Singh, P., Kansal, M., Srivastava, M., & Gupta, M. (2023). Smart Agriculture Resource Allocation and Cost Optimization Using ML in Cloud Computing Environment. In Convergence of Cloud Computing, AI, and Agricultural Science (pp. 152–163). IGI Global. doi:10.4018/979-8-3693-0200-2.ch008

Tao, X., & Fisher, C. B. (2022). Exposure to Social Media Racial Discrimination and Mental Health among Adolescents of Color. *Journal of Youth and Adolescence*, *51*(1), 30–44. doi:10.1007/s10964-021-01514-z PMID:34686952

Tariq, S., Akhtar, N., Afzal, H., Khalid, S., Mufti, M. R., Hussain, S., Habib, A., & Ahmad, G. (2019). A novel co-training-based approach for the classification of mental illnesses using social media posts. *IEEE Access: Practical Innovations, Open Solutions, 7*, 166165–166172. doi:10.1109/ACCESS.2019.2953087

Teague, S. J., Shatte, A. B., Weller, E., Fuller-Tyszkiewicz, M., & Hutchinson, D. M. (2022). Methods and applications of social media monitoring of mental health during disasters: Scoping review. *JMIR Mental Health, 9*(2), e33058. doi:10.2196/33058 PMID:35225815

Verma, G., Bhardwaj, A., Aledavood, T., De Choudhury, M., & Kumar, S. (2022). Examining the impact of sharing COVID-19 misinformation online on mental health. *Scientific Reports, 12*(1), 8045. doi:10.1038/s41598-022-11488-y PMID:35577820

Zeberga, K., Attique, M., Shah, B., Ali, F., Jembre, Y. Z., & Chung, T.-S. (2022). A novel text mining approach for mental health prediction using Bi-LSTM and BERT model. *Computational Intelligence and Neuroscience, 2022*, 1–18. https://www.hindawi.com/journals/cin/2022/7893775/. doi:10.1155/2022/7893775 PMID:35281185

Zhang, T., Schoene, A. M., Ji, S., & Ananiadou, S. (2022). Natural language processing applied to mental illness detection: A narrative review. *NPJ Digital Medicine, 5*(1), 46. doi:10.1038/s41746-022-00589-7 PMID:35396451

Zheng, A., & Casari, A. (2018). *Feature engineering for machine learning: Principles and techniques for data scientists.* O'Reilly Media, Inc. https://books.google.com/books?hl=en&lr=&id=sthSDwAAQBAJ&oi=fnd&pg=PT24&dq=Zheng,+A.,+%26+Casari,+A.+(2018).+Feature+engineering+for+machine+learning:+principles+and+techniques+for+data+scientists.+%22+O%27Reilly+Media,+Inc.%22&ots=ZPWan_4mu1&sig=nt-jerAemDWDZvj07gudiPkwd_4

Chapter 12
Emerging, Assistive, and Digital Technology in Telemedicine Systems

Shabnam Kumari

SRM Institute of Science and Technology, Chennai, India

Amit Kumar Tyagi

https://orcid.org/0000-0003-2657-8700

National Institute of Fashion Technology, New Delhi, India

Avinash Kumar Sharma

https://orcid.org/0000-0001-6762-6778

Sharda School of Engineering and Technology (SSET), Sharda University, India

ABSTRACT

In the recent decade, emerging, assistive, and digital technologies have revolutionized the field of telemedicine, enabling remote healthcare delivery, improving patient outcomes, and expanding access to medical services. This chapter provides an overview of the advancements and applications of these technologies in telemedicine systems. Today mobile apps provide convenient access to medical services, appointment scheduling, medication reminders, and health education. EHRs store and share patient information securely, enabling seamless collaboration and continuity of care across healthcare settings. Telemedicine apps provide intuitive interfaces for video consultations, remote examinations, and sharing of medical data, facilitating efficient remote diagnosis and treatment. Hence, emerging, assistive, and digital technologies have transformed telemedicine, enhancing healthcare delivery, patient engagement, and access to specialized medical expertise. These technologies have the potential to revolutionize healthcare systems, particularly in remote and underserved areas.

DOI: 10.4018/979-8-3693-2359-5.ch012

1. INTRODUCTION TO TELEMEDICINE, DIGITAL TRANSFORMATION/ DIGITAL TECHNOLOGY

Telemedicine is a swiftly expanding sector in healthcare that leverages digital technology to offer remote medical services and consultations (Amit, Timothy, et al., 2023) (Shankar, Deeba, et al., 2023). This approach enables patients to connect with healthcare professionals and receive medical advice, diagnoses, and treatment without necessitating in-person visits to a healthcare facility. The increasing prominence of telemedicine in recent years can be attributed to advancements in digital technology and the demand for convenient and accessible healthcare services. Key components of telemedicine encompass:

- Communication Technology: Telemedicine utilizes a range of digital communication tools such as video conferencing, audio calls, instant messaging, and email to establish connections between healthcare providers and patients. These technological tools enable real-time interactions and the seamless exchange of medical information.
- Electronic Health Records (EHR): Digital patient records and medical information are central to telemedicine. EHR systems store and manage patient data, making it easily accessible to healthcare professionals during virtual consultations.
- Remote Monitoring: Some telemedicine applications incorporate wearable devices and remote monitoring tools that transmit real-time health data to healthcare providers. This allows for ongoing monitoring of a patient's health status and enables prompt intervention when needed.
- Secure Data Transmission: Ensuring the privacy and security of patient information is paramount in telemedicine. It is crucial to securely transmit and store sensitive health data to uphold patient trust and comply with healthcare regulations.
- Mobile Apps and Online Portals: Many telemedicine services are easily accessible through mobile apps or online portals, providing patients with the convenience of scheduling appointments, accessing medical records, and communicating with healthcare providers effortlessly.

Benefits of Telemedicine:

- Accessibility: By removing geographical barriers, telemedicine makes healthcare services accessible to individuals in remote or underserved areas. Patients can receive specialized care without the necessity of undertaking long-distance travel.
- Convenience: Telemedicine eliminates the need for time-consuming visits to a healthcare facility, reducing waiting times and making healthcare more convenient for patients.
- Cost Savings: Patients and healthcare providers alike can experience savings on transportation costs and office space expenses, contributing to potential cost reductions within the healthcare system.
- Continuity of Care: Telemedicine facilitates enhanced continuity of care, as patients can conveniently follow up with their healthcare providers, resulting in improved management of chronic conditions.
- Digital Transformation and Digital Technology in Healthcare: Digital transformation in healthcare involves incorporating and embracing digital technologies and tools to enhance various facets of the healthcare industry.

This transformation spans various applications, including electronic health records, telemedicine, data analytics, and artificial intelligence. Below are some essential components of the digital transformation in healthcare:

- Electronic Health Records (EHRs): Electronic Health Record (EHR) systems electronically store patient records, providing easy accessibility for healthcare providers. EHRs streamline data management, minimize errors, and improve collaboration among medical professionals.
- Big Data and Analytics: Healthcare organizations utilize big data analytics to extract insights from vast datasets, shedding light on patient outcomes, disease trends, and operational efficiency. Adopting this data-driven approach can result in enhanced decision-making and improved patient care.
- Telehealth and Telemedicine: As mentioned earlier, telehealth and telemedicine are significant components of digital transformation, enabling remote healthcare services through digital technology.
- Artificial Intelligence (AI): AI is employed for diagnostic support, predictive analytics, and process automation (Amit Kumar Tyagi, 2022). AI algorithms possess the capability to analyze medical images, recognize patterns in patient data, and aid healthcare providers in making more precise diagnoses and treatment recommendations.
- Internet of Things (IoT): IoT devices, including wearables and remote monitoring tools, gather real-time health data from patients and transmit it to healthcare providers. This ongoing monitoring has the potential for early intervention and improved disease management.
- Cloud Computing: Cloud-based services enable the secure storage and sharing of medical data, allowing healthcare professionals to access information from anywhere with an internet connection.
- Blockchain: Blockchain technology has the potential to improve data security and integrity in healthcare by creating a tamper-proof and transparent record of transactions and data access
- Mobile Health (mHealth): Mobile apps and devices are used to monitor health, deliver healthcare information, and enable remote consultations.

Therefore, digital technology in healthcare holds the potential to enhance patient outcomes, boost operational efficiency, and decrease costs. Nevertheless, it also presents challenges concerning data privacy, security, and regulatory compliance, requiring careful consideration during the digital transformation process.

1.1 Evolution of Telemedicine

The evolution of telemedicine has been a dynamic journey shaped by technological advancements, changing healthcare needs (Amit Kumar Tyagi and Richa. 2023) (Meghna Manoj Nair and Amit Kumar Tyagi,2023) (Dhakshan Y., Amit Kumar Tyagi, 2023), and evolving healthcare policies. Here's an overview of the key milestones and stages in the evolution of telemedicine:

A. Early Telemedicine Concepts (1920s-1940s):
   ○ The idea of using telecommunication technology for healthcare consultations dates back to the early 20th century.

        ◦   Radiology and electrocardiography were among the first medical fields to explore remote consultation using telegraph and telephone systems.

B.   Telemedicine Via Radio and Television (1950s-1960s):

        ◦   Televised medical consultations and radio broadcasts for medical education began to emerge.

        ◦   NASA played a role in developing telemedicine for space missions to provide remote medical support for astronauts.

C.   Telemedicine in Rural Areas (1970s-1980s):

        ◦   Telemedicine started to address healthcare disparities in rural and underserved areas.

        ◦   The use of closed-circuit television systems connected remote clinics to urban medical centers for consultations.

D.   Growth of Telemedicine Networks (1990s-2000s):

        ◦   Advances in video conferencing and digital imaging technologies allowed for real-time consultations between healthcare providers and patients.

        ◦   Telemedicine networks and programs were established to provide a broader range of services, including teleradiology and telepsychiatry.

E.   Expansion of Telehealth Services (2010s):

        ◦   The terms "telemedicine" and "telehealth" began to be used interchangeably.

        ◦   The advent of mobile devices and high-speed internet connectivity facilitated the growth of telehealth services.

        ◦   Telehealth platforms, mobile health apps, and telemedicine companies started to proliferate.

F.   Telemedicine During the COVID-19 Pandemic (2020s):

        ◦   The COVID-19 pandemic expedited the embrace of telemedicine in response to social distancing measures and the increased demand for remote healthcare services.

        ◦   Regulatory barriers were temporarily relaxed to expand telehealth access, and reimbursement policies were adjusted to support virtual care.

        ◦   Telemedicine saw unprecedented growth in various specialties, including primary care, mental health, and chronic disease management.

G.   Continued Technological Advancements (Ongoing):

        ◦   Telemedicine continues to evolve with advancements in digital technology, AI, remote monitoring, and wearables.

        ◦   Integration of telehealth services with electronic health records (EHRs) and health information exchanges is becoming more common.

H.   International Expansion (Ongoing):

        ◦   Telemedicine is not limited to a single country and has expanded internationally, connecting patients and healthcare providers across borders.

        ◦   Cross-border telemedicine can facilitate second opinions, expert consultations, and medical tourism.

I.   Telemedicine Policies and Regulations (Ongoing):

        ◦   Governments and healthcare regulatory bodies are developing and revising policies to accommodate telemedicine.

        ◦   Regulations related to data security, patient privacy, licensure, and reimbursement are continuously evolving.

Hence, the evolution of telemedicine has been characterized by a shift from early experimental concepts to widespread adoption and integration into the healthcare system. As digital technology continues to advance, and healthcare needs change, telemedicine is expected to play an increasingly vital role in providing accessible and efficient healthcare services.

1.2 Role of Digital Technology in Telemedicine

Digital technology plays an important role in enabling and enhancing telemedicine (Meghna Manoj Nair, Amit Kumar Tyagi, 2023) (Amit Kumar Tyagi, 2023). It provides the infrastructure and tools necessary to connect healthcare providers with patients remotely, providing several benefits for both healthcare delivery and patient care. Here are the key roles of digital technology in telemedicine:

- Communication and Connectivity: Digital technology, including the internet and high-speed data networks, enables real-time communication between healthcare providers and patients. Video conferencing, audio calls, and secure messaging platforms facilitate remote consultations. These digital communication channels allow healthcare professionals to visually assess patients, discuss symptoms, and provide medical advice.
- Electronic Health Records (EHRs): EHR systems are a cornerstone of telemedicine, allowing healthcare providers to access and update patient records remotely. Digital records enable a comprehensive view of a patient's medical history, medications, and previous diagnoses during virtual consultations, improving the quality of care.
- Remote Monitoring: Digital technology, coupled with remote monitoring devices and wearables, enables continuous tracking of a patient's vital signs, chronic conditions, and recovery progress. Data from these devices can be transmitted securely to healthcare providers, facilitating early intervention and personalized care.
- Telemedicine Platforms: Specialized telemedicine platforms and mobile apps have been developed to streamline telehealth services. These platforms provide appointment scheduling, secure video conferencing, and integration with EHR systems, making it convenient for both patients and healthcare providers.
- Medical Imaging: Digital imaging technology allows the secure transmission of medical images, such as X-rays, MRIs, and CT scans, for remote interpretation by specialists. This capability is particularly important for radiology and telecardiology services.
- Artificial Intelligence (AI): AI plays a crucial role in telemedicine by analyzing medical data, diagnosing conditions, and offering treatment recommendations. Additionally, AI-driven chatbots and virtual assistants can assist in answering patient queries and conducting initial assessments.
- Data Security: Digital technology includes robust security measures to protect patient data, ensuring that telemedicine consultations adhere to strict privacy and security standards. Encryption, authentication, and data access controls are integral components of secure telemedicine solutions.
- Mobile Health (mHealth): Mobile devices, including smartphones and tablets, are commonly used for telemedicine interactions. mHealth apps can help patients monitor their health, access medical information, and communicate with healthcare providers.
- Data Analytics: Digital technology enables the gathering and analysis of healthcare data, producing insights that can improve patient outcomes and healthcare operations. Utilizing data analytics,

trends can be identified, the efficacy of treatment plans can be monitored, and disease management can be enhanced.

- Virtual Reality (VR) and Augmented Reality (AR): Emerging technologies like VR and AR are being explored for telemedicine applications, such as virtual consultations and surgical training.

Hence, digital technology in telemedicine has revolutionized the way healthcare is delivered, providing convenient access to medical services, improving patient engagement, and expanding healthcare reach. It has become especially important during times of crisis, such as the COVID-19 pandemic, when in-person interactions were limited. As technology continues to advance, telemedicine is expected to evolve further, providing even more sophisticated and accessible healthcare solutions.

1.3 Benefits and Challenges of Digital Transformation in Telemedicine

Digital transformation in telemedicine (Adebiyi, Afolayan, et al., 2023) (Deekshetha, Tyagi, 2023) provides several benefits while also presenting certain challenges. Understanding both the advantages and the obstacles is essential for healthcare organizations and policymakers. Here's a breakdown of the benefits and challenges of digital transformation in telemedicine:

Benefits:

- Improved Access to Healthcare: Telemedicine enhances access to healthcare, especially for individuals in remote or underserved areas, reducing geographical barriers.
- Convenience and Efficiency: Patients can conveniently receive medical care from the comfort of their homes, reducing the time and effort needed for in-person visits.
- Cost Savings: Telemedicine can lower healthcare costs by reducing travel expenses and the need for physical infrastructure. It may also reduce no-show rates for appointments.
- Continuity of Care: Telemedicine allows for ongoing monitoring of patients with chronic conditions and follow-up care, improving care coordination and long-term outcomes.
- Enhanced Patient Engagement: Digital health tools and remote monitoring can empower patients to take an active role in their health and well-being.
- Expanded Specialized Care: Patients can access specialized medical services from experts located far away, providing access to the best care available.
- Reduced Healthcare Disparities: Telemedicine has the potential to bridge healthcare disparities by providing care to underserved populations, including those in rural areas.
- Data-Driven Decision-Making: The process of digital transformation facilitates the gathering and analysis of healthcare data, resulting in more informed decisions and the delivery of more personalized care.
- Scalability and Flexibility: Telemedicine platforms are scalable, allowing healthcare organizations to adapt quickly to changing demands, such as during public health crises.
- Innovation and Research: Digital transformation supports innovation in healthcare, enabling research and development in areas like artificial intelligence and remote monitoring.

Challenges:

- Data Privacy and Security: Ensuring the privacy and security of patient data in telemedicine is a important challenge, and breaches can have serious consequences.
- Regulatory and Licensing Hurdles: Telemedicine services must navigate complex regulations and licensure requirements, which can vary by location.
- Healthcare Disparities: While telemedicine can reduce disparities, it can also create new ones due to disparities in access to technology and internet connectivity.
- Technology Barriers: Patients who are not tech-savvy or lack access to digital devices may struggle to use telemedicine effectively.
- Lack of Physical Examination: Some medical conditions require in-person physical examinations, making it challenging to provide a comprehensive assessment through telemedicine.
- Quality of Care and Misdiagnosis: The quality of care can be compromised when healthcare providers are not physically present, potentially leading to misdiagnoses or inadequate treatment.
- Reimbursement and Financial Challenges: The financial model for telemedicine reimbursement can be complex and may vary by payer and jurisdiction.
- Internet Reliability and Infrastructure: Telemedicine is dependent on internet connectivity, which can be unreliable in some regions or during disasters.
- Provider Workload and Burnout: An increased workload, especially during the COVID-19 pandemic, has led to provider burnout and fatigue.
- Patient-Provider Relationship: Establishing a robust patient-provider relationship can be more challenging in a virtual setting, potentially influencing trust and communication.

Hence, effective implementation of digital transformation in telemedicine requires addressing these challenges to ensure that patients receive safe, high-quality care and that healthcare providers can fully use the advantages of telemedicine. Policymakers, healthcare organizations, and technology companies must work together to strike a balance between the benefits and challenges while fostering innovation and improving healthcare accessibility.

2. DIGITAL TWIN BASED SMART HEALTHCARE SERVICES FOR NEXT GENERATION SOCIETY

Digital twin-based smart healthcare services represent an innovative approach to healthcare in the next generation society (Tyagi, Kukreja, et al., 2023) (Madhav A.V.S., Tyagi A.K. (2022) (Sheth, H.S.K., Tyagi, A.K., 2022) (Varsha Jayaprakash, Amit Kumar Tyagi,). A digital twin is a virtual replica or representation of a physical entity, in this case, a patient's health, medical devices, and healthcare systems. These digital twins are created by collecting and integrating real-time data from various sources, such as sensors, medical records, wearables, and imaging technologies. The concept of digital twins in healthcare can revolutionize how healthcare is delivered, monitored, and personalized. Here are some key aspects of digital twin-based smart healthcare services for the next generation society:

- Personalized Healthcare: Digital twins allow for the creation of highly personalized healthcare profiles for individuals. These profiles incorporate data on a person's genetics, medical history, lifestyle, and real-time health metrics.

- Early Disease Detection: By continuously monitoring health parameters and analyzing the data using AI and machine learning, digital twins can provide early warnings of health issues, allowing for timely interventions and preventive measures.
- Treatment Optimization: Digital twins can simulate the effects of different treatment options on a patient's virtual representation, helping healthcare providers make informed decisions about treatment plans.
- Remote Patient Monitoring: Patients can be continuously monitored through wearable devices and remote sensors, with data fed into their digital twin. Healthcare providers can receive alerts and monitor changes in health status, reducing the need for frequent in-person visits.
- Chronic Disease Management: Digital twins play an important role in managing chronic conditions. They enable healthcare providers to monitor patients with conditions like diabetes, hypertension, or heart disease more effectively, adjusting treatment plans as needed.
- Virtual Consultations and Telehealth: Healthcare professionals can conduct virtual consultations with patients based on real-time data from their digital twins, providing remote care and guidance.
- Predictive Analytics: Using historical and real-time data, digital twins can predict disease trajectories, medication responses, and the likelihood of health complications.
- Medical Device Integration: Digital twins can incorporate data from various medical devices, such as glucose monitors, ECG sensors, and smart inhalers, providing a holistic view of a patient's health.
- Healthcare System Optimization: Digital twins can also be applied to optimize healthcare systems. Hospitals and clinics can create digital twins of their facilities to monitor resource utilization, patient flow, and equipment maintenance.
- Security and Privacy: Securing and preserving the privacy of patient data within digital twin systems is of utmost importance. It requires robust data encryption, stringent access controls, and compliance with healthcare regulations.
- Patient Empowerment: Patients have access to their own digital twins and can actively participate in their healthcare by tracking their health data, setting goals, and receiving personalized recommendations.
- Research and Drug Development: Digital twins can accelerate medical research and drug development by providing a virtual platform for simulating the effects of new drugs and therapies on a diverse range of patient profiles.

Note that the implementation of digital twin-based smart healthcare services brings forth both opportunities and challenges. It holds the potential to revolutionize healthcare delivery, making it more patient-centered, data-driven, and efficient. However, it also introduces concerns regarding data security, ethical utilization of patient data, and the necessity for robust regulatory frameworks to govern these advanced technologies. As healthcare continues to evolve, digital twin-based healthcare services are poised to play a significant role in shaping the future of medical care.

3. ROLE OF EMERGING TECHNOLOGIES IN TELEMEDICINE IN ERA OF SMART HEALTH

Emerging technologies play an important role in advancing telemedicine and smart health in the modern era. They facilitate the creation of innovative solutions that enhance healthcare access, quality, and efficiency. Here are some pivotal roles of emerging technologies in the realm of telemedicine and smart health:

- Artificial Intelligence (AI) and Machine Learning: AI can analyze large amounts of medical data (Tyagi, Aswathy., et al., 2021) (Sai, G.H., Tripathi, K., Tyagi, A.K. (2023) to assist in diagnosing diseases, identifying patterns, and predicting patient outcomes. Machine learning algorithms can optimize treatment plans and improve decision support for healthcare providers. AI-powered chatbots and virtual assistants enhance patient engagement and provide instant medical information.
- Internet of Things (IoT): IoT devices, including wearable fitness trackers and remote monitoring sensors, gather real-time health data and transmit it to healthcare providers. The use of IoT allows for ongoing monitoring of patients with chronic conditions, thereby decreasing hospital readmissions and enhancing the quality of care.
- 5G Connectivity: 5G networks provide low-latency, high-bandwidth connectivity, facilitating real-time video consultations, remote surgeries, and the transmission of large medical images.
- Blockchain Technology: Blockchain ensures secure, transparent, and tamper-proof storage of medical records and data, enhancing data integrity and patient privacy. It can also support consent management, enabling patients to have control over who accesses their health information.
- Virtual Reality (VR) and Augmented Reality (AR): Virtual Reality (VR) and Augmented Reality (AR) technologies find applications in medical training, surgical planning, and patient education. These technologies facilitate virtual consultations, simulating in-person experiences for both remote patients and healthcare providers.
- 3D Printing: 3D printing is used for creating personalized medical devices, prosthetics, and even human tissue. It allows for the customization of healthcare solutions, improving patient outcomes and comfort.
- Genomics and Precision Medicine: Genomic data analysis and precision medicine provide individualized treatment plans based on a patient's genetic makeup. This technology can identify the most effective therapies and reduce adverse drug reactions.
- Robotics: Precision and minimally invasive procedures are facilitated through robotic-assisted surgery, resulting in reduced patient recovery times and complications. Teleoperated robotic systems further enable remote surgery, empowering experts to perform procedures across significant distances.
- Biometric Authentication and Wearables: Biometric authentication ensures secure access to telemedicine platforms and health records. Wearable devices track vital signs, exercise, sleep, and other health metrics, promoting wellness and early intervention.
- Telepathology and Teledermatology: Emerging technologies enable the remote examination of tissue samples and skin conditions, allowing for expert consultations and diagnoses from afar.
- Predictive Analytics and Big Data: The analysis of large datasets helps in identifying health trends, predicting disease outbreaks, and enhancing patient outcomes. It supports population health management and resource allocation.

- Smart Health Apps and Mobile Health (mHealth): Smart health apps provide health education, medication reminders, symptom tracking, and real-time communication with healthcare providers. Note that mHealth apps play a role in preventive care and wellness management.
- Voice and Natural Language Processing: Voice recognition technology enables hands-free access to medical information and telemedicine services. Natural language processing aids in converting spoken or written patient information into structured data for EHRs.

Hence, emerging technologies are instrumental in expanding the capabilities of telemedicine and smart health, improving healthcare access, and enabling more personalized and efficient care delivery. However, their implementation should be guided by robust security measures, ethical issues, and regulatory compliance to ensure the privacy and safety of patient data.

4. ROLE OF ASSISTIVE TECHNOLOGIES IN TELEMEDICINE TODAY'S SMART ERA

Assistive technologies play a significant role in telemedicine, especially in today's smart era (Kute; Tyagi, 2021) (Kute; Tyagi, 2021), by enhancing the accessibility of healthcare services and improving the quality of care for individuals with various needs and conditions. Here are some key roles of assistive technologies in telemedicine:

- Accessibility and Inclusivity: Assistive technologies, including screen readers, voice recognition software, and alternative input devices, ensure the accessibility of telemedicine platforms and health information for individuals with disabilities.
- Remote Monitoring for Chronic Conditions: Patients, including those with chronic conditions, can utilize wearable devices and remote monitoring tools to monitor vital signs, medication adherence, and various health metrics from the comfort of their homes. This data can then be shared with healthcare providers for real-time monitoring.
- Video Interpreting Services: For individuals who are deaf or hard of hearing, video interpreting services provide sign language interpretation during virtual healthcare consultations.
- Braille Displays and Tactile Feedback: Telemedicine platforms can integrate braille displays and tactile feedback devices to make digital health information accessible to individuals with visual impairments.
- Voice Assistants and Speech-to-Text: Voice-controlled devices and speech-to-text technology allow individuals with mobility impairments or limited dexterity to interact with telemedicine platforms and communicate with healthcare providers.
- Remote Consultation for Mobility-Impaired Patients: Telemedicine eliminates the need for travel, making healthcare consultations more accessible for individuals with mobility issues or those living in remote locations.
- Assistive Apps for Medication Management: Mobile apps and reminder systems assist individuals with cognitive impairments or memory issues in managing their medication schedules.
- Cognitive Support Tools: Cognitive assistive technologies, such as virtual assistants and reminder apps, help individuals with cognitive disabilities organize appointments and remember important healthcare information.

- Virtual Reality (VR) and Augmented Reality (AR) for Rehabilitation: VR and AR can be used in telemedicine for physical and occupational therapy, providing engaging and interactive rehabilitation exercises for patients recovering from injuries or surgeries.
- Telepsychiatry and Mental Health Support: Telepsychiatry services, when combined with cognitive-behavioral therapy apps and digital mood trackers, provide individuals with mental health challenges greater access to care and self-management tools.
- Teleaudiology and Hearing Tests: Remote audiology services provide individuals with hearing impairments access to hearing tests and consultations with audiologists, allowing for hearing aid adjustments and support.
- Assistive Navigation and Wayfinding Apps: Mobile apps with GPS and indoor navigation functionalities help individuals with mobility impairments navigate healthcare facilities for in-person visits.
- Patient and Caregiver Education: Assistive technologies can provide accessible educational materials and instructions for both patients and caregivers, ensuring that they have the information needed for care and self-management.

Note that assistive technologies empower individuals with disabilities and healthcare needs to access and benefit from telemedicine services in the smart era. They promote inclusivity, independence, and self-management, while also reducing barriers to healthcare access and improving overall healthcare outcomes. It's essential for telemedicine platforms and healthcare providers to embrace these technologies and ensure that their services are accessible to all.

5. DIGITAL TOOLS, SOLUTIONS, AND SIMULATORS AVAILABLE IN TELEMEDICINE IN THIS SMART ERA

In the smart era of telemedicine, a wide range of digital tools, solutions, and simulators are available to healthcare providers and patients (Kumari, Muthulakshmi, Agarwal, 2022) (Kute, Tyag, Aswathy, 2022). These technologies enhance the delivery of medical services, improve patient engagement, and provide valuable training and educational resources. Here are some of the key digital tools, solutions, and simulators in telemedicine:

- Telemedicine Platforms and Apps: Telemedicine platforms and mobile apps enable virtual consultations between patients and healthcare providers. They often feature appointment scheduling, secure video conferencing, and electronic health record (EHR) integration.
- Electronic Health Records (EHRs): Electronic Health Record (EHR) systems store and manage patient health information, providing easy accessibility to healthcare providers during telemedicine consultations. They contribute to improved care coordination and enhanced patient data security.
- Remote Monitoring Devices: Wearable devices, remote sensors, and health monitoring tools collect real-time patient data, including vital signs, sleep patterns, and medication adherence, enabling continuous monitoring and timely interventions.
- Telehealth Kiosks: Telehealth kiosks are equipped with video conferencing technology and medical devices, allowing patients to have virtual consultations in public spaces, pharmacies, or clinics.

- Health Chatbots and Virtual Assistants: Chatbots and virtual assistants powered by AI offer patients medical information, symptom assessment, appointment scheduling, and general healthcare guidance.
- Video Conferencing Tools: Video conferencing platforms such as Zoom and Microsoft Teams have become indispensable for conducting virtual medical consultations and telehealth appointments.
- Telepathology Solutions: Telepathology enables the remote examination and diagnosis of tissue samples, making it easier for pathologists to provide expert consultations from a distance.
- Teledermatology Apps and Imaging Tools: Teledermatology apps allow patients to capture images of skin conditions and share them with dermatologists for remote diagnosis and treatment recommendations.
- Remote Radiology Platforms: These platforms enable the secure transmission of medical images, such as X-rays, MRIs, and CT scans, for interpretation by radiologists.
- 3D Printing for Medical Models: 3D printing technology is used to create physical models of organs or anatomical structures, which assist in preoperative planning and medical education.
- VR and AR Medical Simulators: Medical training, surgical planning, and patient education benefit from the use of virtual reality (VR) and augmented reality (AR) simulators. These technologies offer immersive experiences, enhancing the learning process.
- Teleaudiology Tools: Teleaudiology platforms enable remote hearing tests, hearing aid adjustments, and consultations with audiologists for individuals with hearing impairments.
- Remote Patient Education and Engagement: Digital tools and interactive patient education materials provide patients with resources for self-management, dietary guidance, medication reminders, and exercise programs.
- AI-Assisted Diagnostic Tools: Diagnostic tools powered by AI analyze medical data, images, and patient history, aiding healthcare providers in making more precise diagnoses and treatment recommendations.
- Genomics and Precision Medicine Software: Genomics tools and software help healthcare providers analyze genetic data to develop personalized treatment plans based on an individual's genetic makeup.
- Simulation Software for Medical Training: Virtual simulation software allows medical professionals to practice surgical procedures, clinical skills, and decision-making in a risk-free environment.
- Mental Health and Telepsychiatry Platforms: Telepsychiatry platforms provide remote mental health services, including video consultations, secure messaging, and digital mental health assessments.

Hence, these digital tools, solutions, and simulators are transforming healthcare and telemedicine by improving access, efficiency, and quality of care. As technology continues to advance, telemedicine will continue to evolve, providing even more sophisticated and innovative solutions to address a wide range of medical needs.

6. INTEGRATION OF EMERGING, ASSISTIVE, AND DIGITAL TECHNOLOGIES IN TELEMEDICINE

The integration of emerging, assistive, and digital technologies in telemedicine is key to delivering comprehensive, efficient, and patient-centered healthcare services (Kute, Tyag, Aswathy, 2022) (Nair, Kumari, Tyagi, Sravanthi, 2021). By combining these technologies, healthcare providers can enhance the quality of care, expand accessibility, and improve patient outcomes. Here's how these technologies can be integrated into telemedicine:

- AI-Powered Decision Support: Healthcare providers can be supported in diagnosing and treating patients through the analysis of medical data by artificial intelligence. AI algorithms can assist in interpreting medical images, suggesting treatment options, and predicting patient outcomes.
- Remote Monitoring with Wearables and IoT: Real-time health data, including heart rate, blood pressure, and glucose levels, is collected by wearable devices and IoT sensors. This information is subsequently transmitted to healthcare providers, enabling them to monitor patients' health status and intervene as needed.
- Assistive Technologies for Accessibility: Integrate assistive technologies like screen readers, voice recognition software, and braille displays to guarantee accessibility of telemedicine platforms for individuals with disabilities.
- Telepsychiatry and Mental Health Support: Integrate telepsychiatry platforms with AI-driven mental health assessments and chatbots that can provide immediate support and resources for individuals with mental health issues.
- Teleaudiology and Hearing Tests: Combine teleaudiology services with assistive technologies for hearing-impaired individuals, such as video interpreting services and hearing aid adjustment apps.
- Blockchain for Secure Data Sharing: Utilize blockchain technology to ensure the security and integrity of patient data, allowing secure sharing of health records and information among healthcare providers and patients.
- Virtual Reality (VR) for Training and Simulation: Virtual Reality (VR) finds application in medical training, enabling healthcare professionals to practice complex procedures in a simulated environment. Additionally, VR can offer virtual patient education for understanding treatment plans and surgeries.
- Remote Radiology and Teledermatology: Integrate remote radiology and teledermatology solutions with AI image analysis for quicker and more accurate diagnosis and treatment recommendations.
- Biometric Authentication for Security: Incorporate biometric authentication methods, such as fingerprint or facial recognition, to safeguard the security of telemedicine platforms and ensure the protection of patient information.
- 3D Printing for Custom Medical Devices: 3D printing technology can be used to create custom medical devices, prosthetics, and anatomical models for surgical planning.
- Mobile Health Apps for Self-Management: Mobile health apps, combined with wearable devices, can assist patients in tracking their health metrics, managing chronic conditions, and receiving personalized health recommendations.
- Voice and Natural Language Processing: Integrate voice-activated commands and natural language processing to allow hands-free interaction with telemedicine platforms, making it easier for individuals with mobility impairments to use the technology.

- Genomics and Precision Medicine Integration: Integrate genomics and precision medicine tools with Electronic Health Records (EHRs) to provide personalized treatment plans tailored to an individual's genetic makeup and medical history.
- Cognitive Support Tools: Use cognitive assistive technologies to provide individuals with cognitive impairments easy access to appointment reminders and healthcare information.
- Remote Patient Education and Engagement: Implement digital tools for patient education, ensuring that patients have access to informative materials for self-management and wellness promotion.

Hence, by integrating these emerging, assistive, and digital technologies, telemedicine can provide comprehensive care that meets the diverse needs of patients, enhances healthcare access, and improves overall healthcare quality. Healthcare providers and technology developers should continue to collaborate to create more innovative and inclusive telemedicine solutions.

7. TELEMEDICINE AND REMOTE HEALTHCARE DELIVERY FOR TODAY'S GENERATION

Telemedicine and remote healthcare delivery have become increasingly relevant and essential for today's generation (Shabnam Kumari, P. Muthulakshmi, 2023) (Amit Kumar Tyagi, V. Hemamalini, Gulshan Soni, 2023) (Sajidha S. A, Rishik, 2023) (A. Deshmukh, N. Sreenath, 2022). These approaches to healthcare delivery use digital technology to provide convenient, accessible, and efficient medical services. Here are some key aspects of telemedicine and remote healthcare delivery for today's generation:

- Convenience and Accessibility: The current generation prioritizes convenience and immediate access to services. Telemedicine enables patients to engage with healthcare providers using smartphones, tablets, or computers from the convenience of their homes or workplaces, eliminating the necessity for travel and reducing waiting times.
- Virtual Consultations: Telemedicine offers virtual consultations with healthcare professionals, delivering a broad spectrum of services such as primary care, mental health support, specialist consultations, and prescription renewals.
- Remote Monitoring: Wearable devices, sensors, and mobile health apps enable remote monitoring of vital signs, chronic conditions, and medication adherence. This continuous monitoring ensures that patients receive timely interventions and personalized care.
- Mental Health Support: Telemedicine has become a lifeline for addressing mental health issues among today's generation. Online therapy and counseling services are readily accessible, providing support for individuals facing anxiety, depression, and stress.
- Digital Health Records: Electronic Health Records (EHRs) simplify the accessibility and secure sharing of medical information for both patients and healthcare providers. This streamlining of the healthcare process fosters coordinated care.
- Telehealth Apps and Portals: Mobile health apps and online patient portals allow patients to schedule appointments, view test results, communicate with healthcare providers, and access health education materials.

- Prescription Refills and Medication Management: Telemedicine platforms provide prescription renewals and medication management, allowing patients to receive ongoing treatment without in-person visits.
- Telepediatrics: Parents can access pediatric care and consultations online for their children, including addressing common childhood illnesses and developmental issues.
- Telepharmacy Services: Telepharmacy services enable patients to consult with pharmacists, receive medication counseling, and get prescription refills via telemedicine.
- Telestroke and Telecardiology: Telemedicine plays a important role in delivering immediate care for stroke and heart-related emergencies, improving the chances of recovery and survival.
- Chronic Disease Management: Individuals with chronic conditions, such as diabetes, hypertension, or asthma, can benefit from telemedicine's remote monitoring and ongoing care, reducing hospitalizations and complications.
- Specialist Access: Telemedicine bridges geographical gaps, giving patients access to specialists who might not be available locally. This is particularly valuable for rare or complex medical conditions.
- Preventive Care and Health Education: Telemedicine platforms often provide preventive care services, wellness programs, and health education resources to help patients make informed lifestyle choices.
- Emergency Medical Services: In some cases, telemedicine is used to provide initial assessment and guidance during emergencies, supporting timely decisions for seeking in-person care or guiding first responders.
- Global Reach: Telemedicine services are not limited to specific regions, providing the potential for international medical consultations, second opinions, and medical tourism.
- Crisis Response: During public health crises, such as the COVID-19 pandemic, telemedicine has been instrumental in delivering care while minimizing the risk of viral transmission.

In summary, telemedicine and remote healthcare delivery have transformed the healthcare landscape for today's generation by aligning with their preferences for technology-driven, convenient, and accessible healthcare solutions. However, it's important to address challenges such as data security, regulatory compliance, and equitable access to ensure that these services meet the diverse healthcare needs of this generation.

8. IMPACT OF EMERGING, ASSISTIVE, AND DIGITAL TECHNOLOGY ON TELEMEDICINE WITH RESPECT TO SMART HEALTHCARE

The impact of emerging, assistive, and digital technology on telemedicine, particularly in the context of smart healthcare, is profound and transformative. These technologies are driving the evolution of telemedicine and are poised to revolutionize healthcare delivery in several ways. Here's an overview of their impact:

- Enhanced Accessibility and Convenience: Emerging technologies, such as mobile health apps and wearable devices, are making healthcare more accessible and convenient for patients. Smart healthcare solutions allow individuals to monitor their health, access medical information, and consult with healthcare providers from the comfort of their homes or on the go.

- Personalized Healthcare: The integration of digital tools and AI-driven algorithms allows for the delivery of personalized healthcare services. Patients can receive tailored treatment plans and recommendations based on their health data, genetic information, and medical history.

- Early Disease Detection and Prevention: Remote monitoring devices and predictive analytics enable the early detection of health issues and the implementation of preventive measures. Patients can be alerted to potential health risks, allowing for timely interventions and lifestyle adjustments.

- Telemedicine Expansion: Telemedicine, supported by digital technology, is extending beyond traditional video consultations. It now includes remote monitoring, telepsychiatry, teleaudiology, and virtual specialty care, providing comprehensive healthcare services to patients in various medical domains.

- Improved Clinical Decision Support: AI-driven diagnostic tools aid healthcare providers in achieving more precise and timely diagnoses. These tools analyze patient data, medical images, and lab results, contributing to informed clinical decision-making.

- Better Management of Chronic Conditions: Remote monitoring, wearable devices, and mobile health apps play a important role in managing chronic conditions. Patients can track their health metrics, receive medication reminders, and share data with healthcare providers, leading to better disease management.

- Telehealth for Mental Health: Telepsychiatry and mental health apps provide essential mental health support and therapy options. They provide a safe and convenient way for individuals to seek help for anxiety, depression, and other mental health issues.

- Patient Empowerment and Engagement: Digital tools and assistive technologies empower patients to play an active role in their healthcare. Patients can retrieve their health data, establish health goals, and communicate with their healthcare providers, fostering a sense of engagement and control.

- Data Security and Privacy: Emerging technologies emphasize data security and privacy. Blockchain technology, in particular, provides a secure and transparent means of protecting patient data, ensuring compliance with privacy regulations like HIPAA.

- Healthcare Ecosystem Integration: Smart healthcare solutions allow for the integration of various components of the healthcare ecosystem, such as EHRs, telemedicine platforms, wearables, and remote monitoring devices. This interconnectedness streamlines the flow of patient information and supports coordinated care.

- Telemedicine during Crises: The COVID-19 pandemic demonstrated the important role of telemedicine in crisis response. Telemedicine platforms enabled healthcare services to continue while minimizing the risk of viral transmission, showcasing their adaptability and resilience.

- Global Healthcare Reach: Telemedicine, powered by digital technology, breaks down geographical barriers, enabling patients to access expert care and second opinions from specialists worldwide, leading to global healthcare collaborations and knowledge sharing.

Thus, the influence of emerging, assistive, and digital technology on telemedicine within the framework of smart healthcare is extensive. These technologies are propelling healthcare into a new era characterized by enhanced accessibility, personalization, and connectivity, ultimately contributing to improved patient outcomes and overall care quality. Nevertheless, challenges associated with data security, interoperability, and equitable access must be addressed as these technologies continue to evolve.

9. TECHNICAL, ETHICAL, LEGAL, AND REGULATORY ISSUES IN TELEMEDICINE WITH RESPECT TO SMART HEALTHCARE

Telemedicine in the context of smart healthcare presents a range of technical, ethical, legal, and regulatory challenges that need to be addressed to ensure its successful and responsible implementation. Here's an overview of these issues:

A. Technical Issues:
   - Data Security and Privacy: Protecting patient data is a paramount issue. Secure transmission, storage, and access control measures are necessary to safeguard sensitive health information.
   - Interoperability: Ensuring that different telemedicine platforms, EHR systems, and medical devices can seamlessly exchange data is essential for providing comprehensive and coordinated care.
   - Technology Accessibility: Not all patients have access to the necessary digital devices or internet connectivity. Ensuring equitable access to telemedicine services is a significant challenge.
   - Data Accuracy and Quality: Remote monitoring devices and AI-powered tools must provide accurate and reliable data to support medical decisions and diagnoses.
   - Scalability and Reliability: Telemedicine platforms need to be scalable to handle a growing user base and reliable to provide uninterrupted services.
   - Digital Divide: Bridging the digital divide is important, as disparities in technology access can result in unequal access to healthcare services.

B. Ethical Issues:
   - Informed Consent: Patients must be fully informed about the benefits and risks of telemedicine services. Obtaining informed consent for remote consultations is an ethical imperative.
   - Patient Autonomy: Patients should have the autonomy to choose between in-person and telemedicine care. Ethical issues include respecting patients' preferences and providing alternatives when necessary.
   - Quality of Care: Ensuring that telemedicine services meet the same quality and standard of care as in-person services is essential. Ethical standards should not be compromised in virtual consultations.
   - Confidentiality and Trust: Establishing and maintaining trust between patients and healthcare providers is vital. Patients should feel confident that their health information is secure and will not be misused.
   - Ethical Use of AI: The ethical use of AI in telemedicine involves transparency, accountability, and ensuring that AI algorithms prioritize patient well-being over commercial interests.

C. Legal and Regulatory Issues:
   - Licensure and Telehealth Regulations: Telemedicine services are subject to regulations that vary by jurisdiction. Licensing and reimbursement policies can be complex and may require ongoing updates to keep pace with technological advances.

- ○ Malpractice and Liability: The allocation of liability in telemedicine, particularly in cases of misdiagnosis or errors in remote care, is a legal issue that requires clarity and standardization.
- ○ Telemedicine Prescribing: Regulations governing the prescription of medication through telemedicine vary by location. Compliance with prescription laws is a significant legal issue.
- ○ Cross-Border Telemedicine: Providing telemedicine services across international borders can be legally complex, as different countries have their own regulations and licensure requirements.
- ○ Intellectual Property: Intellectual property rights related to telemedicine software, algorithms, and medical data need to be clearly defined to avoid legal disputes.

D. Regulatory Compliance:
- ○ HIPAA and Data Security: Healthcare providers in the United States are required to adhere to the regulations outlined in the Health Insurance Portability and Accountability Act (HIPAA) to safeguard patient data and privacy.
- ○ Telehealth Reimbursement: Regulatory frameworks for reimbursement vary by country and even within states or regions. Ensuring that telemedicine services are reimbursed appropriately is an important challenge.
- ○ FDA Approval: Regulatory approval or clearance from agencies like the U.S. Food and Drug Administration (FDA) may be necessary for medical devices and software utilized in telemedicine.
- ○ Data Protection Regulations: Ensuring compliance with data protection regulations, such as the General Data Protection Regulation (GDPR) in Europe, is crucial to safeguarding patient privacy.

Hence, addressing these technical, ethical, legal, and regulatory issues is important for the responsible implementation of telemedicine within the context of smart healthcare. Healthcare organizations, policymakers, and technology providers must work together to establish clear guidelines, ensure patient safety, and support equitable access to telemedicine services while upholding ethical standards and legal requirements.

10. FUTURE OPPORTUNITIES TOWARDS TELEMEDICINE WITH RESPECT TO SMART HEALTHCARE

The future of telemedicine within the context of smart healthcare holds significant opportunities for improving healthcare access, quality, and efficiency. Here are several future opportunities and trends in telemedicine:

- Advanced Telehealth Platforms: Future telehealth platforms will be more user-friendly and feature-rich. They will provide high-definition video, seamless EHR integration, and AI-driven clinical decision support.
- IoT-Enabled Remote Monitoring: Incorporating the Internet of Things (IoT) will facilitate continuous remote monitoring of patients with chronic conditions in real-time, enabling proactive interventions and personalized care.

- 5G Connectivity: The widespread deployment of 5G networks will provide low-latency, high-bandwidth connectivity, enabling high-quality video consultations, remote surgeries, and the rapid transmission of large medical images.
- AI and Machine Learning: AI and machine learning are poised to assume a more significant role in telemedicine, encompassing disease diagnosis, patient outcome prediction, and the optimization of treatment plans.
- Digital Twins for Personalized Medicine: Digital twin technology will create virtual replicas of patients, facilitating personalized treatment plans and medication optimization.
- Telemedicine for Mental Health: Telepsychiatry and mental health apps will expand, addressing the growing need for mental health support and therapy.
- Telemedicine in Emergency Response: Telemedicine will play a important role in emergency response, providing remote medical assistance during natural disasters and crises.
- Telepharmacy Services: Telepharmacy services will become more common, allowing patients to consult with pharmacists, receive medication counseling, and obtain prescription refills remotely.
- Global Telemedicine Services: Telemedicine will facilitate international collaboration among healthcare providers and researchers, enabling second opinions from specialists worldwide.
- Genomics and Precision Medicine: Genomic data will be integrated with telemedicine platforms to provide personalized treatment plans based on patients' genetic profiles.
- Telehealth in Elderly Care: Telemedicine will support elderly care by providing remote monitoring, medication management, and social interaction for seniors.
- Teleaudiology and Remote Hearing Tests: Teleaudiology platforms will enable individuals with hearing impairments to access hearing tests and consultations with audiologists.
- Digital Health Literacy Programs: Education and training programs will help patients and healthcare providers improve digital health literacy, ensuring effective and responsible use of telemedicine.
- Telemedicine for Underserved Areas: Telemedicine will help bridge healthcare disparities by providing services to underserved rural and remote areas, improving healthcare access.
- Integration with Smart Homes: Telemedicine will become seamlessly integrated with smart home technologies, allowing for easy access to healthcare services and remote monitoring within the home environment.
- Telemedicine and Wearable Tech: Wearable devices will become more sophisticated and integrated with telemedicine, enhancing health tracking and remote monitoring.
- Telehealth for Preventive Care: Telemedicine will increasingly focus on preventive care, providing wellness programs, lifestyle guidance, and early intervention for potential health issues.
- Virtual Surgical Consultations and Training: Surgeons will use telemedicine for virtual consultations, surgical planning, and training, potentially enabling remote surgeries with the help of robotics.
- Telemedicine for Pediatrics: Telepediatrics will provide pediatric care and consultations online, addressing common childhood illnesses and developmental issues.
- Regulatory Advancements: Policymakers and regulatory bodies will work to create clear and consistent regulations for telemedicine, ensuring patient safety and standardization.

Hence, the future of telemedicine in the realm of smart healthcare promises to be dynamic and transformative, providing innovative solutions to address healthcare challenges while promoting patient-centered care and enhancing overall well-being.

10.1 The Future of Telemedicine and Digital Healthcare Transformation

The future of telemedicine and digital healthcare transformation is promising and likely to reshape the way healthcare is delivered, accessed, and experienced. Here are some key trends and insights that define the future of telemedicine and digital healthcare transformation:

- AI-Powered Healthcare: Artificial intelligence and machine learning will play an increasingly significant role in healthcare. AI algorithms will assist in disease diagnosis, predict patient outcomes, personalize treatment plans, and automate administrative tasks.
- Telemedicine Integration: Telemedicine will become seamlessly integrated into healthcare systems, providing a continuum of care that blends in-person visits with virtual consultations, remote monitoring, and follow-up care.
- Data-Driven Medicine: Data analytics and big data will support evidence-based medicine and population health management. Real-time patient data from wearables, sensors, and electronic health records will be used for personalized care and health insights.
- Blockchain for Health Records: The utilization of blockchain technology will witness a growing trend in secure and interoperable health data storage and sharing, ensuring the integrity and privacy of patient records.
- Genomics and Precision Medicine: Patient care will incorporate genomic information, enabling personalized treatment plans based on an individual's genetic makeup. The integration of precision medicine is set to revolutionize the treatment of various diseases.
- Wearable Health Tech: Wearable devices and smart clothing will continue to advance, monitoring vital signs, chronic conditions, and fitness metrics. They will be integral to preventive care and early disease detection.
- 5G and IoT: The widespread deployment of 5G networks and the expansion of the Internet of Things will enable real-time, high-quality telemedicine services, remote monitoring, and the interconnection of medical devices.
- Virtual and Augmented Reality: Virtual and augmented reality technologies will be used for medical training, surgical planning, patient education, and enhancing the patient experience during telehealth consultations.
- Digital Twins: Digital twins will create virtual replicas of patients, enabling more accurate simulations and predictions for treatment planning and medical research.
- Remote Surgery and Robotics: Telemedicine will support remote surgery, with the assistance of robotic systems and surgical robots controlled by expert surgeons from distant locations.
- Telepsychiatry and Mental Health Support: Mental health services provided through telepsychiatry will continue to grow, addressing the increasing demand for mental health support and counseling.
- AI Chatbots and Virtual Health Assistants: Chatbots and virtual health assistants powered by AI will furnish instantaneous medical information, aid in appointment scheduling, and offer medication reminders and health guidance.

- Patient-Generated Health Data: Patients will actively participate in their healthcare by sharing self-generated health data, allowing for more personalized treatment and wellness recommendations.
- Telehealth for Rural and Underserved Areas: Telemedicine will bridge healthcare disparities by reaching rural and underserved populations, improving healthcare access and reducing healthcare inequities.
- Digital Health Literacy: Education and training programs will focus on improving digital health literacy for both patients and healthcare providers, promoting responsible and effective use of digital healthcare tools.
- Regulatory and Legal Frameworks: Policymakers will work to establish clear and consistent regulations for telemedicine, addressing issues related to licensure, reimbursement, malpractice, and data privacy.

Note that the future of telemedicine and digital healthcare transformation promises to be patient-centered, data-driven, and highly accessible. It will foster more proactive and personalized healthcare, enable earlier disease detection, and empower individuals to take greater control of their health and well-being. As technology and healthcare continue to evolve, the potential for positive and transformative changes in the industry is large.

11. CONCLUSION

This chapter presents information on emerging, assistive, and digital technologies that are driving innovation and transformation in the realm of telemedicine. These technologies have significantly reshaped healthcare delivery, making it more accessible, efficient, and patient-centered.

Firstly, emerging technologies like artificial intelligence (AI) and machine learning (ML) have revolutionized telemedicine by facilitating automated diagnostics, intelligent triaging, and predictive analytics. AI algorithms analyze various medical data, including images, lab results, and patient history, to deliver accurate diagnoses and personalized treatment plans. ML algorithms predict disease progression and identify high-risk patients, enabling proactive interventions and optimal resource allocation.

Secondly, assistive technologies such as wearable devices, remote monitoring systems, and telehealth platforms have facilitated continuous patient monitoring and remote consultations. Wearable devices, including smartwatches and biosensors, capture real-time physiological data, which can be transmitted to healthcare providers for remote monitoring and early detection of abnormalities.

Note that Remote monitoring systems enable the management of chronic conditions, post-operative care, and elderly care from a distance. Telehealth platforms facilitate virtual consultations, video conferencing, and secure communication between patients and healthcare professionals. Lastly, digital technologies like mobile applications, electronic health records (EHRs), and telemedicine apps have streamlined the telemedicine workflow and improved the patient experience. In this dynamic landscape, the continued collaboration of healthcare providers, technology developers, and policymakers is essential to harness the full potential of emerging, assistive, and digital technologies in telemedicine. By embracing these technologies responsibly, healthcare systems can provide more accessible, patient-centric, and data-driven care that enhances the overall well-being of patients and contributes to the advancement of healthcare as a whole.

REFERENCES

Adebiyi, M. O., Afolayan, J. O., Arowolo, M. O., Tyagi, A. K., & Adebiyi, A. A. (2023). Breast Cancer Detection Using a PSO-ANN Machine Learning Technique. In A. Tyagi (Ed.), *Using Multimedia Systems, Tools, and Technologies for Smart Healthcare Services* (pp. 96–116). IGI Global. doi:10.4018/978-1-6684-5741-2.ch007

Deshmukh, A., Sreenath, N., Tyagi, A. K., & Eswara Abhichandan, U. V. (2022). Blockchain Enabled Cyber Security: A Comprehensive Survey. *2022 International Conference on Computer Communication and Informatics (ICCCI)*, (pp. 1-6). IEEE. 10.1109/ICCCI54379.2022.9740843

Kumari, S., Muthulakshmi, P., & Agarwal, D. (2022). Deployment of Machine Learning Based Internet of Things Networks for Tele-Medical and Remote Healthcare. In V. Suma, X. Fernando, K. L. Du, & H. Wang (Eds.), *Evolutionary Computing and Mobile Sustainable Networks. Lecture Notes on Data Engineering and Communications Technologies* (Vol. 116). Springer. doi:10.1007/978-981-16-9605-3_21

Kute, S. (2021). Building a Smart Healthcare System Using Internet of Things and Machine Learning. Big Data Management in Sensing: Applications in AI and IoT. River Publishers.

Kute, S. (2021). Research Issues and Future Research Directions Toward Smart Healthcare Using Internet of Things and Machine Learning. Big Data Management in Sensing: Applications in AI and IoT. River Publishers.

Kute, S. S., Tyagi, A. K., & Aswathy, S. U. (2022). Industry 4.0 Challenges in e-Healthcare Applications and Emerging Technologies. In A. K. Tyagi, A. Abraham, & A. Kaklauskas (Eds.), *Intelligent Interactive Multimedia Systems for e-Healthcare Applications*. Springer. doi:10.1007/978-981-16-6542-4_14

Kute, S. S., Tyagi, A. K., & Aswathy, S. U. (2022). Security, Privacy and Trust Issues in Internet of Things and Machine Learning Based e-Healthcare. In A. K. Tyagi, A. Abraham, & A. Kaklauskas (Eds.), *Intelligent Interactive Multimedia Systems for e-Healthcare Applications*. Springer. doi:10.1007/978-981-16-6542-4_15

Madhav, A. V. S., & Tyagi, A. K. (2022). The World with Future Technologies (Post-COVID-19): Open Issues, Challenges, and the Road Ahead. In A. K. Tyagi, A. Abraham, & A. Kaklauskas (Eds.), *Intelligent Interactive Multimedia Systems for e-Healthcare Applications*. Springer. doi:10.1007/978-981-16-6542-4_22

Nair, M. M., Kumari, S., Tyagi, A. K., & Sravanthi, K. (2021) Deep Learning for Medical Image Recognition: Open Issues and a Way to Forward. In: Goyal D., Gupta A.K., Piuri V., Ganzha M., Paprzycki M. (eds) *Proceedings of the Second International Conference on Information Management and Machine Intelligence. Lecture Notes in Networks and Systems*. Springer, Singapore. 10.1007/978-981-15-9689-6_38

Nair, M. M., & Tyagi, A. K. (2023). AI, IoT, blockchain, and cloud computing: The necessity of the future. Rajiv Pandey, Sam Goundar, Shahnaz Fatima, Distributed Computing to Blockchain. Academic Press. doi:10.1016/B978-0-323-96146-2.00001-2

Prabu Shankar, K. C., & Deeba, K. (2023). *Machine Learning-Based Big Data Analytics for IoT-Enabled Smart Healthcare Systems, in the book: AI-Based Digital Health Communication for Securing Assistive Systems*. IGI Global. doi:10.4018/978-1-6684-8938-3.ch004

Sai, G. H., Tripathi, K., & Tyagi, A. K. (2023). Internet of Things-Based e-Health Care: Key Challenges and Recommended Solutions for Future. In: Singh, P.K., Wierzchoń, S.T., Tanwar, S., Rodrigues, J.J.P.C., Ganzha, M. (eds) *Proceedings of Third International Conference on Computing, Communications, and Cyber-Security. Lecture Notes in Networks and Systems.* Springer, Singapore. 10.1007/978-981-19-1142-2_37

Sai Dhakshan, Y. (2023). Introduction to Smart Healthcare: Healthcare Digitization. 6G-Enabled IoT and AI for Smart Healthcare. CRC Press.

Sajidha, S. A. (2023). Robust and Secure Evidence Management in Digital Forensics Investigations Using Blockchain Technology. AI-Based Digital Health Communication for Securing Assistive Systems. IGI Global. doi:10.4018/978-1-6684-8938-3.ch010

Shabnam Kumari, P. (2023). *Effective Deep Learning-Based Attack Detection Methods for the Internet of Medical Things, in the book: AI-Based Digital Health Communication for Securing Assistive Systems.* IGI Global. doi:10.4018/978-1-6684-8938-3.ch008

Sheth, H. S. K., & Tyagi, A. K. (2022). Mobile Cloud Computing: Issues, Applications and Scope in COVID-19. In A. Abraham, N. Gandhi, T. Hanne, T. P. Hong, T. Nogueira Rios, & W. Ding (Eds.), *Intelligent Systems Design and Applications. ISDA 2021. Lecture Notes in Networks and Systems* (Vol. 418). Springer. doi:10.1007/978-3-030-96308-8_55

Tyagi, A. (2021, October). AARIN: Affordable, Accurate, Reliable and INnovative Mechanism to Protect a Medical Cyber-Physical System using Blockchain Technology. *IJIN, 2,* 175–183.

Tyagi, A., Kukreja, S., Nair, M. M., & Tyagi, A. K. (2022). Machine Learning: Past, Present and Future. *NeuroQuantology : An Interdisciplinary Journal of Neuroscience and Quantum Physics, 20*(8). doi:10.14704/nq.2022.20.8.NQ44468

Tyagi, V. (2023). Hemamalini, Gulshan Soni, Digital Health Communication With Artificial Intelligence-Based Cyber Security. AI-Based Digital Health Communication for Securing Assistive Systems. IGI Global. doi:10.4018/978-1-6684-8938-3.ch009

Tyagi, A. (2023). Decentralized everything: Practical use of blockchain technology in future applications, Editor(s): Rajiv Pandey, Sam Goundar, Shahnaz Fatima, Distributed Computing to Blockchain. Academic Press. doi:10.1016/B978-0-323-96146-2.00010-3

Tyagi, A. (2022). Using Multimedia Systems, Tools, and Technologies for Smart Healthcare Services. IGI Global. doi:10.4018/978-1-6684-5741-2

Chapter 13
Lung Cancer Classification Using Deep Learning Hybrid Model

Sachin Jain
ⓘ https://orcid.org/0000-0002-2948-7858
Ajay Kumar Garg Engineering College, Ghaziabad, India

Preeti Jaidka
ⓘ https://orcid.org/0000-0002-4978-2192
JSS Academy of Technical Education, India

ABSTRACT

Abnormal growths in the lungs caused by disease. The classification of CT scans is accomplished by applying machine learning strategies. Classification methods based on deep learning, such as support vector machines, can categorize a wide variety of image datasets and produce segmentation results of the highest caliber. In this work, we suggested a method for deep feature extraction from images by altering SVM and CNN and then applying the hybrid model resulting from those modifications (NNSVLC). For this investigation, the Kaggle dataset will be utilized. The proposed method was found to be accurate 91.7% of the time, as determined by the results of the experiments.

1. INTRODUCTION

Lung cancer poses a substantial risk to people's health worldwide for several reasons, including its high death rate, widespread prevalence, and unknown origin (khoddam et al., 2024). It is one of the cancers diagnosed the most frequently, and it is the primary reason people die from cancer worldwide. There is a significant geographical difference in incidence; higher rates are observed in regions with high cigarette consumption and environmental pollution. The presence of numerous histological subtypes, most notably small cell lung cancer (SCLC) and non-small cell lung cancer (NSCLC), further complicates the pathophysiology of lung cancer(Gayap & Akhloufi, 2024): small cell lung cancer (SCLC) and non-small

DOI: 10.4018/979-8-3693-2359-5.ch013

cell lung cancer (NSCLC). When detecting lung cancer, imaging studies such as computed tomography (CT) and positron emission tomography (PET) scans are only one piece of the puzzle; the histological evaluation of biopsy specimens provides the last piece. Deep learning is a sort of machine learning that has shown promising results when used to detect lung cancer in medical imaging (Asuntha & Srinivasan, 2020; Bhatia et al., 2019; Das & Majumder, 2020). Deep learning models, particularly convolutional neural networks (CNNs), have demonstrated their ability to automatically learn and extract complex patterns from medical pictures(Dodia et al., 2022; Wani et al., 2024). This paves the way for diagnoses that are both more accurate and more reliable.

We aim to develop a model that can differentiate between malignant and benign lung nodules with high accuracy. This would allow radiologists and oncologists to diagnose and treat patients with incredible speed and certainty. We have high hopes that our research will contribute to the development of medical AI and improve the diagnosis and treatment of lung cancer in patients.

Following the main text of the report are additional resources, which include the dataset, method, and models utilized in diagnosing lung cell cancer. In the latter part of this chapter, we compare the hybrid model to three alternative models for 5, 10, and 20 folds.

2. LITERATURE SURVEY

The two most common forms of lung cancer are small-cell lung cancer (SCLC) and non-small cell lung cancer (NSCLC). The non-small cell lung cancer (NSCLC) subtype accounts for 75% of all lung cancer diagnoses. Adenocarcinoma (LUAD) and squamous cell carcinoma (LUSC) are the two most common subtypes within this cancer subtype. kilanje(Ayalew et al., 2024; Bushara A. R. et al., 2023; Kim et al., 2024; Lanjewar et al., 2024) In medicine, techniques such as computer-aided diagnostics (CAD) are utilized to diagnose diseases at an earlier stage. Several cancers, such as those of the lung, the skin, and the prostate, can be challenging to diagnose in the early stages (Abunasser et al., 2023). When getting solid results from a CT scan, the only option available is manual identification (Ahmed & MOHAMMED, 2023). However, a method based on artificial intelligence (AI) is necessary to identify lung cancer in its early, benign stages. Two different approaches can be taken in order to identify lung nodules. Before the CT picture can be analysed for the presence of minute nodules in the chest caused by the pulmonary vasculature, the lung endothelium must be eliminated. Deep learning algorithms perform exceptionally well in picture identification tasks such as categorization and detection; hence, these algorithms are frequently employed in medical images and as computer-aided diagnosis tools for various reasons, including those listed above. Convolutional neural networks, often CNNs, are the current industry standard for computer vision (Gudur et al., n.d.; Liu et al., 2024; Poonkodi & Kanchana, 2024; Qian et al., 2024; Rao et al., 2024). A convolutional neural network, also known as a CNN, is a specific kind of deep learning model (Nafisah & Muhammad, 2024)that imitates a network of neurons by employing a processing layer. (Shah & Parveen, 2023) separated the lungs using an upgraded version of the profuse clustering technique after first performing denoising on the photos to improve the overall image quality. Following this step, a neural network is next taught to recognize lung cancer. The authors of (Abdullah et al., 2023) proposed a DL model to evaluate the accuracy of lung cancer prediction using CT scans. U-Net and 3D CNN were successfully utilized to screen for FP nodules, and suggested a DL model. The segmentation issue is resolved thanks to this model's marker-controlled watershed segmentation. According to a classification system developed by (Bishnoi et al., 2023), lung cancer can be benign or malignant.

The system determines the Region of Interest (ROI) using historical data with the House field Unit (HU).

During the training and classification processes of the support vector machine, various form features are recovered, and various statistical parameters are evaluated for textural aspects. This is done to determine whether the nodule is benign or cancerous. As seen in Table 1, the published works are arranged according to the precision of the datasets and the research methodologies. Table 2 is a list of the abbreviations used in the literature review.

Table 1. Summarized literature review

Reference	Performance	Used Database	Approach
(Chen et al., 2022)	Sensitivity: 94.9% CPM score: 94.7%	LUNA16, LIDC-IDRI	3D CNN
(Nam et al., 2019)	Sensitivity 69.9%	Seoul National University Hospital	Deep learning automatic detection algorithm (DLAD)
(Masood et al., 2018)	Accuracy: 84.6%	LIDC-IDRI	SVM-LASSO
(Jin et al., 2017)	Accuracy 87.5% [28]	KDSB17, Kaggle dataset base	3D CNN
(Kumar et al., 2015)	Accuracy75.01%	LIDC-IDRI	Lung nodule classification
(Setio et al., 2016)	detection sensitivities of 85.4% and 90.1%	LIDC-IDRI	Computer-Aided Detection (CAD) 2-D ConvNets
(Shen et al., 2015)	Accuracy: 86.84%	LIDC-IDRI	Multi-scale CNN
(Ciompi et al., 2017)	Accuracy: 85.6%	LIDC-IDRI	ConvNets 1 scale
(Rani & Jawhar, 2020)	Accuracy: 97.3%	LIDC	DCNN
(Fu et al., 2022)	Sensitivity: 96.2	LIDC-IDRI	CNN-based multi-task learning (CNN-MTL) Multiple deep convolutional neural networks (CNNs)
(Thamilarasi & Roselin, 2021)	Accuracy: 86.67%	JSRT	CNN
(Zhang et al., 2019)	Accuracy: 84.0% SingleCNN 81.7%	LIDC-IDRI	Ensemble CNN
(Nasrullah et al., 2019)	Sensitivity: 93.4%	LIDC	CNN
(Matsuyama & Tsai, 2018)	Accuracy: 91.9%	448 images include four categories	Wavelet-Based CNN
(Ramachandran et al., 2018)	Sensitivity: 87	Kaggle Data Science Bow	CNN
(Mao et al., 2018)	Accuracy: 93.9%	ELCAP	Feature Representation Using Deep Autoencoder

According to the review of relevant research, the state-of-the-art CNN model performs admirably when categorizing and diagnosing lung cancer in CT scans.

Table 2. Abbreviation used in literature

Dataset	Details
ECLAP	Programme for the Early Action on Lung Cancer
LUNA-16	Examination of Lung Nodules
KDSB	Kaggle Data Science Bow
LIDC	Image archive provided by the Lung Image Database Consortium
LIDCIDRI	Images from Lung Image Database Consortium Resource image database initiative
JSRT	The Radiological Technology Society of Japan

3. THE DATASET, METHODOLOGY, AND ALGORITHM

This section is subdivided into three subsections.

3.1 Dataset

The paper makes use of data available on the Kaggle platform.

There are 613 CT scans of lung cancer in this collection, labelled a, b, c, and d.

66% of the data set is used for training, whereas 34% is for evaluating the model. All four types of images are represented in Table 3.

3.2 Methodology

The ensemble technique improves the efficiency and precision of conventional classifiers. SVM and CNN are only two examples of classifiers that can be combined in an ensemble deep learning setup. The proposed strategy for lung cancer classification is depicted in Figure 1.

3.3 Proposed Algorithm (SVNNLC)

The model is briefly described below.

Step (1) As an input dataset, there are a total of 613 observations used.

Step (2) The data set is broken up into a training portion of 66% and a testing portion of 34%.

Step (3) Images saved in the RGB color space have their initial width and height reduced to 224 pixels.

Step (4) Five-fold, ten-fold, and twenty-fold cross-validation were performed to assess the reliability of the results.

Step (5) The CNN (Inception V3) and Linear SVM models served as the foundation for the generation of the hybrid classifier that was created.

Step (6) The Inception V3 network of the CNN Model is used for feature extraction. This model has fully connected layers and uses the Relu activation function. The dropout rate is set to 0.1.

Step (7) The final classification is determined by averaging all of the relevant scores.

Table 3. Data set used in the study

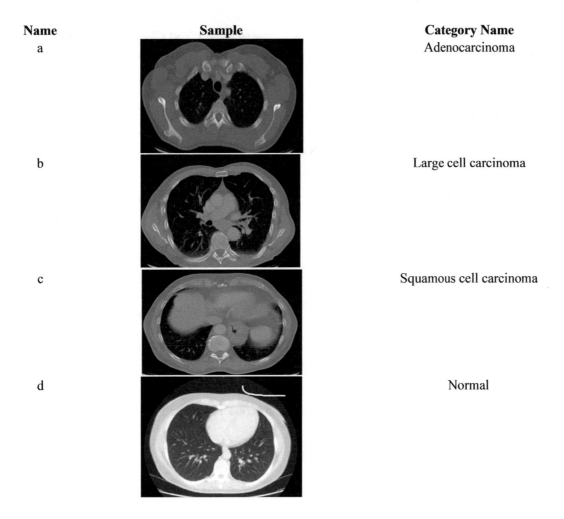

Name	Sample	Category Name
a		Adenocarcinoma
b		Large cell carcinoma
c		Squamous cell carcinoma
d		Normal

Figure 1. Flow Chart of proposed methodology

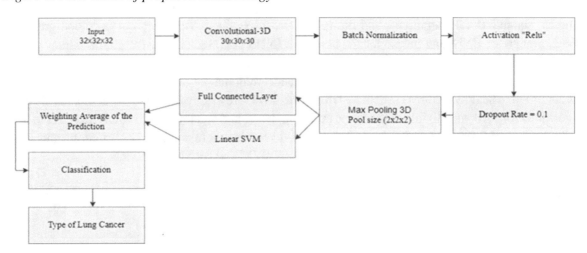

3. ANALYSIS OF RESULTS

The subsequent matrices are employed for the assessment of the SVNNLC's performance.

Accuracy: The accuracy, denoted by Acc, is denoted by the first equation.

$$Acc = \frac{TP + TN}{TP + TN + FP + FN} \tag{1}$$

Whhere abbreviations such as "TP," "TN," "FP," and "FN" stand for "true positive," "true negative," "false positive," and "false negative," respectively.

Precision: The suggested model's precision, denoted by the symbol "Pre," can be seen in equation number 2.

$$Pre = \frac{TP}{TP + FP} \tag{2}$$

Recall: The equation number 3 demonstrates the suggested model's recall, abbreviated as Re.

$$Re = \frac{TP}{TP + FN} \tag{3}$$

F1-Score: The F1-Score for the model that has been proposed can be found in equation number 4.

$$F1 - Score = \frac{Pre.Re}{Pre + Re} \tag{4}$$

4. RESULTS AND DISCUSSIONS

Accuracy, as measured by a factor of 20, is depicted in Figures 2-5 for adenocarcinoma, large cell carcinoma, squamous cell carcinoma, and normal tissue, respectively. Accuracy curve colors: green for SVM, orange for CNN, and purple for the ensemble (NNSVLC) technique. Ten-fold accuracy curves for adenocarcinoma, large cell carcinoma, squamous cell carcinoma, and healthy pictures are shown in Figures 6–9. The five-fold accuracy curve for adenocarcinoma, large cell carcinoma, squamous cell carcinoma, and healthy pictures are depicted in Figures 10–17, respectively. Table 5-7 compares different algorithms for 5,10, and 20 folds for adenocarcinoma, large, and squamous cell carcinoma. Table 8-10 indicates the confusion matrix for fivefold, Table 11-13 for the confusion matrix for tenfold, and Table 14-16 for the confusion matrix for twentyfold for CNN SVM and SVNNLC models.

Table 4. Comparison of different algorithms for 5, 10 and 20 folds

K Folds	Model	AUC	CA	F1	Precision	Recall	MCC
5	CNN	97.7	89.1	89.0	89.2	89.1	85.3
5	SVM	97.7	86.5	86.5	87.7	86.5	82.0
5	SVNNLC	97.8	90.0	90.0	90.2	90.0	86.6
10	CNN	98.0	90.0	90.0	90.0	90.0	86.6
10	SVM	98.1	88.7	88.8	89.3	88.7	84.9
10	SVNNLC	98.3	90.2	90.2	90.2	90.2	86.8
20	CNN	98.4	91.4	91.3	91.3	91.4	88.3
20	SVM	98.5	90.4	90.4	90.7	90.4	87.1
20	SVNNLC	98.5	91.7	91.7	91.6	91.7	88.8

Table 5. Comparison of different algorithms for 5, 10 and 20 folds adenocarcinoma

K Folds	Model	AUC	CA	F1	Precision	Recall	MCC
5	CNN	96.2	90.4	85.4	82.7	88.2	78.3
5	SVM	96.5	86.9	81.6	74.1	90.8	72.5
5	SVNNLC	97.0	91.0	86.3	84.0	88.7	79.7
10	CNN	96.6	91.7	87.2	85.6	88.7	81.0
10	SVM	97.2	89.2	84.1	79.5	89.2	76.3
10	SVNNLC	97.6	91.2	86.3	85.4	87.2	79.8
20	CNN	97.3	92.7	88.5	87.9	89.2	83.2
20	SVM	98.0	91.0	86.6	82.7	90.8	80.0
20	SVNNLC	98.1	92.7	88.5	88.3	88.7	83.1

Table 6. Comparison of different algorithms for 5, 10 and 20 folds large cell carcinoma

K Folds	Model	AUC	CA	F1	Precision	Recall	MCC
5	CNN	97.3	94.5	84.8	87.2	82.6	81.9
5	SVM	98.0	94.5	83.7	93.5	75.7	81.0
5	SVNNLC	97.6	95.3	87.1	89.1	85.2	84.2
10	CNN	97.5	94.6	85.2	88.0	82.6	82.0
10	SVM	98.4	95.1	85.7	94.7	78.3	83.3
10	SVNNLC	98.2	95.1	86.6	89.0	84.3	83.7
20	CNN	98.4	95.4	87.6	89.2	86.1	84.8
20	SVM	98.9	95.4	86.8	94.8	80.0	84.5
20	SVNNLC	98.5	95.6	88.1	89.3	87.0	85.4

Table 7. Comparison of different algorithms for 5, 10 and 20 folds squamous cell carcinoma

K Folds	Model	AUC	CA	F1	Precision	Recall	MCC
5	CNN	97.9	94	87.6	91	84.5	83.7
5	SVM	96.7	91.7	82.2	89.4	76.1	77.3
5	SVNNLC	97.7	94.3	88.4	91.1	85.8	84.7
10	CNN	98.1	94.2	88.9	90.1	87.7	85.2
10	SVM	97.5	93.5	86.8	88.6	85.2	82.5
10	SVNNLC	98.2	94.5	89	89	89	85.3
20	CNN	98.5	95.4	90.8	92.1	89.7	87.8
20	SVM	98	94.6	89.3	90.1	88.4	85.7
20	SVNNLC	98.3	95.6	91.3	91.6	91	88.3

Table 8. Confusion matrix of CNN model for 5 folds

		Predicted				
		a	b	c	d	Σ
	a	172	10	3	0	195
	b	16	95	1	3	115
Actual	c	0	0	148	10	148
	d	20	4	0	131	155
	Σ	208	109	152	144	613

Table 9. Confusion matrix of SVM model for 5 folds

		Predicted				
		a	b	c	d	Σ
	a	177	4	0	14	195
	b	27	87	0	1	115
Actual	c	0	0	148	0	148
	d	35	2	0	118	155
	Σ	239	93	148	133	613

Table 10. Confusion matrix of SVNNLC model for 5 folds

		Predicted				
		a	b	c	d	Σ
	a	173	10	3	9	195
	b	13	98	0	4	115
Actual	c	0	0	148	0	148
	d	20	2	0	133	155
	Σ	206	110	151	146	613

Table 11. Confusion matrix of CNN model for 10 folds

		Predicted				
		a	b	c	d	Σ
	a	173	9	3	10	195
	b	14	95	1	5	115
Actual	c	0	0	148	0	148
	d	15	4	0	136	155
	Σ	202	108	152	151	613

Table 12. Confusion matrix of SVM model for 10 folds

		Predicted				
		a	b	c	d	Σ
Actual	a	174	3	2	16	195
	b	24	90	0	1	115
	c	0	0	148	0	148
	d	21	2	0	132	155
	Σ	219	95	150	149	613

Table 13. Confusion matrix of NNSVLC model for 10 folds

		Predicted				
		a	b	c	d	Σ
Actual	a	170	10	2	13	195
	b	14	97	0	4	115
	c	0	0	148	0	148
	d	15	2	0	138	155
	Σ	199	109	150	133	613

Table 14. Confusion matrix of CNN model for 20 folds

		Predicted				
		a	b	c	d	Σ
Actual	a	174	9	4	8	195
	b	11	99	1	4	115
	c	0	0	148	0	148
	d	13	3	0	139	155
	Σ	198	111	153	151	613

Table 15. Confusion matrix of SVM model for 20 folds

		Predicted				
		a	b	c	d	Σ
Actual	a	177	3	2	13	195
	b	21	92	0	2	115
	c	0	0	148	0	148
	d	16	2	0	137	155
	Σ	214	97	150	152	613

Table 16. Confusion matrix of NNSVLC model for 20 folds

		Predicted				
		a	b	c	d	Σ
Actual	a	173	10	3	9	195
	b	11	99	0	5	115
	c	0	0	148	0	148
	d	12	2	0	141	155
	Σ	196	111	151	133	613

Figure 2. Accuracy curve of 20 folds adenocarcinoma

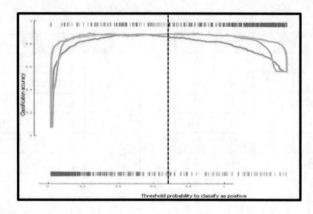

Figure 3. Accuracy curve of 20 folds large cell carcinoma

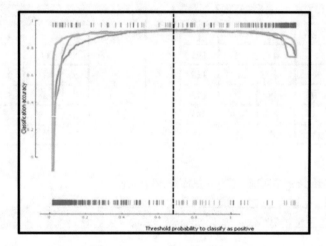

Figure 4. Accuracy curve of 20 folds squamous cell carcinoma

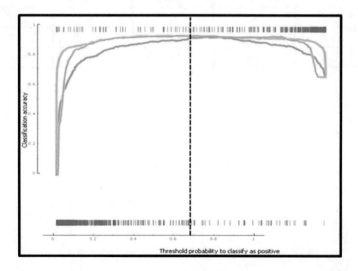

Figure 5. Accuracy curve of 20 folds normal cell

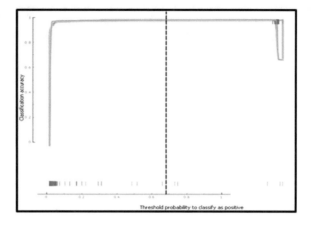

Figure 6. Accuracy curve of 10 folds adenocarcinoma

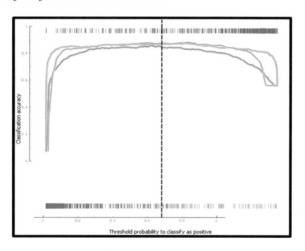

Figure 7. Accuracy curve of 10 folds large cell carcinoma

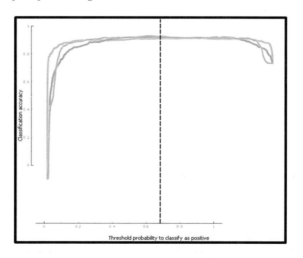

Figure 8. Accuracy curve of 10 folds squamous cell carcinoma

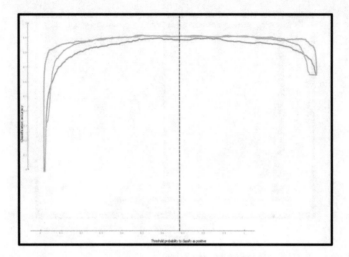

Figure 9. Accuracy curve of 10 folds normal cell

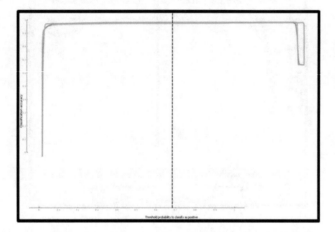

Figure 10. Accuracy curve of 5 folds adenocarcinoma

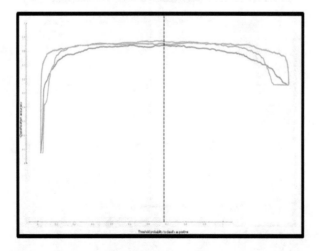

Figure 11. Accuracy curve of 5 folds normal cell

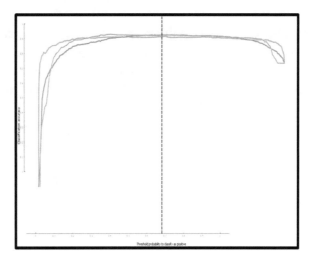

Figure 12. Accuracy curve of 5 folds large cell carcinoma

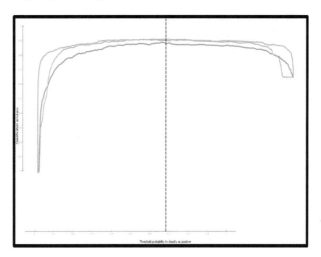

Figure 13. Accuracy curve of 5 folds squamous cell carcinoma

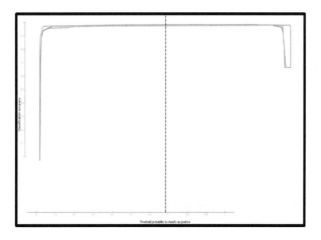

5. CONCLUSION

Automatically categorizing lung cancer is a significant advance in medical science's quest for early diagnosis and treatment. We can reach our goals more efficiently with AI. We suggested automated lung cancer classification. We were grouping deep-learning models. Transfer learning removed the top layers of two-component classifiers (InceptionV3, SVM). Transfer learning removed the top layers of two-component classifiers (InceptionV3 and SVM) to recognize lung cancer CT scan features and connect them to Dense Layers, which were trained with the Relu classifier to classify lung cancer.

The lung cancer dataset was cross-validated 200 times to verify the component classifier's accuracy. We used a weighted aggregate of classifiers to classify using SVNNLC. Test set performance and five, ten, and twenty-fold cross-validation were used to evaluate approaches. The SVNNLC surpassed the most advanced pre-trained models at twenty, ten, and five-fold cross-validation, achieving 91.7%, 90.2%, and 90.0%, as in Table 4.

REFERENCES

Abdullah, M. F., Sulaiman, S. N., Osman, M. K., Karim, N. K. A., Setumin, S., & Ani, A. I. C. (2023). Lung Lesion Identification Using Geometrical Feature and Optical Flow Method from Computed Tomography Scan Images. In Intelligent Multimedia Signal Processing for Smart Ecosystems (pp. 165–193). Springer International Publishing. doi:10.1007/978-3-031-34873-0_7

Abunasser, B., AL-Hiealy, M. R., Zaqout, I., & Abu-Naser, S. (2023). Convolution Neural Network for Breast Cancer Detection and Classification Using Deep Learning. *Asian Pacific Journal of Cancer Prevention*, *24*(2), 531–544. doi:10.31557/APJCP.2023.24.2.531 PMID:36853302

Ahmed, F. M., & Mohammed, D. B. A. D. A. M. A. S. I. S. A. N. I. (2023). Feasibility of Breast Cancer Detection Through a Convolutional Neural Network in Mammographs. *Tamjeed Journal of Healthcare Engineering and Science Technology*, *1*(2), 36–43. doi:10.59785/tjhest.v1i2.24

Asuntha, A., & Srinivasan, A. (2020). Deep learning for lung Cancer detection and classification. *Multimedia Tools and Applications*, *79*(11–12), 7731–7762. doi:10.1007/s11042-019-08394-3

Ayalew, A. M., Bezabih, Y. A., Abuhayi, B. M., & Ayalew, A. Y. (2024). Atelectasis detection in chest X-ray images using convolutional neural networks and transfer learning with anisotropic diffusion filter. *Informatics in Medicine Unlocked*, *45*, 101448. doi:10.1016/j.imu.2024.101448

Bhatia, S., Sinha, Y., & Goel, L. (2019). *Lung Cancer Detection: A Deep Learning Approach.*, doi:10.1007/978-981-13-1595-4_55

Bishnoi, V., Goel, N., & Tayal, A. (2023). Automated system-based classification of lung cancer using machine learning. *International Journal of Medical Engineering and Informatics*, *15*(5), 403–415. doi:10.1504/IJMEI.2023.133130

Bushara A. R., Vinod Kumar R. S., & Kumar S. S. (2023). Classification of Benign and Malignancy in Lung Cancer Using Capsule Networks with Dynamic Routing Algorithm on Computed Tomography Images. Journal of Artificial Intelligence and Technology. doi:10.37965/jait.2023.0218

Chen, Y., Hou, X., Yang, Y., Ge, Q., Zhou, Y., & Nie, S. (2022). A Novel Deep Learning Model Based on Multi-Scale and Multi-View for Detection of Pulmonary Nodules. *Journal of Digital Imaging*, *36*(2), 688–699. doi:10.1007/s10278-022-00749-x PMID:36544067

Ciompi, F., Chung, K., van Riel, S. J., Setio, A. A. A., Gerke, P. K., Jacobs, C., Scholten, E. Th., Schaefer-Prokop, C., Wille, M. M. W., Marchianò, A., Pastorino, U., Prokop, M., & van Ginneken, B. (2017). Towards automatic pulmonary nodule management in lung cancer screening with deep learning. *Scientific Reports*, *7*(1), 46479. doi:10.1038/srep46479 PMID:28422152

Das, S., & Majumder, S. (2020). Lung Cancer Detection Using Deep Learning Network: A Comparative Analysis. *2020 Fifth International Conference on Research in Computational Intelligence and Communication Networks (ICRCICN)*, 30–35. 10.1109/ICRCICN50933.2020.9296197

Dodia, S. B. A., & Mahesh, P. A. (2022). Recent advancements in deep learning based lung cancer detection: A systematic review. *Engineering Applications of Artificial Intelligence*, *116*, 105490. doi:10.1016/j.engappai.2022.105490

Fu, X., Bi, L., Kumar, A., Fulham, M., & Kim, J. (2022). An attention-enhanced cross-task network to analyse lung nodule attributes in CT images. *Pattern Recognition*, *126*, 108576. doi:10.1016/j.patcog.2022.108576

Gayap, H. T., & Akhloufi, M. A. (2024). Deep Machine Learning for Medical Diagnosis, Application to Lung Cancer Detection: A Review. *BioMedInformatics*, *4*(1), 236–284. doi:10.3390/biomedinformatics4010015

Gudur, R., Asif, D., Tamboli, I., Garg, A., & Sharma, M. (n.d.). International Journal of INTELLIGENT SYSTEMS AND APPLICATIONS IN ENGINEERING Optimizing Computed Tomography Image Reconstruction Parameters for Improved Lung Cancer Diagnosis with Grey Wolf Algorithm. In *Original Research Paper International Journal of Intelligent Systems and Applications in Engineering IJISA*. www.ijisae.org

Jin, T., Cui, H., Zeng, S., & Wang, X. (2017). Learning Deep Spatial Lung Features by 3D Convolutional Neural Network for Early Cancer Detection. *2017 International Conference on Digital Image Computing: Techniques and Applications (DICTA)*, (pp. 1–6). IEEE. 10.1109/DICTA.2017.8227454

Kim, K., Oh, S. J., Lee, J. H., & Chung, M. J. (2024). 3D unsupervised anomaly detection through virtual multi-view projection and reconstruction: Clinical validation on low-dose chest computed tomography. *Expert Systems with Applications*, *236*, 121165. doi:10.1016/j.eswa.2023.121165

Kumar, D., Wong, A., & Clausi, D. A. (2015). Lung Nodule Classification Using Deep Features in CT Images. *2015 12th Conference on Computer and Robot Vision*, (pp. 133–138). IEEE. 10.1109/CRV.2015.25

Lanjewar, M. G., Panchbhai, K. G., & Patle, L. B. (2024). Fusion of transfer learning models with LSTM for detection of breast cancer using ultrasound images. *Computers in Biology and Medicine*, *169*, 107914. doi:10.1016/j.compbiomed.2023.107914 PMID:38190766

Liu, Y., Hsu, H. Y., Lin, T., Peng, B., Saqi, A., Salvatore, M. M., & Jambawalikar, S. (2024). Lung nodule malignancy classification with associated pulmonary fibrosis using 3D attention-gated convolutional network with CT scans. *Journal of Translational Medicine*, *22*(1), 51. doi:10.1186/s12967-023-04798-w PMID:38216992

Mao, K., Tang, R., Wang, X., Zhang, W., & Wu, H. (2018). Feature Representation Using Deep Autoencoder for Lung Nodule Image Classification. *Complexity*, *2018*, 1–11. doi:10.1155/2018/3078374

Masood, A., Sheng, B., Li, P., Hou, X., Wei, X., Qin, J., & Feng, D. (2018). Computer-Assisted Decision Support System in Pulmonary Cancer detection and stage classification on CT images. *Journal of Biomedical Informatics*, *79*, 117–128. doi:10.1016/j.jbi.2018.01.005 PMID:29366586

Matsuyama, E., & Tsai, D.-Y. (2018). Automated Classification of Lung Diseases in Computed Tomography Images Using a Wavelet Based Convolutional Neural Network. *Journal of Biomedical Science and Engineering*, *11*(10), 263–274. doi:10.4236/jbise.2018.1110022

Nafisah, S. I., & Muhammad, G. (2024). Tuberculosis detection in chest radiograph using convolutional neural network architecture and explainable artificial intelligence. *Neural Computing & Applications*, *36*(1), 111–131. doi:10.1007/s00521-022-07258-6 PMID:35462630

Nam, J. G., Park, S., Hwang, E. J., Lee, J. H., Jin, K.-N., Lim, K. Y., Vu, T. H., Sohn, J. H., Hwang, S., Goo, J. M., & Park, C. M. (2019). Development and Validation of Deep Learning–based Automatic Detection Algorithm for Malignant Pulmonary Nodules on Chest Radiographs. *Radiology*, *290*(1), 218–228. doi:10.1148/radiol.2018180237 PMID:30251934

Nasrullah, N., Sang, J., Alam, M. S., Mateen, M., Cai, B., & Hu, H. (2019). Automated Lung Nodule Detection and Classification Using Deep Learning Combined with Multiple Strategies. *Sensors (Basel)*, *19*(17), 3722. doi:10.3390/s19173722 PMID:31466261

Poonkodi, S., & Kanchana, M. (2024). Lung cancer segmentation from CT scan images using modified mayfly optimization and particle swarm optimization algorithm. *Multimedia Tools and Applications*, *83*(2), 3567–3584. doi:10.1007/s11042-023-15688-0

Qian, L., Bai, J., Huang, Y., Zeebaree, D. Q., Saffari, A., & Zebari, D. A. (2024). Breast cancer diagnosis using evolving deep convolutional neural network based on hybrid extreme learning machine technique and improved chimp optimization algorithm. *Biomedical Signal Processing and Control*, *87*, 105492. doi:10.1016/j.bspc.2023.105492

Ramachandran, S., George, J., Skaria, S., & V.V., V. (2018). Using YOLO based deep learning network for real time detection and localization of lung nodules from low dose CT scans. In K. Mori & N. Petrick (Eds.), *Medical Imaging 2018: Computer-Aided Diagnosis* (p. 53). SPIE. doi:10.1117/12.2293699

Rani, K. V., & Jawhar, S. J. (2020). Superpixel with nanoscale imaging and boosted deep convolutional neural network concept for lung tumor classification. *International Journal of Imaging Systems and Technology*, *30*(4), 899–915. doi:10.1002/ima.22422

Rao, G. V. E., B, R., Srinivasu, P. N., Ijaz, M. F., & Woźniak, M. (2024). Hybrid framework for respiratory lung diseases detection based on classical CNN and quantum classifiers from chest X-rays. *Biomedical Signal Processing and Control*, *88*, 105567. doi:10.1016/j.bspc.2023.105567

Setio, A. A. A., Ciompi, F., Litjens, G., Gerke, P., Jacobs, C., van Riel, S. J., Wille, M. M. W., Naqibullah, M., Sanchez, C. I., & van Ginneken, B. (2016). Pulmonary Nodule Detection in CT Images: False Positive Reduction Using Multi-View Convolutional Networks. *IEEE Transactions on Medical Imaging*, *35*(5), 1160–1169. doi:10.1109/TMI.2016.2536809 PMID:26955024

Shah, S. N. A., & Parveen, R. (2023). An Extensive Review on Lung Cancer Diagnosis Using Machine Learning Techniques on Radiological Data: State-of-the-art and Perspectives. *Archives of Computational Methods in Engineering*, *30*(8), 4917–4930. doi:10.1007/s11831-023-09964-3

Shen, W., Zhou, M., Yang, F., Yang, C., & Tian, J. (2015). *Multi-scale Convolutional Neural Networks for Lung Nodule Classification.*, doi:10.1007/978-3-319-19992-4_46

Thamilarasi, V., & Roselin, R. (2021). Automatic Classification and Accuracy by Deep Learning Using CNN Methods in Lung Chest X-Ray Images. *IOP Conference Series. Materials Science and Engineering*, *1055*(1), 012099. doi:10.1088/1757-899X/1055/1/012099

Wani, N. A., Kumar, R., & Bedi, J. (2024). DeepXplainer: An interpretable deep learning based approach for lung cancer detection using explainable artificial intelligence. *Computer Methods and Programs in Biomedicine*, *243*, 107879. doi:10.1016/j.cmpb.2023.107879 PMID:37897989

Zhang, B., Qi, S., Monkam, P., Li, C., Yang, F., Yao, Y.-D., & Qian, W. (2019). Ensemble Learners of Multiple Deep CNNs for Pulmonary Nodules Classification Using CT Images. *IEEE Access : Practical Innovations, Open Solutions*, *7*, 110358–110371. doi:10.1109/ACCESS.2019.2933670

Chapter 14
Advancing Healthcare:
Economic Implications of Immediate MRI in Suspected Scaphoid Fractures – A Comprehensive Exploration

Rita Komalasari

https://orcid.org/0000-0001-9963-2363

Yarsi University, Indonesia

ABSTRACT

This study explores the economic implications of immediate magnetic resonance imaging (MRI) in treating suspected scaphoid fractures. Historically, conventional methods have been used, but recent advancements have introduced MRI into acute care settings, challenging established diagnostic paradigms. The study aims to close the empirical-economic evidence gap on the prompt use of MRI in cases with suspected scaphoid fractures, providing insight into cost-effectiveness, resource use, and overall healthcare efficiency. The literature study illuminates the evolution of diagnostic approaches for scaphoid fractures, highlighting the limitations of conventional methods. The findings underscore the pivotal role of MRI in scaphoid fracture management, demonstrating cost-effectiveness and enhanced healthcare outcomes, challenging traditional diagnostic pathways.

1. INTRODUCTION

Traditional diagnostic procedures, especially X-rays, have limitations that have long hampered the identification and treatment of suspected scaphoid fractures (Simon et al., 2020). Misdiagnosis, prolonged treatment, and consequences due to these shortcomings place heavy demands on healthcare budgets and delivery systems (Filip et al., 2022). Since scaphoid fractures are prevalent, particularly after trauma or falls, it is crucial to get a correct diagnosis as soon as possible to minimize long-term problems and lessen the burden on healthcare budgets (Mallee et al., 2020). In the realm of modern healthcare, the integration of cutting-edge technologies has reshaped diagnostic paradigms, challenging conventional

DOI: 10.4018/979-8-3693-2359-5.ch014

methods and ushering in an era of unprecedented precision and efficiency. Magnetic resonance imaging (MRI) is one such development that has revolutionised medical practise, especially with regards to the detection of scaphoid fractures (Chunara et al., 2019). Although traditional methods have formed the backbone of fracture diagnoses for quite some time, advances in MRI technology have raised the bar, particularly in emergencies. This chapter delves into the transformative power of immediate MRI in suspected scaphoid fractures, exploring its economic implications from the perspective of healthcare payers. By delving into the historical evolution of diagnostic methods for scaphoid fractures, scrutinizing the limitations of conventional approaches, and highlighting the pivotal role of MRI in acute care, this study bridges the empirical-economic evidence gap. The purpose is to present a complete knowledge of the financial ramifications of fast MRI use, revealing problems of cost-effectiveness, resource utilization, and healthcare efficiency. The knowledge and information yielded by the research on the economic implications of immediate MRI in suspected scaphoid fractures can significantly benefit several key stakeholders, leading to positive changes and improvements in the present situation within the healthcare system and the broader medical field.

Here are some ways in which various people and organizations may put this new information to use: Orthopaedic surgeons, emergency room doctors, and radiologists in particular, might use the results in their daily work. They may make better judgments about diagnosing and treating suspected scaphoid fractures if they have a thorough understanding of the benefits of immediate MRI, including its lower cost and increased diagnostic accuracy. Better patient outcomes, fewer incorrect diagnoses, and more efficient treatment plans are all possible thanks to this insight. This research will aid in more efficient resource allocation by hospitals and their management and policymakers. They may invest in cutting-edge imaging technology, which guarantees patients get prompt and accurate diagnosis while reaping the financial advantages of instant MRI. These findings can help policymakers advocate for MRI scans whenever a scaphoid fracture is suspected, raising the bar for patient treatment. Statistics from this research on the cost-effectiveness of giving emergency MRIs for suspected scaphoid fractures may be utilized by healthcare providers and payers to make decisions about whether or not to cover the procedure. Understanding the long-term advantages of correct and early diagnoses may lead to the inclusion of MRI treatments in insurance coverage, thereby decreasing total healthcare expenditures by eliminating issues associated with misdiagnosis. Researchers and academics in radiology, orthopedics, and health economics may expand upon the study's results. Patient satisfaction, long-term health outcomes, and quality of life are all areas where further study is required, including how immediate MRI affects these factors. This continuing study has the potential to enhance current diagnostic procedures and healthcare standards. This information may help patients and their supporters understand why it is crucial to have an MRI right away when a scaphoid fracture is suspected. Patients who are well-informed may partner with their doctors in making treatment decisions, such as promoting MRI usage when it is warranted. Patients and their families will benefit from speedier and more accurate diagnoses due to this empowerment, as will the healthcare system. This research helps advance medicine and healthcare by shedding light on how to increase diagnostic precision, standardize care delivery, and make better use of scarce resources. The research lays the path for an improved, patient-centered, and cost-effective method of identifying and treating suspected scaphoid fractures by equipping multiple stakeholders with this important data. The study's findings on the financial benefits of doing an MRI on patients with suspected scaphoid fractures right away may contribute to numerous practice areas and applied research.

Medical professionals may use the findings of this research to guide their choice of diagnostic procedures. The results may help doctors decide whether or not to do an MRI on patients with suspected scaphoid fractures right away. With this information, doctors can provide their patients with the best possible treatment. Findings from this research may inform the creation of more recent emergency room and orthopedic practice policies and recommendations. The diagnostic consistency and quality of treatment delivered to patients by healthcare facilities may be enhanced by including rapid MRI in routine procedures for suspected scaphoid fractures. Clear rules boost the efficiency of healthcare procedures and help to standardize practices. Health economists and policymakers may use the study's financial data to assess the value of urgent MRI. The healthcare system would benefit from more strategic investments in cutting-edge imaging technology if its leaders had a better grasp of the financial ramifications. Allocating funds based on evidence has the potential to reduce waste in healthcare systems and maximize the effectiveness of healthcare expenditures. The results of this study might motivate further investigations and clinical tests in this field.

Further investigation on the financial implications of immediate MRI for other orthopedic disorders or other imaging modalities is warranted. Improvements in clinical practice may be sustained by adding to the existing body of research in diagnostic imaging and healthcare economics. Patients and advocacy organizations may use the research findings to stress the value of an emergency MRI for scaphoid fractures. Well-informed patients can better advocate for themselves and may make informed decisions about the diagnostic procedures they undergo. Such lobbying has the potential to influence healthcare policy and practice, bringing it closer in line with the results of the most recent scientific studies. Medical education curricula and training programs for healthcare workers may incorporate the study's conclusions. Future medical professionals may be prepared to recognize the importance of prompt MRI in scaphoid fracture diagnosis if this knowledge is included in teaching materials. This integration ensures that the next generation of healthcare professionals is equipped with the latest knowledge and best practices. The study's findings have the potential to greatly affect the real world of healthcare by informing clinical choices and procedures, influencing health economics policy, stimulating more study, empowering patients, and bettering healthcare education. Patients with suspected scaphoid fractures, and maybe other medical disorders, might benefit from implementing these results into practice, which can enhance patient outcomes, resource utilization, and the progress of knowledge in applied research.

2. BACKGROUND

Each year, emergency rooms in Indonesia see a high volume of patients with wrist injuries (Suroto et al., 2021). Scaphoid fractures account for 51-90% of carpal fractures and 2-7% of total fractures in this population (Almigdad et al., 2023). Scaphoid fractures are common among young, otherwise healthy people who fall onto their extended hands (Bhashyam & Mudgal, 2023). Existence reports need to be more consistent. Scaphoid fractures ranged from 5% to 50% in a systematic study (Chong et al., 2022). These numbers were obtained from various reference tests, explaining some fluctuation. There may have been discrepancies in the published incidence rates for scaphoid fractures due to changes in the diagnostic procedures used by different hospitals. Despite this doubt, clinical data shows that between 10 and 20 percent of patients who arrive with a suspected fracture have a fractured scaphoid (Daniels et al., 2020). When dealing with patients who may have fractures of the scaphoid, doctors face three primary obstacles: The incidence of true fractures in patients who arrive with symptoms suggesting a break is low. Studies have shown that between 66 and 84 percent of those with ED do not have any bone injuries (Wu et al., 2021). Diagnosing a scaphoid fracture clinically and radiographically was challenging during the lecture. Chang et al., (2022) estimate that 40% of scaphoid fractures may be misdiagnosed and undertreated. That would Scaphoid fractures are often misdiagnosed, which may lead to clinical issues and affect patient outcomes, particularly in young adults. Arthritis of the wrist after non-union and avascular necrosis Better patient outcomes and fewer problems result from prompt diagnosis and treatment. Clinicians may overtreat patients with a suspected scaphoid fracture with splints and plaster casts, even if there is no radiological evidence of a fracture. There are societal costs associated with over-treating scaphoid fractures, such as lost productivity from prolonged plaster cast usage. Using publicly accessible data, Pitros et al., (2020) constructed a decision tree model and discovered that the lowest total cost of care was found with CT scans performed immediately upon presentation. Significant societal costs, such as lost output, make using it impractical. Injuries to the scaphoid account for between 51 and 90 percent of all carpal fractures and 2 to 7 percent of all fractures. The frequency with which people break their scaphoid is estimated to range from 5 percent to 50 percent. Research reveals that between 10 and 20 percent of individuals with a suspected scaphoid fracture have a confirmed incidence value in this range (Swärd et al., 2019). Timely diagnosis and treatment are essential for improving patient outcomes and reducing the risk of future impacts. It is common practice to overtreat patients with suspected scaphoid fractures by applying splints and casts even when there is no radiological evidence of fracture. This might have far-reaching consequences for patients' experiences and quality of life, leading to higher costs for everyone. Patients who appear without a scaphoid fracture may save the healthcare system money by having a computed tomography (CT) scan performed as soon as possible after their first presentation.

A large percentage of all hand-related emergency room visits are due to scaphoid fractures, making it one of the most prevalent wrist injuries. The prevalence of scaphoid fractures has been demonstrated to rise steadily over the years, underscoring the need for speedy and precise diagnosis in order to permit early and suitable interventions (Jørgsholm, et al., 2020). Conventional diagnostic procedures, such as X-rays, have trouble picking up on tiny scaphoid fractures, which may cause them to be ignored or diagnosed late (Sahu et al., 2023). Studies have shown the limitations of conventional methods, highlighting the need to investigate novel imaging modalities like MRI for precise diagnosis. Increased Sensitivity and Specificity of MRI Scaphoid fractures may now be diagnosed with MRI even when there is only a small amount of displacement or when the fracture is only partially healed. When compared to traditional diagnostic approaches, MRI has been shown to have a far higher rate of success in study after study. Non-union, avascular necrosis, and long-term impairment are just some of the problems that may arise from a missed or delayed diagnosis of a scaphoid fracture, all of which add to the financial burden on patients and healthcare providers alike (Sabbagh et al., 2019). Prompt and accurate diagnosis with MRI can potentially mitigate these economic burdens by enabling timely and appropriate management strategies. Efficient utilization of healthcare resources is paramount in modern healthcare systems. Immediate MRI can streamline the diagnostic process, reducing unnecessary follow-up visits, additional imaging tests, and interventions related to missed or delayed diagnoses. This optimized resource utilization aligns with the broader goal of healthcare systems to enhance efficiency and reduce overall costs. Economic statistics for treating suspected scaphoid fractures have been synthesized using modern imaging techniques including computed tomography (CT) and magnetic resonance imaging (MRI) (Conombo et al., 2022). Population/patient, intervention/treatment, and comparison with traditional radiography all played roles in the search approach, which was developed using the PICOS framework. Total expenses associated with advanced imaging for acute therapy of suspected scaphoid fractures are the main result, with secondary outcomes, including economic assessments, also being taken into account. Researchers examined the cost-effectiveness of modern imaging methods for detecting and treating scaphoid fractures. Quantitative studies with patients who may have had a scaphoid fracture were considered for inclusion.

Due to the rarity of official economic assessments before 2019, the study only considered articles published in 2019. Studies focused only on treating scaphoid fractures that had already been identified were also excluded. Database searches yielded 150 documents; after eliminating duplicates, only 99 remained. Twenty-one articles were evaluated for their entire texts, with six records being thrown out for different reasons. There was a comparison of the studies' methodologies, interventions, timings, and monetary outcomes. All the studies were about using MRI to diagnose and treat individuals who may have fractures. However, besides bone scintigraphy, CT, and ultrasound, additional imaging modalities have been used in certain studies as well. The retrieved papers did not lend themselves to a meta-analysis due to differences in research design, follow-up methodologies, imaging modalities, economic/cost data, and economic views. Four British studies and one each from the Netherlands, Spain, Norway, and Denmark made up the five European studies collated. Research from the United States, China, New Zealand, and Australia revealed the remaining evidence.

The structure of this chapter is designed to facilitate a systematic exploration of this intriguing subject matter. First, a detailed review of historical and contemporary sources illuminates the evolution of diagnostic techniques, setting the stage for the emergence of MRI in scaphoid fracture management. This comprehensive literature study serves as the foundation upon which the subsequent analysis is built. The chapter then digs into the technique used in this investigation after briefly reviewing the relevant literature. Methodical data analysis is used to draw conclusions, spot patterns, and locate knowledge gaps in the diagnostic field. In order to provide a solid foundation for the economic assessments that will follow, this methodological rigor is essential. The findings and discussion of this study highlight the need for emergency MRI to manage scaphoid fractures. This study questions the status quo of diagnostic practices by examining the monetary ramifications, which include improved healthcare outcomes and reduced healthcare expenditures. In addition, this study's results aid in the development of well-informed healthcare policy and the improvement of clinical practices. Studying the complete effects of rapid MRI in cases of suspected scaphoid fractures is important for optimizing resource allocation and providing the best possible treatment for patients. In this chapter, we begin our exploration of the financial ramifications of this game-changing technology, illuminating the far-reaching effects it will have on healthcare delivery and individual health outcomes.

3. METHOD

In order to arrive at its conclusions, the approach used rigorous data analysis methods, synthesizing data from a wide range of historical and current sources. A more sophisticated comprehension of the diagnostic landscape was achieved via the identification of patterns and gaps in the available literature. This methodological rigor enabled a thorough examination of existing information, allowing the researchers to identify the limitations of traditional approaches and the benefits of rapid MRI in emergency situations. The critical rise of MRI in acute care settings was a major feature of the literature analysis, demonstrating its potential to solve the limitations of conventional diagnostic techniques. In situations with limited displacement or incomplete fractures, the investigation showed that immediate MRI had greater diagnostic accuracy. Based on this information, additional cost-benefit analyses investigated the financial effects of requiring rapid MRI for all suspected scaphoid fractures. The approaches section's narrative literature analysis established the background for scaphoid fracture therapy and the limits of traditional diagnostic approaches, underlining the need for a paradigm change in this area of medicine. The evaluation paved the way for in-depth data analysis, which in turn allowed for the investigation of immediate MRI as a potentially game-changing option. Relevant information was gathered by doing a targeted search of Google Scholar for terms associated with scaphoid fractures, diagnostic procedures, and MRI. The research set out to fill a vacuum in the literature by systematically analyzing the cost-effectiveness, resource usage, and overall healthcare efficiency of using MRI for suspected scaphoid fractures as soon as possible.

4. THE DEVELOPMENT OF SCAPHOID FRACTURE DIAGNOSTICS

In this section, the author discuss the development of scaphoid fracture diagnostics across time, highlighting the strengths and weaknesses of previous approaches before the advent of more recent imaging technologies. Scaphoid fractures have often been diagnosed via X-rays (Wijetunga et al., 2019). When dealing with small or partial cracks, however, a careful examination of past procedures shows their inherent limitations. X-rays, although beneficial in many diagnostic circumstances, typically prove ineffective in identifying scaphoid fractures owing to their poor sensitivity in collecting minute details of bone structures. Fractures that are very subtle or occur in anatomically complicated places might be difficult to detect on X-ray, increasing the risk of misdiagnosis or delay in treatment. Misdiagnosis may have serious consequences for individuals, including non-union, avascular necrosis, and permanent impairment. With this information in hand, you can better see the pressing need for innovative methods of scaphoid fracture diagnosis. Better imaging methods, especially magnetic resonance imaging (MRI), must be investigated to close the diagnostic gap. By delving into the historical inadequacies, this section sets the stage for the subsequent exploration of MRI's pivotal role in transforming scaphoid fracture management. The development of diagnostic tools has shed light on the need for a paradigm change, ushering in the game-changing age of urgent MRI in suspected scaphoid fractures. Scaphoid fractures are frequent and may be treated with both standard radiography and more sophisticated imaging techniques (CT and MRI). Due to its limited availability, CT is often suggested. However, there is concern that radiation exposure might cause predictable and unexpected health problems. MRI may be used to properly detect scaphoid fractures and other bone fractures in the emergency room since it has a high negative predictive value for such injuries.

4.1 Fast MRI Has Better Diagnostic Accuracy Than Other Methods

The diagnostic process for scaphoid fractures has evolved with the advent of magnetic resonance imaging (MRI) in recent years (Ibrahim et al., 2022). MRI has been demonstrated to be superior to traditional diagnostic modalities for scaphoid fractures. One of the primary characteristics of MRI consists in its remarkable sensitivity and specificity, allowing it to locate scaphoid fractures with unmatched accuracy (Coventry et al., 2023). MRI is superior to X-rays in situations of little displacement or incomplete fractures because it provides a clearer picture of soft tissue and bone structures. Since small scaphoid fractures are often overlooked or misconstrued by standard imaging modalities, this skill is vital in their treatment. Studies comparing MRI and other methods have shown that it is accurate in diagnosing even the smallest fractures. Because of its superior visualization capabilities, a more thorough evaluation may be performed, leading to a more accurate and dependable diagnosis (Hendrix et al., 2021). In cases where immediate intervention is essential, such as suspected scaphoid fractures, the precision offered by MRI is invaluable. Preventing problems, directing proper therapies, and ultimately improving patient outcomes all depend on timely and accurate diagnosis. Since the same imaging modality performed at different times may give varied clinical and economic results, scheduling the diagnostic test at the optimal time was equally as important as the imaging modality itself. Patients were photographed using cutting-edge equipment ranging from two to five days post-injury in three randomized clinical studies. Advanced imaging was analyzed on the day of injury and again two weeks later in certain research, especially those that included economic models. The monetary evidence was sorted into many groups according to study strategy and point of view (healthcare payer vs. society). Snaith et al., (2021) showed that rapid CT was the most cost-effective strategy for treating patients with suspected scaphoid fractures. The differences and similarities between cost-benefit assessments and cost-utility analyses were discussed.

Healthcare payer costs were not significantly different across three randomized controlled trials. Owing to patients spending too much time in bed owing to severe immobilization, only one of the three studies undertaken had sufficient power to detect statistically significant changes in economic results. Magnetic resonance imaging (MRI) and other forms of advanced imaging are either cost-effective or cost-saving. From the standpoint of healthcare payers, the four non-randomized empirical investigations exhibited mixed results, but overall, enhanced imaging was related to higher healthcare expenses. According to the results of investigations, the cost of wrist immobilization without early advanced imaging is lower than that of the technique using advanced imaging (Norimoto et al., 2021). However, statistical analysis of economic effects (p-value or confidence intervals) was not performed in the these studies. Rua et al., (2020) discovered no notable cost variations in scaphoid fracture treatment. Kodumuri et al., (2021) conducted the sole economic assessment of the four quasi-experimental investigations.

The evidence presented in these studies underscores the critical role of immediate MRI in enhancing diagnostic outcomes for suspected scaphoid fractures. By providing a level of precision that conventional methods cannot match, immediate MRI not only reduces the risk of misdiagnosis and delayed treatment but also ensures that patients receive timely and appropriate care. Immediate MRI is a staple of contemporary scaphoid fracture therapy due to its higher diagnostic accuracy, which is in line with the overriding objective of enhancing healthcare efficiency and patient satisfaction. Third, the monetary effects of incorrect diagnoses and postponed treatment: The significant financial cost associated with misdiagnosis and delayed treatment is an important consideration when weighing the financial consequences of early MRI in suspected scaphoid fractures. The long-term expenses caused by problems from untreated or improperly treated scaphoid fractures have been illuminated by studies on this topic. Aside from negatively impacting patients' quality of life, problems including non-union, avascular necrosis, and long-term incapacity also put a heavy financial burden on healthcare systems and individuals.

Scaphoid fractures are rather frequent and may have serious practical and financial consequences. Different findings may be obtained from the same imaging modality when used at different periods, illustrating the significance of timing in diagnosis. The benefits of advanced imaging 2-5 days and 1-3 days after injury were evaluated in three randomized clinical trials. The use of high-tech imaging on the day of injury and up to two weeks after that has also been the subject of cost-benefit analyses. However, it has been shown that when societal expenses like time off work are included, modern imaging, especially MRI, is either cost-saving or cost-effective. Healthcare expenses have been proven to rise in tandem with the use of sophisticated imaging, according to non-randomized empirical investigations.

The average cost of an MRI to rule out a scaphoid fracture was \$692, which was less than the overall hospital charges (Han et al., 2022). Patients with undiagnosed or mismanaged scaphoid fractures often experience complications that necessitate costly interventions, such as surgical procedures to address non-union or prolonged rehabilitation efforts to regain functional abilities. The financial implications of these complications extend beyond the immediate healthcare costs, encompassing expenses related to extended medical treatments, loss of productivity due to disability, and potential long-term care requirements. The emotional and psychological costs to patients and their loved ones also cannot be discounted when considering the repercussions of a missed diagnosis and subsequent delay in treatment. The indirect expenditures associated with scaphoid fractures may be substantial, accounting for as much as 85 percent of overall management expenses (Dean & SUSPECT study group, 2021). The cost-effectiveness of using sophisticated imaging to treat patients with suspected scaphoid fractures was assessed in three trials using economic modeling. The most cost-effective treatments were computed tomography (CT) on the day of injury and magnetic resonance imaging (MRI) on day three. An MRI-based approach to addressing suspected scaphoid fractures was anticipated to be viable and cost-effective, depending on healthcare payers' willingness to pay levels, local institutional costs, and imaging availability.

There have been inconsistent results from previous studies utilizing economic modeling to analyze the cost of adopting sophisticated imaging to treat suspected scaphoid fractures (Stirling et al., 2021). However, the meta-analysis also revealed that there may be no direct comparability between the findings of different studies owing to changes in sample size, sample composition, study design, imaging technology, time post-injury, and economic impacts (Chong et al., 2022).The systematic review uncovered varying economic results depending on the angle of research. When viewed from a societal viewpoint, using cutting-edge imaging techniques is expected to result in financial benefits. The systematic review study, however, did not give concrete monetary statistics if one were to take a healthcare perspective (de Lurdes, 2022). A significant drawback of non-randomized research is the absence of empirical data required to assess the influence of sophisticated imaging on the utilization of healthcare resources. Another is that the economic models used in the studies do not necessarily reflect actual clinical practice. Immediate MRI emerges as a pivotal intervention in mitigating these economic challenges. By enabling timely and accurate diagnoses of scaphoid fractures, MRI is proactive in preventing complications associated with untreated fractures. Early detection allows for prompt initiation of appropriate treatment strategies, reducing the likelihood of complications and their associated costs. The investment in immediate MRI, when compared to the potential long-term expenses incurred by complications, proves to be a cost-effective approach. Furthermore, the cost savings achieved through preventing complications reverberate throughout the healthcare system. Hospitals and healthcare providers experience reduced burdens related to complex surgical procedures and extensive rehabilitation efforts. Patients, on the other hand, benefit from shorter recovery periods, minimizing the impact on their daily lives and livelihoods. Hospital costs were increased by \$692 due to the MRI, however ruling out a scaphoid fracture was worth the extra money (Simón et al., 2022). Finally, two societal investigations indicated that better imaging resulted in reduced societal costs, supporting the findings of the RCT study. Up to 85% of overall management expenses, according to a study by Han et al. (2022), are attributable to indirect costs for workers (due to sick absence). The cost-effectiveness of more sophisticated imaging for suspected scaphoid fractures was assessed in three trials using economic modeling. The cost-effectiveness evaluations indicated that doing CT immediately and MRI on day 3 had the most favorable results. et al. (2015) did a second trial evaluating quality-adjusted life years and concluded that high-tech imaging was superior to sham cast immobilization in a community context. Medical insurance coverage, local healthcare expenditures, and the availability of imaging services all had a role in determining whether or not MRI was a practical treatment option for patients with suspected scaphoid fractures. The third research was carried out by Yoon et al., 2021. Bone scintigraphy saved money by preventing a non-union in one patient who would have needed more X-rays. Costs were analyzed using economic models in five different studies. Advanced imaging for suspected scaphoid fractures was shown to have substantially varying costs in these studies. While one research did not discover a significant price difference, four others did. Könneker et al., (2019) suggested a course of five MRI or bone scintigraphy scans spaced out across the first day, the next four days, and the next two weeks. Advanced imaging may increase or decrease management expenses depending on the imaging modalities used. Performing an MRI on day 1 (or within a few days) and after that, reviewing it on the same day resulted in reduced expenditures. By comparing the costs of MRI screening to traditional immobilization, Asfia et al., (2020) found no significant difference. The price of sophisticated imaging increases when patients need to book appointments on days other than the day of their scans to discuss the results. According to a study by Rua et al. (2019), the cost of treatment for a suspected scaphoid injury was $139 more than that of an MRI. The price of MRI and CT scans, two of the most advanced imaging methods, increased by $225 (£158) and $82 (£58), respectively. Finally, when societal expenses due to missed time from work are included. Utilizing MRI to treat suspected scaphoid fractures increased costs by £242 (£168) but saved an average of $1,655 (£1,151) per patient. Study designs, countries of origin, and modalities of imaging all impacted the timing of imaging and the resulting economic effects. Key limitations of the papers included in this analysis were inadequate reporting, inadequate follow-up, and weak statistical power. Although the three studies' conclusions were different, they shared methodological issues, such as a lack of empirical information required to predict healthcare resource utilization and the use of sophisticated imaging on the day of injury. There must be a comprehensive examination of the evidence. In light of this, Dean et al., (2021) undertook a thorough analysis and discovered economic differences via the use of analytical methods. In the long term, improved imaging could help society save money regardless of when or what shape it takes. The systematic review and randomized trials both failed to identify statistically significant differences in costs, and the results were not persuasive economically. The absence of empirical data to quantify the influence of advanced imaging on healthcare resource utilization, such as the omission of resource use following a negative advanced imaging scan and the utilization of economic models that did not necessarily mirror real-world clinical practice, were significant deficiencies in the non-randomized studies. Scaphoid fractures may be difficult to detect in imaging studies and the clinic. The diagnostic process for GSTT starts with an initial clinical examination on presentation, generally in the ED. However, it may be complicated by the absence of uniform imaging methods for suspected scaphoid fractures across institutions. Four sequential plain radiographs are obtained to exclude the likelihood of a scaphoid fracture. Upon detection of anomalies, patients are provided with a splint and sent to a fracture clinic for further evaluation within 1-2 weeks. Patients presenting with a confirmed scaphoid fracture often get a CT scan (or, less commonly, an MRI scan) at the fracture clinic to assess the degree of displacement. Scaphoid fractures are often managed with the use of cast immobilization for 6-8 weeks or through surgical intervention in cases where the fracture is displaced or involves the proximal pole (van Delft et al., 2019). Patients who have normal results on their first 4-view plain x-ray are sent to a fracture clinic for further assessment. At this juncture, further computed tomography (CT) or magnetic resonance imaging (MRI) scans are conducted alongside repeated conventional radiographs (often four-view plain X-rays). The MRI findings dictate the subsequent course of action for the patient, which may include discharge, surgical intervention, or application of a cast. As previously stated, GSTT uses normal radiography as well as more sophisticated imaging techniques like CT and, to a lesser degree, MRI for the management of scaphoid fractures. If the 4-view plain x-ray yields no abnormal findings, although the patient continues to have symptoms, a computed tomography (CT) scan will be conducted at the subsequent follow-up visit. CT was probably employed rather than MRI because MRI was unavailable. A CT scan may be ordered and analyzed by the referring physician on the day of the fracture clinic session. The non-stochastic and stochastic risks of radiation exposure to patients receiving CT or any other radiation-based imaging method are real. The recommended action for emergency department clinicians who suspect scaphoid fractures is to get an MRI immediately. Because of its superior accuracy and lack of radiation, MRI has largely replaced CT as the diagnostic method of choice for scaphoid fractures. Scaphoid and other bone fractures were identified in the "positive" (i.e., abnormal) results of the first MRI. Scaphoid fractures have been demonstrated to be easily ruled in with MRI. Hence, it has been hypothesized that MRI will correctly identify additional bone fractures brought to the ED. If an MRI was negative or the patient's injuries were relatively modest, the ER would send them home without further care. Some patients may still have wrist discomfort two weeks after injury, even if there are no fractures apparent; these patients should be evaluated and treated. The idea was that the high specificity of MRI in excluding scaphoid fractures among suspected fractures would enable the safe release of patients without scaphoid or other bone fractures. The use of high-fidelity imaging in the assessment of suspected fractures has been substantiated by three randomized controlled trials, two quasi-experimental studies, and several economic modeling studies. Magnetic resonance imaging (MRI) has never been used as the principal diagnostic tool in examining an abrupt occurrence. The benefits of having an MRI performed right when a patient arrives at the emergency department were investigated in this research. This method appears novel to me, and it might easily become the de facto norm throughout the nation and the world. The financial impact of incorrect diagnosis and delayed treatment emphasizes the need for prompt MRI scans in cases with suspected scaphoid fractures. Expediting MRI scans not only improves patient outcomes but also contributes to substantial cost savings in the long run by diminishing the probability of complications and the financial burden associated with them. This proactive approach aligns with efficient resource allocation, patient-centered care, and overall healthcare sustainability, making immediate MRI a valuable asset in scaphoid fracture management.

4.2 Streamlined Healthcare Processes and Resource Utilization

Immediate MRI is a beacon of efficiency in the realm of suspected scaphoid fractures, reshaping healthcare processes and optimizing resource utilization. This section explores how immediate MRI, by streamlining the diagnostic pathway, brings forth a paradigm shift in healthcare operations, ensuring rapid and accurate diagnoses while minimizing unnecessary interventions and follow-up visits. One of the primary advantages of immediate MRI lies in its ability to provide rapid and precise results, offering clinicians valuable insights into scaphoid fractures promptly. Due to unclear findings or postponed diagnoses, patients of traditional medicine are sometimes required to return for many follow-up visits and further imaging tests; however, with instantaneous MRI, these unnecessary procedures are no longer necessary. With the detailed information provided by an MRI scan, doctors can make educated judgments quickly, allowing them to begin effective treatments and interventions sooner. The streamlined diagnostic pathway facilitated by immediate MRI translates into substantial time savings for both patients and healthcare professionals. Patients experience reduced waiting times, ensuring that their diagnostic journey is expedited, and the subsequent treatment can commence promptly. Additionally, healthcare professionals benefit from the efficiency of immediate MRI, enabling them to allocate their time and expertise more effectively, addressing other critical healthcare needs. Furthermore, the optimized resource utilization achieved through immediate MRI has profound implications for cost savings within the healthcare system. By minimizing the need for multiple diagnostic procedures and interventions, unnecessary healthcare expenditures are curtailed. This not only conserves financial resources but also frees up healthcare facilities and personnel, allowing them to focus on other essential aspects of patient care and medical services. The enhanced efficiency brought about by immediate MRI aligns seamlessly with the overarching goal of healthcare systems— to provide excellent medical care that is both efficient and affordable. By reducing the burden of misdiagnoses, unnecessary interventions, and prolonged waiting periods, immediate MRI ensures that resources are channeled judiciously, optimizing the overall healthcare experience for both patients and providers. In essence, the streamlined healthcare processes and resource utilization facilitated by immediate MRI not only save costs but also enhance overall healthcare efficiency. This section underscores the transformative impact of immediate MRI on the diagnostic pathway, emphasizing its role in improving patient outcomes, maximizing healthcare resources, and contributing to a more effective and patient-centric healthcare system.

4.3 Alignment With Patient-Centered Care

At the heart of modern healthcare lies the principle of patient-centered care, where the focus is on delivering personalized, timely, and effective services tailored to meet the unique needs of individual patients. Immediate MRI emerges as a beacon of patient-centricity, aligning seamlessly with these fundamental principles by prioritizing accurate and timely diagnoses. In this article, we will discuss how instantaneous MRI may improve patient-centered treatment, resulting in higher levels of patient satisfaction, less anxiety, and better outcomes for patients as a whole. When dealing with possible scaphoid fractures, having access to reliable diagnostic data as soon as possible is crucial. Immediate MRI reduces patients' stress and uncertainty throughout the diagnostic procedure. The existence and severity of scaphoid fractures may be determined quickly and accurately by MRI as opposed to the time-consuming and potentially inaccurate procedures used traditionally (Daniels et al., 2020). Patients benefit from this quick turnaround since it shortens their overall experience with the healthcare system and decreases their time spent waiting. Patients are spared the physical agony and mental suffering that comes with extended medical procedures thanks to rapid MRI, which reduces the need for unneeded treatments and follow-up visits. Patients are spared the trauma of having to undergo several tests and invasive procedures, giving them more time to concentrate on getting well. Not only can eliminating needless medical procedures improve the quality of care provided to patients, but it also gives them more agency in shaping their treatment plans. Immediate MRI has a demonstrable, favorable effect on patients' attitudes toward their treatment generally. Patients are more likely to have a positive experience with their treatment if they are given a timely and correct diagnosis. This optimistic outlook affects their confidence in healthcare practitioners and facilities beyond the first diagnostic phase. The trust between a patient and their healthcare practitioner is crucial to successful treatment and good health. Quick MRI is a cornerstone of patient-centered treatment because it exemplifies the values of precision, efficiency, and empathy. Patient satisfaction is increased, anxiety is decreased, and the number of interventions required is cut down significantly thanks to rapid MRI. The healthcare system benefits from its alignment with patient-centered care principles because it encourages a more compassionate, trustworthy, and high-performing workforce. The significance of early MRI for suspected scaphoid fractures has been highlighted, along with its revolutionary effect on healthcare delivery, resource allocation, and patient satisfaction. This section has offered a thorough overview of the many advantages of immediate MRI by diving into its historical limits, showing its greater diagnostic accuracy, investigating its economic consequences, and emphasizing its alignment with patient-centered treatment. With its capacity to enhance diagnostic pathways, optimum resource utilization, and elevate patient-centered care, rapid MRI is fast becoming a cornerstone in managing scaphoid fractures. The healthcare system benefits from its rapid and accurate diagnosis, which is consistent with the system's goals of precision, economy, and compassion.

5. SOLUTIONS AND RECOMMENDATIONS

Given the overwhelming evidence, hospitals and governments must begin routinely ordering MRIs for patients with suspected scaphoid fractures. Policy suggestions should incorporate instantaneous MRI into established diagnostic methods, providing prompt and accurate patient diagnoses. In addition, insurance coverage and reimbursement regulations should be revised to make instant MRI more widely available to patients by considering the savings and long-term advantages it provides.

6. FUTURE RESEARCH DIRECTIONS

Future research endeavors should focus on expanding the scope of immediate MRI applications in orthopedic diagnostics, exploring its potential to detect other subtle fractures and injuries. Comparative studies between immediate MRI and other advanced imaging modalities can further refine our understanding of its diagnostic superiority. Additionally, longitudinal studies assessing the long-term impact of immediate MRI on patient outcomes, healthcare costs, and overall healthcare system efficiency would provide valuable insights into its sustained benefits.

7. CONCLUSION

In conclusion, immediate MRI stands at the intersection of innovation and patient care, reshaping the landscape of scaphoid fracture management. Embracing this technology not only leads to more accurate and timely diagnoses but also paves the way for a patient-centered, efficient, and cost-effective approach to orthopedic diagnostics. Through informed policy decisions and continued research efforts, integrating immediate MRI into standard practice promises to enhance healthcare quality, optimize resource allocation, and improve patients' lives affected by suspected scaphoid fractures.

REFERENCES

Almigdad, A., Al-Zoubi, A., Mustafa, A., Al-Qasaimeh, M., Azzam, E., Mestarihi, S., ... Almanasier, G. (2023). A review of scaphoid fracture, treatment outcomes, and consequences. *International Orthopaedics*, 1–8. doi:10.1007/s00264-023-06014-2 PMID:37880341

Amrami, K. K., Frick, M. A., & Matsumoto, J. M. (2019). Imaging for acute and chronic scaphoid fractures. *Hand Clinics*, *35*(3), 241–257. doi:10.1016/j.hcl.2019.03.001 PMID:31178083

Asfia, A., Novak, J. I., Mohammed, M. I., Rolfe, B., & Kron, T. (2020). A review of 3D printed patient specific immobilisation devices in radiotherapy. *Physics and Imaging in Radiation Oncology*, *13*, 30–35. doi:10.1016/j.phro.2020.03.003 PMID:33458304

Bhashyam, A. R., & Mudgal, C. (2023). Scaphoid and Carpal Bone Fracture: The Difficult Cases and Approach to Management. *Hand Clinics*, *39*(3), 265–277. Advance online publication. doi:10.1016/j.hcl.2023.02.003 PMID:37453756

Chang, M. T. K., Price, M., Furness, J., Kemp-Smith, K., Simas, V., Pickering, R., & Lenaghan, D. (2022). The current management of scaphoid fractures in the emergency department across an Australian metropolitan public health service: A retrospective cohort study. *Medicine*, *101*(28), e29659. doi:10.1097/MD.0000000000029659 PMID:35839014

Chong, H. H., Kulkarni, K., Shah, R., Hau, M. Y., Athanatos, L., & Singh, H. P. (2022). A meta-analysis of union rate after proximal scaphoid fractures: Terminology matters. *Journal of Plastic Surgery and Hand Surgery*, *56*(5), 298–309. doi:10.1080/2000656X.2021.1979016 PMID:34550858

Chunara, M. H., McLeavy, C. M., Kesavanarayanan, V., Paton, D., & Ganguly, A. (2019). Current imaging practice for suspected scaphoid fracture in patients with normal initial radiographs: UK-wide national audit. *Clinical Radiology*, *74*(6), 450–455. doi:10.1016/j.crad.2019.02.016 PMID:30952360

Conombo, B., Guertin, J. R., Tardif, P. A., Gagnon, M. A., Duval, C., Archambault, P., Berthelot, S., Lauzier, F., Turgeon, A. F., Stelfox, H. T., Chassé, M., Hoch, J. S., Gabbe, B., Champion, H., Lecky, F., Cameron, P., & Moore, L. (2022). Economic Evaluation of In-Hospital Clinical Practices in Acute Injury Care: A Systematic Review. *Value in Health*, *25*(5), 844–854. doi:10.1016/j.jval.2021.10.018 PMID:35500953

Coventry, L., Oldrini, I., Dean, B., Novak, A., Duckworth, A., & Metcalfe, D. (2023). Which clinical features best predict occult scaphoid fractures? A systematic review of diagnostic test accuracy studies. *Emergency Medicine Journal*, *40*(8), 576–582. Advance online publication. doi:10.1136/emermed-2023-213119 PMID:37169546

Daniels, A. M., Bevers, M. S. A. M., Sassen, S., Wyers, C. E., Van Rietbergen, B., Geusens, P. P. M. M., Kaarsemaker, S., Hannemann, P. F. W., Poeze, M., van den Bergh, J. P., & Janzing, H. M. J. (2020). Improved detection of scaphoid fractures with high-resolution peripheral quantitative CT compared with conventional CT. *The Journal of Bone and Joint Surgery. American Volume*, *102*(24), 2138–2145. doi:10.2106/JBJS.20.00124 PMID:33079896

de Lurdes, P. M. M. (2022). *Surgical versus conservative treatment of undisplaced or minimally-displaced acute scaphoid waist fractures: a systematic review and meta-analysis.*

Dean, B. J.SUSPECT study group. (2021). The management of suspected scaphoid fractures in the UK: A national cross-sectional study. *Bone & Joint Open*, *2*(11), 997–1003. doi:10.1302/2633-1462.211.BJO-2021-0146 PMID:34839716

Filip, R., Gheorghita Puscaselu, R., Anchidin-Norocel, L., Dimian, M., & Savage, W. K. (2022). Global challenges to public health care systems during the COVID-19 pandemic: A review of pandemic measures and problems. *Journal of Personalized Medicine*, *12*(8), 1295. doi:10.3390/jpm12081295 PMID:36013244

Han, S. M., Cao, L., Yang, C., Yang, H. H., Wen, J. X., Guo, Z., Wu, H.-Z., Wu, W.-J., & Gao, B. L. (2022). Value of the 45-degree reverse oblique view of the carpal palm in diagnosing scaphoid waist fractures. *Injury*, *53*(3), 1049–1056. doi:10.1016/j.injury.2021.10.023 PMID:34809925

Hendrix, N., Scholten, E., Vernhout, B., Bruijnen, S., Maresch, B., de Jong, M., Diepstraten, S., Bollen, S., Schalekamp, S., de Rooij, M., Scholtens, A., Hendrix, W., Samson, T., Sharon Ong, L.-L., Postma, E., van Ginneken, B., & Rutten, M. (2021). Development and validation of a convolutional neural network for automated detection of scaphoid fractures on conventional radiographs. *Radiology. Artificial Intelligence*, *3*(4), e200260. doi:10.1148/ryai.2021200260 PMID:34350413

Ibrahim, B., Baker, P., Jeyakumar, G., & Ali, K. (2022). MRI as gold standard for scaphoid fracture diagnosis. *Clinical Radiology*, *77*, e28–e29. doi:10.1016/j.crad.2022.09.086

Jørgsholm, P., Ossowski, D., Thomsen, N., & Björkman, A. (2020). Epidemiology of scaphoid fractures and non-unions: A systematic review. *Handchirurgie· Mikrochirurgie· Plastische Chirurgie*, *52*(05), 374-381. doi:10.1055/a-1250-8190

Kodumuri, P., McDonough, A., Lyle, V., Naqui, Z., & Muir, L. (2021). Reliability of clinical tests for prediction of occult scaphoid fractures and cost benefit analysis of a dedicated scaphoid pathway. [European Volume]. *The Journal of Hand Surgery*, *46*(3), 292–296. doi:10.1177/1753193420979465 PMID:33323009

Könneker, S., Krockenberger, K., Pieh, C., von Falck, C., Brandewiede, B., Vogt, P. M., Kirschner, M. H., & Ziegler, A. (2019). Comparison of SCAphoid fracture osteosynthesis by MAGnesium-based headless Herbert screws with titanium Herbert screws: Protocol for the randomized controlled SCAMAG clinical trial. *BMC Musculoskeletal Disorders*, *20*(1), 1–11. doi:10.1186/s12891-019-2723-9 PMID:31387574

Mallee, W. H., Walenkamp, M. M. J., Mulders, M. A. M., Goslings, J. C., & Schep, N. W. L. (2020). Detecting scaphoid fractures in wrist injury: A clinical decision rule. *Archives of Orthopaedic and Trauma Surgery*, *140*(4), 575–581. doi:10.1007/s00402-020-03383-w PMID:32125528

Norimoto, M., Yamashita, M., Yamaoka, A., Yamashita, K., Abe, K., Eguchi, Y., Furuya, T., Orita, S., Inage, K., Shiga, Y., Maki, S., Umimura, T., Sato, T., Sato, M., Enomoto, K., Takaoka, H., Hozumi, T., Mizuki, N., Kim, G., & Ohtori, S. (2021). Early mobilization reduces the medical care cost and the risk of disuse syndrome in patients with acute osteoporotic vertebral fractures. *Journal of Clinical Neuroscience*, *93*, 155–159. doi:10.1016/j.jocn.2021.09.011 PMID:34656240

Pitros, P., O'Connor, N., Tryfonos, A., & Lopes, V. (2020). A systematic review of the complications of high-risk third molar removal and coronectomy: Development of a decision tree model and preliminary health economic analysis to assist in treatment planning. *British Journal of Oral & Maxillofacial Surgery*, *58*(9), e16–e24. doi:10.1016/j.bjoms.2020.07.015 PMID:32800608

Polo Simón, F., García Medrano, B., & Delgado Serrano, P. J. (2020). Diagnostic and Therapeutic Approach to Acute Scaphoid Fractures. *Revista Iberoamericana de Cirugía de la Mano*, *48*(02), 109–118. doi:10.1055/s-0040-1718457

Rua, T., Gidwani, S., Malhotra, B., Vijayanathan, S., Hunter, L., Peacock, J., Turville, J., Razavi, R., Goh, V., McCrone, P., & Shearer, J. (2020). Cost-effectiveness of immediate magnetic resonance imaging in the management of patients with suspected scaphoid fracture: Results from a randomized clinical trial. *Value in Health*, *23*(11), 1444–1452. doi:10.1016/j.jval.2020.05.020 PMID:33127015

Sabbagh, M. D., Morsy, M., & Moran, S. L. (2019). Diagnosis and management of acute scaphoid fractures. *Hand Clinics*, *35*(3), 259–269. doi:10.1016/j.hcl.2019.03.002 PMID:31178084

Sahu, A., Kuek, D. K., MacCormick, A., Gozzard, C., Ninan, T., Fullilove, S., & Suresh, P. (2023). Prospective comparison of magnetic resonance imaging and computed tomography in diagnosing occult scaphoid fractures. *Acta Radiologica*, *64*(1), 201–207. doi:10.1177/02841851211064595 PMID:34918571

Snaith, B., Walker, A., Robertshaw, S., Spencer, N. J. B., Smith, A., & Harris, M. A. (2021). Has NICE guidance changed the management of the suspected scaphoid fracture: A survey of UK practice. *Radiography*, *27*(2), 377–380. doi:10.1016/j.radi.2020.09.014 PMID:33011069

Stirling, P. H., Strelzow, J. A., Doornberg, J. N., White, T. O., McQueen, M. M., & Duckworth, A. D. (2021). Diagnosis of suspected scaphoid fractures. *JBJS Reviews*, *9*(12), e20. doi:10.2106/JBJS.RVW.20.00247 PMID:34879033

Suroto, H., Antoni, I., Siyo, A., Steendam, T. C., Prajasari, T., Mulyono, H. B., & De Vega, B. (2021). Traumatic brachial plexus injury in Indonesia: An experience from a developing country. *Journal of Reconstructive Microsurgery*, *38*(07), 511–523. doi:10.1055/s-0041-1735507 PMID:34470060

Swärd, E. M., Schriever, T. U., Franko, M. A., Björkman, A. C., & Wilcke, M. K. (2019). The epidemiology of scaphoid fractures in Sweden: A nationwide registry study. [European Volume]. *The Journal of Hand Surgery*, *44*(7), 697–701. doi:10.1177/1753193419849767 PMID:31106681

van Delft, E. A., van Gelder, T. G., de Vries, R., Vermeulen, J., & Bloemers, F. W. (2019). Duration of cast immobilization in distal radial fractures: A systematic review. *Journal of Wrist Surgery*, *8*(05), 430–438. doi:10.1055/s-0039-1683433 PMID:31579555

Wijetunga, A. R., Tsang, V. H., & Giuffre, B. (2019). The utility of cross-sectional imaging in the management of suspected scaphoid fractures. *Journal of Medical Radiation Sciences*, *66*(1), 30–37. doi:10.1002/jmrs.302 PMID:30160062

Wu, A. M., Bisignano, C., James, S. L., Abady, G. G., Abedi, A., Abu-Gharbieh, E., Alhassan, R. K., Alipour, V., Arabloo, J., Asaad, M., Asmare, W. N., Awedew, A. F., Banach, M., Banerjee, S. K., Bijani, A., Birhanu, T. T. M., Bolla, S. R., Cámera, L. A., Chang, J.-C., & Vos, T. (2021). Global, regional, and national burden of bone fractures in 204 countries and territories, 1990-2019: A systematic analysis from the Global Burden of Disease Study 2019. *The Lancet. Healthy Longevity*, *2*(9), e580–e592. doi:10.1016/S2666-7568(21)00172-0 PMID:34723233

Yoon, A. P., Lee, Y. L., Kane, R. L., Kuo, C. F., Lin, C., & Chung, K. C. (2021). Development and validation of a deep learning model using convolutional neural networks to identify scaphoid fractures in radiographs. *JAMA Network Open*, *4*(5), e216096–e216096. doi:10.1001/jamanetworkopen.2021.6096 PMID:33956133

ADDITIONAL READINGS

Komalasari, R. (2022). A Social Ecological Model (SEM) to Manage Methadone Programmes in Prisons. In Handbook of Research on Mathematical Modeling for Smart Healthcare Systems (pp. 374-382). IGI Global. doi:10.4018/978-1-6684-4580-8.ch020

Komalasari, R. (2023). The Relationship Between Cybersecurity and Public Health. In *Handbook of Research on Current Trends in Cybersecurity and Educational Technology* (pp. 78–91). IGI Global., doi:10.4018/978-1-6684-6092-4.ch005

Komalasari, R. (2023). Postnatal Mental Distress: Exploring the Experiences of Mothers Navigating the Healthcare System. In Perspectives and Considerations on Navigating the Mental Healthcare System (pp. 159-181). IGI Global. doi:10.4018/978-1-6684-5049-9.ch007

Komalasari, R. (2023). Designing Health Systems for Better, Faster, and Less Expensive Treatment. In *Exploring the Convergence of Computer and Medical Science Through Cloud Healthcare* (pp. 1–13). IGI Global. doi:10.4018/978-1-6684-5260-8.ch001

Komalasari, R. (2023). The Ethical Consideration of Using Artificial Intelligence (AI) in Medicine. In Advanced Bioinspiration Methods for Healthcare Standards, Policies, and Reform (pp. 1-16). IGI Global. doi:10.4018/978-1-6684-5656-9.ch001

Komalasari, R. (2023). Healthcare for the Elderly With Digital Twins. In Digital Twins and Healthcare: Trends, Techniques, and Challenges (pp. 145-156). IGI Global. doi:10.4018/978-1-6684-5925-6.ch010

Komalasari, R. (2023). Cloud Computing's Usage in Healthcare. In Recent Advancements in Smart Remote Patient Monitoring, Wearable Devices, and Diagnostics Systems (pp. 183-194). IGI Global. doi:10.4018/978-1-6684-6434-2.ch009

Komalasari, R. (2023). History and Legislative Changes Governing Medical Cannabis in Indonesia. In Medical Cannabis and the Effects of Cannabinoids on Fighting Cancer, Multiple Sclerosis, Epilepsy, Parkinson's, and Other Neurodegenerative Diseases (pp. 274-284). IGI Global. doi:10.4018/978-1-6684-5652-1.ch012

Komalasari, R. (2023). Ambient Assisted Living (AAL) Systems to Help Older People. In Exploring Future Opportunities of Brain-Inspired Artificial Intelligence (pp. 84-99). IGI Global. doi:10.4018/978-1-6684-6980-4.ch006

Komalasari, R. (2023). Telemedicine in Pandemic Times in Indonesia: Healthcare Professional's Perspective. In Health Informatics and Patient Safety in Times of Crisis (pp. 138-153). IGI Global. doi:10.4018/978-1-6684-5499-2.ch008

Komalasari, R. (2023). Cloud Computing's Usage in Healthcare. In Recent Advancements in Smart Remote Patient Monitoring, Wearable Devices, and Diagnostics Systems (pp. 183-194). IGI Global. doi:10.4018/978-1-6684-6434-2.ch009

Komalasari, R. (2023). The Relationship Between Cybersecurity and Public Health. In *Handbook of Research on Current Trends in Cybersecurity and Educational Technology* (pp. 78–91). IGI Global., doi:10.4018/978-1-6684-6092-4.ch005

Komalasari, R. (2023). Treatment of Menstrual Discomfort in Young Women and a Cognitive Behavior Therapy (CBT) Program. In Perspectives on Coping Strategies for Menstrual and Premenstrual Distress (pp. 194-211). IGI Global. doi:10.4018/978-1-6684-5088-8.ch011

Komalasari, R. (2023). Healthcare for the Elderly With Digital Twins. In Digital Twins and Healthcare: Trends, Techniques, and Challenges (pp. 145-156). IGI Global. doi:10.4018/978-1-6684-5925-6.ch010

Komalasari, R. (2023). Telemedicine in Pandemic Times in Indonesia: Healthcare Professional's Perspective. In Health Informatics and Patient Safety in Times of Crisis (pp. 138-153). IGI Global. doi:10.4018/978-1-6684-5499-2.ch008

Komalasari, R. (2023). Regulatory Shift Healthcare Applications in Industry 5.0. In Advanced Research and Real-World Applications of Industry 5.0 (pp. 149-165). IGI Global. doi:10.4018/978-1-7998-8805-5.ch008

Komalasari, R. (2023). Exploring Pedagogies Of Affect In Secondary School Physical Education For Enhanced Emotional Well-Being. *Pedagogik: Jurnal Pendidikan Guru Sekolah Dasar*, *11*(2), 117–127. doi:10.33558/pedagogik.v11i2.7374

Komalasari, R. (2023). Integrating Sport education model and the athletics challenges approach for transformative physical education in Indonesian Middle Schools. *Motion: Jurnal Riset Physical Education*, *13*(2), 118–135. doi:10.33558/motion.v13i2.7372

Komalasari, R. (2023). Rancangan Program Bagi Keberhasilan Gerakan Mencuci Tangan Yang Sehat Bagi Para Ibu Dan Anak. *Sulolipu: Media Komunikasi Sivitas Akademika dan Masyarakat*, *23*(1), 55-60. doi:10.32382/sulolipu.v23i1.3103

Komalasari, R. (2023). Culture as A Catalyst: Unveiling the Nexus Between Health Services Performance Management and National Identity. *Journal of Business and Political Economy: Biannual Review of The Indonesian Economy*, *5*(1).

Komalasari, R. (2023). Exploring Pedagogies Of Affect In Secondary School Physical Education For Enhanced Emotional Well-Being. *Pedagogik: Jurnal Pendidikan Guru Sekolah Dasar*, *11*(2), 117–127. doi:10.33558/pedagogik.v11i2.7374

Komalasari, R. (2023). Integrating sport education model and the athletics challenges approach for transformative physical education in Indonesian Middle Schools. *Motion: Jurnal Riset Physical Education*, *13*(2), 118–135. doi:10.33558/motion.v13i2.7372

Komalasari, R. (2023). Efek Ganja Medis pada Pasien Parkinson: A Literature Review of Clinical Evidence. *Journal of Islamic Pharmacy*, *8*(1), 44–48. doi:10.18860/jip.v8i1.17832

Komalasari, R. (2023). Rancangan Program Bagi Keberhasilan Gerakan Mencuci Tangan Yang Sehat Bagi Para Ibu Dan Anak. *Sulolipu: Media Komunikasi Sivitas Akademika dan Masyarakat, 23*(1), 55-60. doi:10.32382/sulolipu.v23i1.3103

Komalasari, R. (2024). Unravelling the Veil: Exploring the Nexus of Insecure Attachment and Functional Somatic Disorders in Adults. In *Discourses, Inquiries, and Case Studies in Healthcare, Social Sciences, and Technology*. IGI Global. doi:10.4018/979-8-3693-3555-0.ch001

Komalasari, R. (2024). Medical Educators (ME) and their Continuous Professional Development (CPD). In The Lifelong Learning Journey of Health Professionals: Continuing Education and Professional Development. IGI Global.

Komalasari, R. (2024). Advancing Healthcare: Economic Implications of Immediate MRI in Suspected Scaphoid Fractures - A Comprehensive Exploration. In *Future of AI in Medical Imaging*. IGI Global.

Komalasari, R. (2024). Women's perceptions of midlife mothering during perimenopause: the impact on health and well-being through life's transitions. In *Utilizing AI Techniques for the Perimenopause to Menopause Transition*. IGI Global.

Komalasari, R. (2024). Machine Learning in Health Information Security: Unraveling Patterns, Concealing Secrets, and Mitigating Vulnerabilities. In *Enhancing Steganography Through Deep Learning Approaches*. IGI Global.

Komalasari, R. (2024). Navigating Complexity: Unraveling the IVHM Requirements Puzzle in Unmanned Aerial Systems Through Innovative IVHM-RD Methodology and Rigorous Data Analysis. In *Ubiquitous Computing and Technological Innovation for Universal Healthcare*. IGI Global.

Komalasari, R. (2024). Trust Dynamics in Remote Patient-Expert Communication: Unraveling the Role of ICT in Indonesia's Private Healthcare Sector. In *Improving Security, Privacy, and Connectivity Among Telemedicine Platforms*. IGI Global.

Komalasari, R. (2024). Cyberbullying in the Healthcare Workplace: How to Find Your Way Through the Digital Maze. In M. Aslam, Y. Kim, & Q. Linchao (Eds.), *Workplace Cyberbullying and Behavior in Health Professions* (pp. 84–112). IGI Global. doi:10.4018/979-8-3693-1139-4.ch004

Komalasari, R. (2024). Harmonizing Minds and Machines: A Transformative AI-Based Mental Health Care Framework in Medical Tourism. In *Impact of AI and Robotics on the Medical Tourism Industry*. IGI Global.

Komalasari, R. (2024). Navigating the Future of Healthcare: A User-Centric Approach to Designing Lucrative Business Models for the IoMT. In *Lightweight Digital Trust Architectures in the Internet of Medical Things (IoMT)*. IGI Global.

Komalasari, R. (2024). Biospheric Reverie: Unraveling Indoor Air Quality through Bio-Inspired Textiles, Awareness, and Decision-Making. In *Intelligent Decision Making Through Bio-Inspired Optimization*. IGI Global.

Komalasari, R. (2024). An Integrated Approach to Next-Generation Telemedicine and Health Advice Systems through AI Applications in Disease Diagnosis. In *AI-Driven Innovations in Digital Healthcare: Emerging Trends, Challenges, and Applications*. IGI Global.

Komalasari, R. (2024). Transformative Insights: Harnessing Artificial Intelligence for Enhanced Ovarian Cancer Prediction and Prognosis. In *Biomedical Research Developments for Improved Healthcare*. IGI Global.

Komalasari, R. (2024). Bridging the Gap: Theory of Change Guided Digital Health Implementation in Indonesian Primary Care. In *Analyzing Current Digital Healthcare Trends Using Social Networks*. IGI Global.

Komalasari, R. (2024). Navigating the Digital Frontier: A Socio-Technical Review of Indonesia's NHS E-Health Strategy and the Path to Seamless Healthcare Transformation. In *Inclusivity and Accessibility in Digital Health*. IGI Global.

Komalasari, R. (2024). *Pursuit of Excellence: A Comprehensive Framework for Ensuring Quality in Digital Health Apps. In Multi-Sector Analysis of the Digital Healthcare Industry*. IGI Global.

Komalasari, R. (2024). Fostering Transparency in AI for Disease Detection: Exploring Meaningful Explanations and Interactive Modalities in Healthcare. In *Federated Learning and Privacy-Preserving in Healthcare AI*. IGI Global.

Komalasari, R. (2024). Predictive Pioneers: Bridging the Mental Health Gap in Older Adults through Advanced Digital Technologies. In *Using Machine Learning to Detect Emotions and Predict Human Psychology*. IGI Global. doi:10.4018/979-8-3693-1910-9.ch005

Komalasari, R. (2024). Unravelling the Veil: Exploring the Nexus of Insecure Attachment and Functional Somatic Disorders in Adults. In *Discourses, Inquiries, and Case Studies in Healthcare, Social Sciences, and Technology*. IGI Global. doi:10.4018/979-8-3693-3555-0.ch001

Komalasari, R. (2024). Cyberbullying in the Health Care Workplace: How to Find Your Way Through the Digital Maze. In *Workplace Cyberbullying and Behavior in Health Professions*. IGI Global. doi:10.4018/979-8-3693-1139-4.ch004

Komalasari, R. (2024). Navigating Mental Health Crises: Understanding Pivotal Phases, Health Campaigns, and Community Resilience for Recovery and Reform. In *The Role of Health Literacy in Major Healthcare Crises*. IGI Global.

Komalasari, R. (2024). Decoding the Genomic and Proteomic Landscape: Dissemination and Mechanisms of Antibiotic Resistance in Environmental Staphylococci. In *Contemporary Approaches to Mitigating Antibacterial Drug Resistance*. IGI Global.

Komalasari, R. (2024). Unveiling the Future: Blockchain-Powered Digital Twins for Personalized Privacy Preservation in Metaverse Healthcare Data. In D. Burrell (Ed.), *Innovations, Securities, and Case Studies Across Healthcare, Business, and Technology* (pp. 321–342). IGI Global., doi:10.4018/979-8-3693-1906-2.ch017

Komalasari, R. (2024). Safeguarding the Future: Cutting-Edge Time-Stamping Services and Blockchain Technologies for Maintaining EHR Data Integrity Over the Long Term. In *Blockchain and IoT Approaches for Secure Electronic Health Records (EHR)*. IGI Global.

Komalasari, R. (2024). Empowering Informed Healthcare Choices in Rural Areas: SIKDA - A Novel Model for Enhancing Patient Access to Reliable Consumer Health Information in Indonesia. In *Emerging Technologies for Health Literacy and Medical Practice*. IGI Global.

Komalasari, R. (2024). Advancing Trauma Care: Contemporary Cranio-Maxillo-Facial Surgery in Indonesia and Beyond. In *Contemporary Cranio-Maxillo-Facial Surgery: From Trauma to Reconstruction*. IGI Global.

Komalasari, R. (2024). Innovations in Neurodegenerative Disease Diagnosis: Unraveling the Transformative Potential of Deep Learning and MRI Integration. In *Deep Learning Approaches for Early Diagnosis of Neurodegenerative Diseases*. IGI Global.

Komalasari, R. (2024). Secure and privacy-preserving federated learning with explainable artificial intelligence for smart healthcare systems. In *Federated Learning and AI for Healthcare 5.0*. IGI Global.

Komalasari, R. (2024) Optimizing Prostate Cancer Radiotherapy: Advanced Machine Learning in Virtual Patient-Specific Plan Verification. *Indonesian Journal of Cancer*.

Komalasari, R. (2024). Optimizing Prostate Cancer Radiotherapy: Advanced Machine Learning in Virtual Patient-Specific Plan Verification. *Indonesian Journal of Cancer*.

Komalasari, R. (2024). Bridging Uncertainties: Exploring the Lived Experiences of Pediatric Long-COVID-19 Through ME/CFS Caregiver Narratives. In G. Rao & S. Dhamdhere-Rao (Eds.), *Clinical Practice and Post-Infection Care for COVID-19 Patients* (pp. 207–227). IGI Global. doi:10.4018/978-1-6684-6855-5.ch009

Komalasari, R., & Mustafa, C. (2023). Combating International Cyber Conflict: A Healthy Just War and International Law Analysis of NATO and Indonesian Policies. Jurnal Pertahanan: Media Informasi tentang Kajian & Strategi Pertahanan yang Mengedepankan Identity. *Nasionalism & Integrity*, 9(3), 559–570. doi:10.33172/jp.v9i2.16794

Komalasari, R., & Mustafa, C. (2023). Analysis Of The Propulsion And Maneuvering Characteristics Of Autonomous Underwater Vehicles And Their Strategic Defense. *Propeller Jurnal Permesinan*, 1(2).

Komalasari, R., & Mustafa, C. (2023). Amphibious Forces in the Total War Age: Exploring Indonesia's Multifaceted Contributions to Statecraft in the Asia-Pacific Region. *Jurnal Strategi Pertahanan Laut*, 9(2), 62–77. doi:10.33172/spl.v9i2.12606

Komalasari, R., & Mustafa, C. (2023). The Evolution and Institutionalization of the Naval Partnership between Indonesia and ASEAN. *Jurnal Strategi Pertahanan Laut*, 9(2), 1–18. doi:10.33172/spl.v9i2.12576

Komalasari, R., & Mustafa, C. (2023). A Healthy Game-Theoretic Evaluation of NATO and Indonesia's Policies in the Context of International Law. Jurnal Pertahanan: Media Informasi tentang Kajian & Strategi Pertahanan yang Mengedepankan Identity. *Nasionalism & Integrity*, 9(2), 333–349. doi:10.33172/jp.v9i2.16794

Komalasari, R., & Mustafa, C. (2023) Combating International Cyber Conflict: A Healthy Just War and International Law Analysis of NATO and Indonesian Policies. *Jurnal Pertahanan: Media Informasi tentang Kajian & Strategi Pertahanan yang Mengedepankan Identity, Nasionalism & Integrity, 9*(3).

Komalasari, R., & Mustafa, C. (2023). A Healthy Game-Theoretic Evaluation of NATO and Indonesia's Policies in the Context of International Law. *Jurnal Pertahanan: Media Informasi tentang Kajian & Strategi Pertahanan yang Mengedepankan Identity. Nasionalism & Integrity, 9*(2), 333–349. doi:10.33172/jp.v9i2.16794

Komalasari, R., & Mustafa, C. (2024). Strengthening National Security Through Integrated Farming Systems: A Comprehensive Assessment and Strategic Outlook. *Jurnal Pertanian Terpadu, 1*(1), 19–33.

Komalasari, R., & Mustafa, C. (2024). Dimensi Sosial-Ekologi Pengelolaan Danau Tropis Berkelanjutan: Pelajaran Dari Danau Toba, Indonesia. *Wrasse Jurnal Perikanan dan Kelautan Nusantara, 1*(1).

Komalasari, R., & Mustafa, C. (2024) Rehabilitasi Pengguna Narkoba: Tantangan dan Peluang. *Arena Hukum, 14*(4)

Komalasari, R., & Mustafa, C. (2024). *Healthy Competition Policy Dynamics: the Influence of Domestic-Specific Factors in a Globalized Landscape.* Jurnal Persaingan Usaha.

Komalasari, R., & Mustafa, C. (2024). *Comparative Analysis of Healthy Electoral Fraud Legislation in Established Democracies.* Jurnal Adhyasta Pemilu.

Komalasari, R., Nurhayati, N., & Mustafa, C. (2022). Enhancing the Online Learning Environment for Medical Education: Lessons From COVID-19. In Policies and procedures for the implementation of safe and healthy eaducational environments: Post-COVID-19 perspectives (pp. 138-154). IGI Global. doi:10.4018/978-1-7998-9297-7.ch009

Komalasari, R., Nurhayati, N., & Mustafa, C. (2022). Insider/outsider issues: Reflections on qualitative research. *The Qualitative Report, 27*(3), 744–751. doi:10.46743/2160-3715/2022.5259

Komalasari, R., Nurhayati, N., & Mustafa, C. (2022). Professional Education and Training in Indonesia. In *Public Affairs Education and Training in the 21st Century* (pp. 125–138). IGI Global. doi:10.4018/978-1-7998-8243-5.ch008

Komalasari, R., Nurhayati, N., & Mustafa, C. (2022). Professional Education and Training in Indonesia. In *Public Affairs Education and Training in the 21st Century* (pp. 125–138). IGI Global. doi:10.4018/978-1-7998-8243-5.ch008

Komalasari, R., Wilson, S., & Haw, S. (2021). A systematic review of qualitative evidence on barriers to and facilitators of the implementation of opioid agonist treatment (OAT) programmes in prisons. *The International Journal on Drug Policy, 87*, 102978. doi:10.1016/j.drugpo.2020.102978 PMID:33129135

Komalasari, R., Wilson, S., & Haw, S. (2021). A social ecological model (SEM) to exploring barriers of and facilitators to the implementation of opioid agonist treatment (OAT) programmes in prisons. *International Journal of Prisoner Health, 17*(4), 477–496. doi:10.1108/IJPH-04-2020-0020

Komalasari, R., Wilson, S., Nasir, S., & Haw, S. (2020). Multiple burdens of stigma for prisoners participating in Opioid Antagonist Treatment (OAT) programmes in Indonesian prisons: A qualitative study. *International Journal of Prisoner Health*, *17*(2), 156–170. doi:10.1108/IJPH-03-2020-0018

Mustafa, C. (2020). The influence of sunni islamic values on rehabilitation as judicial decision for minor drug users in Indonesian court. *Ijtihad: Jurnal Wacana Hukum Islam dan Kemanusiaan*, *20*(1), 79-96. doi:10.18326/ijtihad.v20i1.79-96

Mustafa, C. (2021). Qualitative Method Used in Researching the Judiciary: Quality Assurance Steps to Enhance the Validity and Reliability of the Findings. *The Qualitative Report*, *26*(1), 176–185. doi:10.46743/2160-3715/2021.4319

Mustafa, C. (2021). Key Finding: Result of a Qualitative Study of Judicial Perspectives on the Sentencing of Minor Drug Offenders in Indonesia: Structural Inequality. *The Qualitative Report*, *26*(5), 1678–1692. doi:10.46743/2160-3715/2021.4436

Mustafa, C. (2021). The view of judicial activism and public legitimacy. *Crime, Law, and Social Change*, *76*(1), 23–34. doi:10.1007/s10611-021-09955-0

Mustafa, C. (2021). The News Media Representation of Acts of Mass Violence in Indonesia. In *Mitigating Mass Violence and Managing Threats in Contemporary Society* (pp. 127–140). IGI Global., doi:10.4018/978-1-7998-4957-5.ch008

Mustafa, C. (2021). The Challenges to Improving Public Services and Judicial Operations: A unique balance between pursuing justice and public service in Indonesia. In Handbook of research on global challenges for improving public services and government operations (pp. 117-132). IGI Global. doi:10.4018/978-1-7998-4978-0.ch007

Mustafa, C., Malloch, M., & Hamilton Smith, N. (2020). Judicial perspectives on the sentencing of minor drug offenders in Indonesia: Discretionary practice and compassionate approaches. *Crime, Law, and Social Change*, *74*(3), 297–313. doi:10.1007/s10611-020-09896-0

Suhariyanto, B. (2023). Contradiction Over The Application Of Corporate Liability In Corruption Court Decisions In Indonesia. *Indonesia Law Review*, *13*(1), 8.

Suhariyanto, B., Mustafa, C., & Santoso, T. (2021). Liability incorporate between transnational corruption cases Indonesia and the United States of America. *J. Legal Ethical & Regul. Isses*, *24*, 1.

KEY TERMS AND DEFINITIONS

Cost-Effectiveness: Cost-effectiveness refers to measuring the efficiency of a healthcare intervention, treatment, or technology and its cost. It assesses whether the benefits gained from a specific intervention justify the resources (both monetary and non-monetary) invested in it. In the context of healthcare, a cost-effective intervention provides significant benefits in improving health outcomes while utilizing resources efficiently and economically.

Diagnostic Accuracy: The diagnostic accuracy of a test or treatment is its reliability in determining whether or not a patient has a certain illness or condition. It measures the precision of a diagnostic tool, indicating how well it distinguishes between patients with the condition and those without. High diagnostic accuracy implies that the test provides reliable and consistent results, minimizing the chances of false positives or false negatives.

Healthcare Efficiency: Healthcare efficiency refers to the optimal use of resources, time, and effort within the healthcare system to achieve the best possible outcomes. It involves maximizing the quality and quantity of healthcare services delivered while minimizing waste, reducing costs, and enhancing patient satisfaction. Efficient healthcare systems ensure timely access to appropriate care, effective utilization of medical technologies, and streamlined processes, ultimately leading to improved patient outcomes.

Immediate MRI: When talking about diagnostic procedures, "immediate MRI" means using magnetic resonance imaging (MRI) without any additional waits. Scaphoid fractures are sometimes misdiagnosed as other types of injuries. Therefore, it is important to have a quick and correct diagnosis so that the patient may get the care they need as soon as possible.

Scaphoid Fractures: Fractures of the scaphoid, a carpal bone in the wrist and one of the tinier bones in the human body, are common. These fractures commonly result from falls or trauma to the hand and wrist area. Scaphoid fractures are significant due to their prevalence and potential complications, including delayed healing, non-union, and long-term disability if not diagnosed and treated promptly and accurately.

Chapter 15
Digital Twin–Based Smart Healthcare Services for the Next Generation Society

V. Hemamalini

SRM Institute of Science and Technology, Chennai, India

Firas Armosh

https://orcid.org/0009-0006-6458-3331

De Montfort University, Dubai, UAE

Amit Kumar Tyagi

https://orcid.org/0000-0003-2657-8700

National Institute of Fashion Technology, New Delhi, India

ABSTRACT

In today's smart era, the healthcare landscape is rapidly evolving, driven by advancements in technology and the growing healthcare needs of an aging and increasingly interconnected society. To address these challenges, the concept of digital twins has emerged as a promising solution to transform healthcare services for the next generation. This work provides an overview of the key aspects and benefits of digital twin-based smart healthcare services and their potential to revolutionize the healthcare industry. DWT involves creating a digital replica or model of a physical entity, in this case, an individual's health and medical data. By harnessing real-time data from various sources, including wearable devices, electronic health records, and medical imaging, Digital Twins provide a holistic view of an individual's health status, treatment history, and predictive analytics for future health outcomes. This work provides information about data-driven approach enables healthcare providers to make more informed decisions and tailor personalized treatment plans/ improving patient outcomes.

DOI: 10.4018/979-8-3693-2359-5.ch015

1. INTRODUCTION TO DIGITAL TWIN, SMART HEALTHCARE AND NEXT GENERATION SOCIETY

In recent years, the convergence of cutting-edge technologies (Amit Kumar Tyagi, 2022) (Amit Kumar Tyagi and Richa., 2023) has given rise to transformative concepts that hold great promise for the future of healthcare and society as a whole. Among these concepts, Digital Twins, Smart Healthcare, and the vision of a Next-Generation Society are at the forefront, each playing an important role in reshaping the way we manage and deliver healthcare services, and how we envision the society of tomorrow.

- Digital Twin: Digital Twin technology is a paradigm-shifting innovation that involves creating a virtual, data-driven replica of a physical object, system, or process. In the context of healthcare, Digital Twins are applied to individuals, capturing and continuously updating their health-related data. This digital replica integrates information from various sources, including electronic health records, wearable devices, genetic information, and medical imaging. As a result, it provides a comprehensive, real-time representation of a person's health status, medical history, and predictive analytics for future health outcomes. The concept of Digital Twins is revolutionizing how healthcare is personalized, monitored, and managed, with profound implications for diagnosis, treatment, and prevention.
- Smart Healthcare: Intelligent Healthcare spans a wide range of inventive solutions leveraging technology to elevate the standard, effectiveness, and availability of healthcare services. This incorporates the utilization of Internet of Things (IoT) devices, artificial intelligence, telemedicine, and data analytics to establish a cohesive healthcare network. The objective of Smart Healthcare is to enhance patient results, diminish healthcare expenditures, and elevate overall patient contentment. It encompasses functionalities like remote patient surveillance, wearable health gadgets, telehealth appointments, and data-informed decision-making, collectively fostering a healthcare system that is more patient-focused and streamlined.
- Next-Generation Society: The concept of a Next-Generation Society envisions a future in which technology, particularly digital innovation, plays a central role in shaping various aspects of human life, including healthcare, education, transportation, and governance. It reflects a society that embraces technological advances, emphasizes sustainability, and focuses on improving the well-being and quality of life for its citizens. Next-generation societies are characterized by connectivity, data-driven decision-making, and a commitment to addressing complex societal challenges through technological solutions.

The intersection of Digital Twins, Smart Healthcare, and the vision of a Next-Generation Society (Nair and Tyagi, 2023) has the capacity to transform healthcare services. Through the integration of data, automation, and artificial intelligence, healthcare can evolve into a more personalized, predictive, and efficient system, ultimately resulting in improved patient outcomes and a more interconnected and healthier society. Nevertheless, this transformation comes with challenges such as data privacy, security, ethical concerns, and the necessity for regulatory frameworks to ensure responsible implementation. In this context, it is crucial for healthcare professionals, policymakers, and technology innovators to collaboratively navigate the complexities and ethical implications associated with these advancements, unlocking their full potential. The journey towards a Next-Generation Society, facilitated by Digital

Twins and Smart Healthcare, envisions a future where healthcare is more patient-centric, data-driven, and sustainable, bringing us closer to the realization of healthier, more interconnected communities.

1.1 Background

Digital Twin, Smart Healthcare, and the vision of a Next-Generation Society are interrelated concepts that have evolved in response to the rapid advancement of technology, changing demographics, and societal demands. Understanding their background provides insight into how these ideas have developed and their potential impact on the future.

- Digital Twin: The concept of a Digital Twin has its roots in industrial processes and manufacturing. It was first coined and developed by Dr. Michael Grieves at the University of Michigan in the early 2000s. Digital Twins were initially used to create digital replicas of physical machinery and systems, enabling real-time monitoring, analysis, and optimization. Over time, this concept has expanded beyond manufacturing into various domains, including healthcare. In healthcare, Digital Twins provide a way to represent and monitor an individual's health status and medical data. The concept has gained prominence due to advancements in data collection, artificial intelligence, and the increasing importance of personalized medicine.
- Smart Healthcare: The idea of Smart Healthcare (Amit Kumar Tyagi, 2023) has grown alongside the broader movement of "Smart Cities" and "Smart Technologies." These concepts emerged in response to the challenges of urbanization and the need for more efficient and sustainable urban living. Smart Healthcare uses technology to create a more connected, data-driven, and patient-centered healthcare system. It has its roots in the use of electronic health records (EHRs), telemedicine, and the Internet of Things (IoT) to improve healthcare delivery and reduce costs. As healthcare systems worldwide faced increasing demands, especially during the COVID-19 pandemic, the need for more agile and tech-driven healthcare became apparent, further propelling the concept of Smart Healthcare.
- Next-Generation Society: The notion of a Next-Generation Society emerges from the broader context of societal evolution. It is driven by the recognition that technology is becoming increasingly integrated into all aspects of our lives. Factors such as demographic shifts, urbanization, climate change, and technological innovation are pushing society toward a transformation. In this context, the Next-Generation Society aims to use digital advancements, environmental sustainability, and societal well-being as central pillars. It envisions a society that harnesses the power of data, automation, and connectivity to address complex challenges and create a more inclusive and efficient future.

Hence, the convergence of Digital Twin technology and Smart Healthcare represents a significant step toward achieving the goals of the Next-Generation Society. As healthcare becomes more personalized, data-driven, and interconnected, it aligns with the broader vision of a society that embraces digital transformation for the betterment of its citizens. However, realizing this vision also comes with challenges related to data security, privacy, and ethics, which must be addressed to ensure responsible and equitable implementation. In summary, the backgrounds of Digital Twin, Smart Healthcare, and the Next-Generation Society are deeply intertwined with the evolution of technology, changing societal needs, and the quest for more efficient, sustainable, and patient-centric healthcare systems. These concepts collectively represent a vision of a future where technology serves as a cornerstone for societal well-being and progress.

1.2 The Evolution of Healthcare Services in previous decade

The transformation of healthcare services in the last ten years has witnessed notable progress in technology, alterations in healthcare delivery models, and changes in patient expectations (Gomathi, Mishra, and Tyagi, 2023) (Adebiyi, Afolayan, et al., 2023). Here are several noteworthy trends and advancements that have shaped the evolution of healthcare services in the preceding decade:

- Telemedicine and Telehealth: Over the last decade, telemedicine and telehealth services have experienced explosive growth. The widespread availability of high-speed internet and the development of secure, user-friendly telehealth platforms have made it easier for patients to access medical consultations, receive remote monitoring, and even access mental health services from the comfort of their homes. This transformation was accelerated during the COVID-19 pandemic, making telehealth a cornerstone of modern healthcare delivery.

- Electronic Health Records (EHRs): The adoption of EHR systems became nearly universal across healthcare providers during the past decade. EHRs have improved patient record-keeping, data sharing, and overall efficiency in healthcare. They enable healthcare professionals to access patient information more readily, reduce errors, and provide more coordinated care.

- Healthcare Analytics and Data Science: The healthcare industry has increasingly embraced data analytics and data science to improve patient care and outcomes. Big data analytics and machine learning have been used to predict disease outbreaks, identify high-risk patients, and optimize treatment plans. These data-driven information are transforming healthcare decision-making.

- Precision Medicine: The prominence of genomics and personalized medicine has increased significantly. Customizing treatment plans according to an individual's genetic makeup and health history has become more widespread. This personalized approach results in more effective treatments with reduced side effects.

- Patient-Centered Care: The concept of patient-centered care has become a central focus. Healthcare providers are increasingly involving patients in their care decisions, emphasizing shared decision-making and patient empowerment. This shift in approach aims to improve patient satisfaction and health outcomes.

- Wearable Health Technology: Wearable devices, such as fitness trackers and smartwatches, have become ubiquitous. They provide users with real-time health data, promote physical activity, and can be integrated into clinical care for remote patient monitoring. The use of health-related mobile apps has also become more prevalent.

- Value-Based Care: The transition from fee-for-service models to value-based care models has garnered momentum. Healthcare providers now receive rewards based on the quality of care delivered rather than the quantity of services provided. This approach promotes improved patient outcomes and cost-effective healthcare.

- AI and Robotics: The application of artificial intelligence (AI) and robotics in healthcare has witnessed a growing trend. AI is employed for activities such as image analysis, early disease detection, and predictive analytics. Meanwhile, robots find application in surgery, rehabilitation, and patient care, enhancing precision and efficiency.

- Mental Health Integration: Recognizing the importance of mental health, there has been a greater integration of mental health services into overall healthcare. Teletherapy, mental health apps, and destigmatization efforts have all contributed to improving mental health care accessibility.
- Health Policy Changes: Changes in healthcare policies, exemplified by the Affordable Care Act (ACA) in the United States, have significantly influenced access to healthcare services. Globally, endeavors to broaden healthcare coverage and enhance affordability have played a pivotal role in shaping the healthcare landscape.

In summary, the previous decade has seen remarkable progress in healthcare services, driven by technology, changing patient expectations, and the need for more accessible, cost-effective, and patient-centric care. The evolution is ongoing, with continuous advancements in healthcare technology and delivery models shaping the healthcare landscape for the next decade and beyond.

1.3 The Role of Digital Twins in Healthcare

The role of Digital Twins in healthcare (Deekshetha, Tyagi, 2023), is undergoing swift evolution and carries significant potential for industry transformation. Serving as virtual replicas of physical objects, systems, or, in healthcare's context, individual patients, Digital Twins are generated through the assimilation of real-time data. These digital counterparts play a crucial role in enhancing patient care, facilitating research, and streamlining healthcare management. Here are some pivotal functions that Digital Twins fulfill in the healthcare sector:

- Personalized Medicine: Digital Twins provide a detailed and real-time representation of an individual's health status. By continuously monitoring and updating data from various sources, including electronic health records, wearable devices, and genetic information, healthcare providers can create highly personalized treatment plans. This tailored approach to care allows for more effective treatments and medications, minimizing adverse effects.
- Early Disease Detection: With the ability to track an individual's health over time, Digital Twins can identify subtle changes or anomalies that may indicate the early stages of diseases. This early detection is invaluable for improving patient outcomes and potentially preventing the progression of certain conditions.
- Remote Patient Monitoring: Digital Twins facilitate constant remote monitoring of patients' health, offering particular advantages for individuals managing chronic conditions, recovering from surgery, or requiring ongoing care. Through proactive intervention triggered by abnormal readings or trends detected by the Digital Twin, healthcare providers can effectively minimize hospital readmissions and enhance the overall well-being of patients.
- Treatment Optimization: Digital Twins provide the optimization of treatment plans. By simulating different treatment scenarios and predicting their outcomes based on the patient's unique health data, healthcare providers can make more informed decisions about the most effective course of action. This reduces trial-and-error approaches and enhances treatment success rates.
- Drug Development and Testing: Digital Twins are used in pharmaceutical research and drug development. They enable the simulation of the effects of new drugs on virtual patient avatars, allowing researchers to understand potential outcomes, side effects, and efficacy before conducting clinical trials. This can expedite drug development and reduce costs.

- Chronic Disease Management: For patients with chronic diseases such as diabetes, heart disease, and hypertension, Digital Twins provide a means to closely monitor their health status and adherence to treatment plans. They can also predict exacerbations or complications, enabling timely interventions.
- Data Security and Privacy: Digital Twins prioritize data security and privacy by employing technologies like blockchain. Patients can assert more control over their health data, feeling confident that it is securely stored and accessible only with their explicit consent.
- Population Health Management: Digital Twins play a role in population health management by gathering and analyzing data from a broad spectrum of patients. This allows healthcare organizations to discern health trends, allocate resources efficiently, and implement preventive measures on a population-wide scale.

Note that digital twins are used to revolutionize healthcare by delivering more patient-centered, data-driven, and proactive care. However, their implementation requires careful consideration of data privacy, ethical issues, and regulatory compliance. As the technology continues to advance, Digital Twins have the potential to significantly improve healthcare outcomes and the overall healthcare experience for individuals.

1.4 Issues and Challenges in Traditional Healthcare

Traditional healthcare, while providing important services, faces several issues and challenges that impact the quality, accessibility, and cost of care. Some of the key issues and challenges in traditional healthcare include:

- Access Disparities: Access to healthcare services is not equitable, with disparities based on socio-economic status, geography, race, and ethnicity. Many underserved and rural populations struggle to access essential healthcare services due to limited healthcare infrastructure and resources.
- Cost of Care: Healthcare costs have been steadily rising, making it unaffordable for many individuals, even in developed countries. This can lead to financial barriers that prevent people from seeking necessary medical care.
- Inefficient Healthcare Delivery: The traditional healthcare system can be cumbersome and inefficient. Long wait times, administrative red tape, and fragmented care coordination often hinder the patient experience and impede timely care delivery.
- Medical Errors: Medical errors, including misdiagnoses, medication errors, and healthcare-associated infections, are significant issues in traditional healthcare. These errors can result in harm to patients and even fatalities.
- Fragmented Care: Traditional healthcare is often delivered by various providers and specialties, resulting in fragmented care. Poor communication and coordination among healthcare providers can lead to suboptimal patient outcomes and unnecessary costs.
- Limited Preventive Care: The traditional healthcare system has historically focused on treating illnesses rather than preventing them. This reactive approach can lead to higher healthcare costs and more significant health issues.

- Health Information Exchange: Data sharing and interoperability among healthcare systems, providers, and electronic health records can be challenging. Incomplete patient information and a lack of standardized data formats can hinder care coordination and decision-making.
- Aging Population: Demographic changes, including an aging population, place increased demands on healthcare systems. Aging individuals often have complex health needs, and healthcare systems must adapt to provide comprehensive geriatric care.
- Healthcare Workforce Shortages: Numerous regions are grappling with shortages of healthcare professionals, encompassing doctors, nurses, and allied health workers. This scarcity can result in overburdened healthcare providers, extended wait times, and diminished access to care.
- Mental Health Stigma: Even as the significance of mental health gains acknowledgment, a substantial stigma persists around mental health issues. This stigma has the potential to deter individuals from seeking necessary mental health treatment and support.
- Patient Engagement: Engaging patients in their own care can be a challenge. Many patients may not fully understand their health conditions or treatment options, leading to non-compliance with treatment plans and poor health outcomes.
- Lack of Preventive Measures: Traditional healthcare systems often underinvest in preventive care and public health initiatives. Focusing more on preventing diseases and promoting healthy lifestyles can reduce the burden of chronic conditions.
- Healthcare Inequalities: Healthcare inequalities persist, with marginalized and vulnerable populations experiencing poorer health outcomes and reduced access to care. This includes disparities in maternal and child health, chronic disease management, and access to quality healthcare facilities.

Hence, addressing these issues and challenges in traditional healthcare requires a multifaceted approach that includes healthcare policy reform, investment in health infrastructure, improved healthcare delivery models, increased focus on preventive care, and efforts to reduce healthcare disparities. Transitioning to more patient-centered, value-based care models and using technology can also help mitigate some of these challenges.

2. THE NEED FOR DIGITAL TRANSFORMATION IN HEALTHCARE

Digital transformation in healthcare is important for several reasons (Tyagi, Swetta Kukreja, Meghna Manoj Nair, Amit Kumar Tyagi,2023) (Madhav A.V.S., Tyagi A.K. 2022) (Sheth, H.S.K., Tyagi, A.K. 2022), as it has the potential to significantly improve patient care, streamline operations, and enhance overall efficiency in the healthcare industry. Here are some key reasons why there is a need for digital transformation in healthcare:

A. Improved Patient Care and Outcomes:
   ◦ Digital technologies empower healthcare providers to access real-time patient data, fostering improved and more informed decision-making.
   ◦ Centralizing patient information, Electronic Health Records (EHRs) offer a comprehensive overview of a patient's medical history, medications, and treatment plans. This has the potential to improve the coordination of care among various healthcare providers.

B. Enhanced Efficiency and Workflow:
  ◦ Automation of routine tasks and administrative processes can reduce the burden on health-care professionals, allowing them to focus more on patient care.
  ◦ Digital tools such as telemedicine and remote monitoring enable healthcare providers to deliver care outside traditional clinical settings, improving access and convenience for patients.
C. Data Analytics and Population Health Management:

Digital transformation enables the collection and analysis of large datasets (A. K. Tyagi, S. Chandrasekaran and N. Sreenath, 2022) (A. Deshmukh, N. Sreenath, A. K. Tyagi and U. V, 2022)

- , leading to information that can improve population health management.
- Predictive analytics can help identify at-risk populations, allowing for proactive and preventive interventions.
  D. Interoperability and Information Sharing:
- Interoperable systems ensure that different healthcare entities can share and access patient information seamlessly, promoting continuity of care.
- Health Information Exchanges (HIEs) facilitate the secure sharing of patient data across different healthcare organizations.
  E. Patient Engagement and Empowerment:
- Digital tools, such as mobile apps and patient portals, empower individuals to actively participate in their healthcare management.
- Telehealth services enable remote consultations, making healthcare more accessible to individuals who may face geographical or mobility challenges.
  F. Cost Reduction and Resource Optimization:
- Automation and streamlining of processes can lead to cost savings for healthcare organizations.
- Preventive care and early intervention facilitated by digital technologies can reduce the overall cost of healthcare by preventing more expensive treatments later.

Hence, such areas discuss the use of Digital Transformation in Healthcare (in this modern era) in detail.

3. DIGITAL TWIN BASICS, BENEFITS, AND ITS APPLICATIONS IN HEALTHCARE IN THIS SMART ERA

A Digital Twin is a virtual representation or duplicate of a physical entity, system, or process. It is constructed using real-time data, sensors, and information from its physical counterpart, which could be an object, system, or even a living organism, such as a patient in healthcare. The Digital Twin is continually updated to mirror changes in the physical entity, serving as a valuable tool for analysis, prediction, and decision-making. In healthcare, Digital Twins can be employed to model and monitor individual patients, capturing their health data, medical history, and more in a digital format. These representations play a crucial role in personalized medicine, predictive analytics, and optimizing patient care.

3.1 Benefits of Digital Twins in Healthcare

- Personalized Medicine: Leveraging Digital Twins allows healthcare providers to customize treatments and care plans for individual patients, taking into account their distinctive health data, genetics, and medical history.
- Early Disease Detection: By continuously monitoring and analyzing a patient's health data, Digital Twins can detect early signs of diseases or health abnormalities, leading to quicker intervention and better outcomes.
- Remote Patient Monitoring: Digital Twins facilitate remote monitoring, allowing patients to be observed and cared for outside of traditional healthcare settings, reducing the need for frequent hospital visits.
- Treatment Optimization: Healthcare providers can use Digital Twins to simulate various treatment scenarios, allowing for informed decisions and improved treatment outcomes.
- Drug Development: Within pharmaceutical research, Digital Twins have the capability to simulate the impact of new drugs on virtual patient avatars. This accelerates the drug development process and results in cost reductions.
- Interdisciplinary Collaboration: Digital Twins encourage collaboration among healthcare professionals and specialists, leading to more integrated and comprehensive care.
- Data Security and Privacy: Emphasizing data security and privacy, Digital Twins ensure that patient data is securely stored and can only be accessed with explicit consent.

3.2 Applications of Digital Twins in Healthcare

- Personal Health Monitoring: Digital Twins can represent an individual's health status, enabling real-time monitoring of important signs, activity levels, and chronic conditions. This information aids in the management of chronic diseases and proactive health maintenance.
- Disease Modeling: Researchers and healthcare providers can use Digital Twins to model specific diseases, such as cancer, to understand disease progression, response to treatment, and the impact of interventions.
- Surgical Simulation: Surgeons can practice complex procedures using Digital Twins of patients, improving surgical precision and reducing the risk of complications.
- Drug Discovery and Testing: Pharmaceutical companies use Digital Twins to simulate drug interactions and effects on virtual patient avatars before clinical trials, saving time and resources.
- Mental Health Support: Digital Twins can be used to monitor and provide support for individuals with mental health conditions by analyzing data related to mood, behavior, and other indicators.
- Preventive Healthcare: Digital Twins can help identify health risks early and promote preventive measures, such as lifestyle changes and immunizations, to reduce the occurrence of diseases.
- Geriatric Care: Digital Twins play a important role in managing the complex health needs of aging populations by continuously monitoring their health and providing early intervention when required.

Hence, Digital Twins are increasingly becoming a fundamental part of healthcare, providing the potential for more personalized, data-driven, and proactive care. However, their implementation must consider data security, ethical issues, and regulatory compliance to ensure responsible and equitable use in the healthcare industry

3.3 Building a Healthcare Digital Twin for Modern Society

Today Building a Healthcare Digital Twin for Modern Society is a complex and multifaceted endeavor that requires careful planning, technological infrastructure, data management, and collaboration among various consumers/ users (Deshmukh, Sreenath, Tyagi and U. V., 2022). Here are the key steps and considerations to build an effective Healthcare Digital Twin for the modern era:

- Define the Purpose and Scope: Determine the specific goals and objectives of your Healthcare Digital Twin. Decide what aspects of healthcare it will encompass, whether it's focused on individual patient management, disease modeling, drug development, or a combination of these and more.
- Data Integration and Collection: Collect and amalgamate varied sources of health-related data, encompassing electronic health records (EHRs), information from wearable devices, genetic data, and other healthcare databases. Prioritize data quality, security, and compliance with pertinent regulations, such as HIPAA in the United States.
- Patient Engagement and Informed Consent: Establish clear guidelines for obtaining informed consent from patients whose data will be used to create their Digital Twins. It's essential to engage patients in the process and ensure they understand how their data will be used to benefit their healthcare.
- Digital Twin Creation: Develop the technology and algorithms to create accurate and real-time Digital Twins. This may involve creating virtual models of patients, diseases, or healthcare systems, depending on the intended application.

3.4 Data Analytics and Machine Learning

Implementing data analytics/ machine learning tools to analyze the data and derive information from the Digital Twins is essential (Varsha Jayaprakash, Amit Kumar Tyagi,
    Amit Kumar Tyagi, Aswathy S U, G Aghila, N Sreenath, 2021)(Sai, G.H., Tripathi, K., Tyagi, A.K. 2023). These information may include predictive modeling, early disease detection, and treatment optimization.

- Remote Monitoring and IoT Devices: Enable remote monitoring by integrating Internet of Things (IoT) devices for real-time data collection, such as wearable health trackers and sensors, which can continuously update the Digital Twins.
- Interoperability and Standards: Ensure interoperability between different healthcare systems and data sources by adhering to health data exchange standards like HL7 and FHIR. This allows for seamless data sharing and integration.
- Security and Privacy: Enforce strong security measures to safeguard patient data and adhere to data privacy regulations like GDPR or HIPAA. Crucial components include data encryption, access controls, and audit trails.

- Collaboration and Interdisciplinary Teams: Healthcare Digital Twins require collaboration among healthcare professionals, data scientists, software engineers, and regulatory experts. Interdisciplinary teams can ensure the success and ethical use of Digital Twins.
- Regulatory Compliance: Understand and adhere to healthcare regulations and standards relevant to your region, ensuring that your Healthcare Digital Twin project complies with local laws and requirements.
- Testing and Validation: Thoroughly test and validate the Digital Twins' accuracy, performance, and security. Conduct rigorous clinical trials and assessments to ensure that the technology is safe and effective.
- Scaling and Adoption: Plan for scalability and adoption across healthcare institutions, encouraging the widespread use of Healthcare Digital Twins for improved patient care and research.
- Continuous Improvement and Updates: Healthcare Digital Twins should be continuously updated and improved as new data and technologies become available. Regular assessments of their effectiveness and patient outcomes should guide further enhancements.

Note that Building a Healthcare Digital Twin for modern society is a dynamic and evolving process. It requires a commitment to data-driven, patient-centered care and a focus on ethical, secure, and compliant practices to ensure the best possible outcomes for patients and healthcare systems.

4. DIGITAL TWINS AND IOT DEVICE ROLE IN IN SMART HEALTHCARE

Digital Twins and IoT devices play significant roles in the advancement of Smart Healthcare (Kute; Tyagi; et al.,2021) Kute; Tyagi; Nair, 2021) (Kumari, Muthulakshmi, Agarwal2022). They complement each other, creating a symbiotic relationship that enhances patient care, healthcare management, and overall health outcomes. Here's how Digital Twins and IoT devices contribute to Smart Healthcare:

4.1 Role of Digital Twins in Smart Healthcare

Role of Digital Twins in Smart Healthcare can be discussed as:

- Patient-Centric Care: Digital Twins allow the creation of virtual representations of individual patients, incorporating their health data, medical history, and real-time health metrics. This enables highly personalized, patient-centric care that considers each patient's unique needs and conditions.
- Early Disease Detection: Digital Twins continuously monitor and analyze a patient's health data, enabling the early detection of deviations or abnormalities. This can lead to timely intervention and preventive measures to manage chronic conditions or detect diseases at an earlier, more treatable stage.
- Treatment Optimization: Healthcare providers can use Digital Twins to simulate different treatment scenarios, allowing for data-driven decisions about the most effective and efficient treatment plans. This reduces trial-and-error approaches and enhances treatment outcomes.
- Remote Patient Monitoring: Digital Twins facilitate remote monitoring of patients' health. By integrating data from IoT devices, healthcare providers can track patients' important signs, medica-

tion adherence, and overall health status. In case of anomalies, timely interventions can be made, reducing the need for frequent in-person visits.

- Data-Driven Decision-Making: Digital Twins offer healthcare professionals a comprehensive perspective on a patient's health, enabling data-driven decision-making. This results in more precise diagnoses, streamlined treatment plans, and enhanced patient outcomes.

4.2 Role of IoT Devices in Smart Healthcare

Role of IoT Devices in Smart Healthcare can be discussed as:

- Continuous Data Collection: Internet of Things (IoT) devices, including wearable health trackers, sensors, and remote monitoring devices, gather real-time health data such as heart rate, blood pressure, glucose levels, and more. This data is seamlessly integrated into a patient's Digital Twin.
- Telehealth and Telemedicine: IoT devices enable remote patient monitoring and telehealth consultations. Patients can have virtual visits with healthcare providers, share health data, and receive real-time feedback, enhancing access to healthcare services, especially in remote or underserved areas.
- Chronic Disease Management: IoT devices play a vital role in the management of chronic conditions. Individuals with diabetes, heart disease, or respiratory conditions can utilize these devices to monitor their health, receive timely alerts, and share relevant data with their healthcare providers, ultimately enhancing the management of their diseases.
- Wearable Health Technology: Wearable IoT devices, like fitness trackers and smartwatches, provide users with real-time health data and promote healthy lifestyles. These devices encourage physical activity, monitor sleep patterns, and track overall well-being.
- Medication Adherence: Smart pill dispensers and medication reminder systems enabled by IoT assist patients in adhering to their medication regimens. This is especially crucial for individuals dealing with chronic conditions or intricate medication schedules.
- Public Health and Epidemiology: IoT devices and data analytics are used to monitor population health, track disease outbreaks, and identify trends. This information is important for early intervention and public health decision-making.
- Aging Population Support: IoT devices support aging populations with fall detection, remote monitoring, and health tracking, enabling older individuals to live independently and receive necessary care.

Hence, the convergence between Digital Twins and IoT devices empowers Smart Healthcare by providing a holistic view of a patient's health and enabling remote monitoring, early intervention, personalized care, and data-driven decision-making. This approach not only enhances patient outcomes but also contributes to the efficiency and sustainability of healthcare systems in the modern era.

5. EMERGING TECHNOLOGIES FOR DIGITAL TWIN-BASED HEALTHCARE

Emerging technologies continue to shape and enhance the field of Digital Twin-based healthcare, providing new opportunities for personalized care, predictive analytics, and improved patient outcomes

(Kute Tyagi Aswathy., 2022) (Kute Tyagi Aswathy, 2022). Some of the key emerging technologies in this field include:

- Artificial Intelligence (AI) and Machine Learning: AI and machine learning are instrumental in analyzing large healthcare data for predictive modeling, early disease detection, and personalized treatment plans. AI-powered algorithms can process and interpret data from Digital Twins, assisting healthcare professionals in making data-driven decisions.
- Blockchain Technology: Blockchain ensures the security, privacy, and integrity of healthcare data. By using a decentralized ledger, blockchain technology can help maintain the trustworthiness of patient data in Digital Twins, allowing secure data sharing and consent management.
- 5G Connectivity: The advent of 5G networks enables high-speed, low-latency data transmission, which is essential for real-time monitoring and communication with IoT devices and Digital Twins. It supports the seamless integration of data from various sources.
- Edge Computing: Edge computing entails processing data in proximity to the source, such as IoT devices, rather than solely relying on centralized cloud servers. This methodology diminishes latency and facilitates real-time analytics and decision-making, thereby enhancing the responsiveness of Digital Twins in healthcare.
- Genomic Data Analysis: Advancements in genomics and genomic data analysis play an important role in creating more accurate and personalized Digital Twins. These technologies help healthcare providers understand an individual's genetic makeup and its implications for disease risk and treatment.
- Virtual Reality (VR) and Augmented Reality (AR): VR and AR technologies are applied to enhance surgical simulations, medical training, and patient education. They can be integrated with Digital Twins to provide an immersive experience for healthcare professionals and patients.
- Biotechnology and Nanotechnology: Emerging biotechnology and nanotechnology advancements are applied in drug development and personalized medicine. These innovations enable the creation of precise treatments based on an individual's unique health profile.
- Natural Language Processing (NLP): Natural Language Processing (NLP) technologies empower healthcare providers to extract valuable information from unstructured clinical notes, patient records, and research documents. This capability aids in constructing more comprehensive and accurate Digital Twins.
- Robotic Process Automation (RPA): RPA is used for administrative tasks, such as managing patient records, appointment scheduling, and billing processes. This technology streamlines healthcare operations, reducing administrative burdens.
- Quantum Computing: Although in its nascent phases, quantum computing harbors the potential to swiftly address complex healthcare problems. Its capacity to optimize treatment plans, analyze massive datasets, and expedite drug discovery is particularly noteworthy.
- Biometric Authentication: Biometric authentication methods, including fingerprint and facial recognition, bolster the security and access control of Digital Twins. These methods play a crucial role in ensuring that only authorized individuals can access sensitive healthcare data.
- Immersive Health Monitoring: Wearable IoT devices, combined with augmented reality or smart glasses, can provide healthcare professionals with real-time patient data directly within their field of vision, facilitating better patient care and monitoring.

- Synthetic Biology: Synthetic biology techniques enable the creation of custom-made biological systems for various healthcare applications, including drug production and the development of targeted therapies.
- Voice and Speech Recognition: Voice and speech recognition technology can enhance the ease of accessing and updating patient data in Digital Twins, making healthcare interactions more efficient.

It is essential to recognize that the integration of these emerging technologies with Digital Twins has the potential to revolutionize healthcare. This integration can lead to more precise, personalized, and efficient care, while also enabling predictive and preventive healthcare strategies. As these technologies advance, the future of Digital Twin-based healthcare appears promising, with a primary focus on improving patient outcomes and enhancing the overall patient experience.

5.3 Data Analytics and AI in Healthcare

Data analytics and artificial intelligence (AI) play important roles in healthcare, transforming the way patient care is delivered, clinical decisions are made, and healthcare systems are managed. Here's an overview of the roles of data analytics and AI in healthcare:

Data Analytics in Healthcare:

- Patient Data Analysis: Data analytics plays a pivotal role in thoroughly analyzing patient data, encompassing electronic health records (EHRs), medical histories, and diagnostic images. This process can uncover patterns, trends, and anomalies within patient data, facilitating early disease detection and enhancing treatment planning.
- Predictive Analytics: Healthcare data analytics can predict patient outcomes, such as readmissions, disease progression, and complications. By analyzing historical data, healthcare providers can identify high-risk patients and intervene proactively.
- Population Health Management: Utilizing data analytics tools, healthcare organizations manage the health of entire populations. These tools assist in identifying at-risk groups, allocating resources efficiently, and implementing preventive measures to enhance public health.
- Financial Analysis: Data analytics is employed for financial management, helping healthcare organizations optimize revenue, control costs, and identify billing and coding errors.
- Operational Efficiency: Hospitals and clinics use data analytics to enhance operational efficiency. It can optimize staff scheduling, bed utilization, and inventory management, leading to cost savings and better resource allocation.
- Quality Improvement: Data analytics assists in monitoring healthcare quality and compliance with standards. Healthcare organizations can track performance indicators, identify areas for improvement, and implement quality enhancement initiatives.
- Clinical Research: Data analytics supports clinical research by analyzing data from clinical trials and research studies. It helps researchers identify trends, evaluate treatment effectiveness, and make data-driven conclusions.

AI in Healthcare:

- Disease Diagnosis and Prediction: Algorithms powered by artificial intelligence can analyze medical images, including X-rays and MRIs, aiding in the diagnosis of conditions such as cancer, heart disease, and neurological disorders. Additionally, AI can predict disease risks based on patient data and genetics.
- Treatment Personalization: Artificial intelligence can recommend personalized treatment plans for patients by analyzing their medical history, genetic information, and real-time health data. This approach tailors treatment to the unique needs of each patient.
- Drug Discovery: Artificial intelligence accelerates drug discovery by simulating molecular interactions and predicting the efficacy and safety of potential drugs. This efficient approach saves time and resources in the development of new medications.
- Natural Language Processing (NLP): Natural Language Processing (NLP) algorithms can extract valuable information from unstructured clinical notes and medical literature, providing assistance in medical coding, disease surveillance, and clinical decision support.
- Remote Patient Monitoring: AI powers remote monitoring devices that can continuously track important signs, medication adherence, and other health metrics. AI can analyze this data and trigger alerts if anomalies are detected, allowing for timely intervention.
- Robot-Assisted Surgery: Robotic systems powered by artificial intelligence aid surgeons in conducting minimally invasive and highly precise surgeries, thereby reducing the risk of complications and improving surgical outcomes.
- Chatbots and Virtual Health Assistants: Chatbots and virtual health assistants driven by artificial intelligence offer patients health information, address medical queries, and even provide mental health support. These tools enhance patient engagement and alleviate the burden on healthcare professionals.
- Fraud Detection: AI can identify fraudulent claims and activities in healthcare, helping insurance providers and healthcare organizations prevent financial losses.
- Genomic Analysis: Artificial intelligence analyzes vast amounts of genomic data to pinpoint genetic markers linked to specific diseases, facilitating personalized medicine and targeted therapies.
- Behavioral Health Analysis: AI is used to analyze patient behavior and speech patterns to detect mental health issues and provide early intervention.

Hence, the integration of data analytics and AI in healthcare provides several benefits, including improved patient care, more accurate diagnoses, enhanced research capabilities, and streamlined healthcare operations. However, it also raises important issues, such as data privacy, ethical use of AI, and regulatory compliance, that must be addressed to ensure responsible and secure implementation in the healthcare industry.

5.4 Electronic Health Records (EHR) Importance in smart healthcare

Electronic Health Records (EHR) are important in the context of smart healthcare. They represent a foundational element in the digitization and modernization of healthcare systems, providing several benefits that contribute to the overall advancement of healthcare services. Here's why EHRs are important in smart healthcare:

- Efficient Information Management: EHRs enable healthcare providers to efficiently manage and store patient information, eliminating the need for paper-based records. This makes it easier to access, update, and share patient data among healthcare professionals, leading to improved care coordination.

- Accurate and Up-to-Date Patient Information: EHRs ensure that patient information is accurate and up to date. This is important for making informed clinical decisions and providing appropriate care. Real-time updates and alerts help healthcare professionals stay informed about a patient's condition and needs.

- Interoperability: EHRs support interoperability by allowing the exchange of patient information between different healthcare facilities and systems. This interoperability is important for providing continuity of care, especially in cases where patients seek treatment at multiple facilities or when transferring medical records.

- Remote Access and Telemedicine: EHRs facilitate remote access to patient data, making telemedicine and remote patient monitoring more effective. This is particularly important for smart healthcare initiatives, as it enables virtual consultations and monitoring of patients from a distance.

- Data Analytics and Decision Support: EHRs provide a wealth of data that can be used for data analytics and decision support. Healthcare professionals can use EHR data to identify trends, predict patient outcomes, and make more informed clinical decisions.

- Reduced Medical Errors: EHRs help reduce medical errors, such as illegible handwriting and transcription mistakes. Electronic records are legible and can incorporate alerts and reminders for medication administration, allergy warnings, and more.

- Patient Engagement: EHRs can be accessible to patients, allowing them to view their own medical records, test results, and treatment plans. This promotes patient engagement, empowerment, and self-management of their health.

- Cost Reduction: EHRs can lead to cost reductions in healthcare operations. They minimize the need for paper records, streamline administrative tasks, and reduce the risk of duplicate testing, leading to cost savings.

- Public Health Reporting: EHRs play a role in public health reporting by capturing data on disease outbreaks, trends, and health disparities. This information is valuable for public health organizations in tracking and responding to health crises.

- Research and Innovation: EHRs support medical research and innovation by providing a large dataset for studies and clinical trials. Researchers can access de-identified patient data to advance medical knowledge and develop new therapies and treatments.

- Regulatory Compliance and Reporting: EHRs facilitate compliance with healthcare regulations and reporting requirements, ensuring that healthcare organizations meet legal and quality standards.

- Smart Healthcare Integration: EHRs are a foundational technology in the development of smart healthcare solutions. They provide the necessary infrastructure to integrate and analyze data from various sources, including IoT devices, telemedicine platforms, and digital twin technologies.

- Security and Privacy: Implementing sophisticated security measures is crucial for EHR systems to safeguard patient data, maintaining patient privacy and ensuring data integrity.

Hence in the context of smart healthcare, EHRs serve as the central repository for patient data and are a important enabler of digital transformation and data-driven decision-making. Their adoption and effective use are essential for achieving the goals of modern, patient-centered, and data-driven healthcare systems.

6. INTEGRATION OF EMERGING TECHNOLOGIES WITH MODERN HEALTHCARE IT SYSTEMS

Integrating modern healthcare IT systems with emerging technologies is vital for enhancing patient care, improving operational efficiency, and advancing healthcare services. Here are key areas where the integration of emerging technologies is pivotal in healthcare IT systems:

- Artificial Intelligence (AI) and Machine Learning: AI and machine learning are integrated into healthcare IT systems for tasks such as predictive analytics, diagnostic assistance, treatment recommendations, and personalized medicine. AI-driven chatbots and virtual health assistants also enhance patient engagement.
- IoT Devices and Wearables: Healthcare IT systems incorporate data from IoT devices and wearables for remote monitoring, important signs tracking, and early disease detection. The data collected is analyzed and displayed within EHRs for real-time clinical decision support.
- Telehealth and Telemedicine: Telehealth and telemedicine platforms are integrated with EHRs, allowing healthcare providers to conduct virtual consultations and share patient data seamlessly. These platforms include secure video conferencing, patient portals, and remote monitoring capabilities.
- Blockchain Technology: Blockchain is used to secure electronic health records, ensuring patient data integrity and privacy. It facilitates secure data sharing among authorized parties while maintaining a tamper-proof record of access.
- 5G Connectivity: 5G networks enable high-speed data transmission, allowing healthcare IT systems to support remote monitoring, real-time communication, and the transfer of large medical images, such as MRIs and CT scans.
- Edge Computing: Healthcare IT integrates edge computing to process data closer to the source, thereby reducing latency and enabling real-time analytics. This integration is particularly crucial for applications like remote monitoring and IoT devices.
- Augmented Reality (AR) and Virtual Reality (VR): Augmented Reality (AR) and Virtual Reality (VR) technologies enhance medical training, surgical simulations, and patient education. These technologies are integrated into healthcare IT systems to deliver immersive experiences for healthcare professionals and patients.
- Genomic Data Analysis: Genomic data analysis platforms are integrated with healthcare IT systems to support precision medicine. This integration allows healthcare providers to incorporate genetic information about treatment plans and risk assessments.
- Robotic Process Automation (RPA): RPA is used in healthcare IT systems for administrative tasks, such as claims processing, billing, and scheduling. RPA bots streamline operational workflows and reduce administrative burdens.
- Remote Patient Monitoring: EHRs and healthcare IT systems seamlessly integrate with IoT devices designed for remote patient monitoring to capture real-time patient data. Subsequently, this data is analyzed and presented in a user-friendly interface for healthcare providers.

- Quantum Computing: In the future, quantum computing can be integrated into healthcare IT systems for complex problem solving, such as drug discovery, genomics, and optimizing treatment plans.

- Natural Language Processing (NLP): Healthcare IT systems integrate Natural Language Processing (NLP) algorithms to extract valuable information from unstructured clinical notes, medical records, and research documents. This integration enhances clinical decision support and coding processes.

- Voice and Speech Recognition: Voice and speech recognition technology is integrated into healthcare IT systems for clinical documentation, allowing healthcare professionals to dictate patient notes and interact with EHRs through voice commands.

- Chatbots and Virtual Health Assistants: Chatbots and virtual health assistants are integrated with patient portals and healthcare IT systems to provide patient support, answer medical queries, and schedule appointments.

Note that the integration of emerging technologies with modern healthcare IT systems is a continuous process, designed to enhance patient care, streamline operations, and support data-driven decision-making. These integrations are essential for creating more efficient, patient-centered, and advanced healthcare systems.

7. APPLICATIONS OF DIGITAL TWINS IN SMART HEALTHCARE

Digital Twins have a wide range of applications in smart healthcare, revolutionizing patient care, healthcare management, and medical research. Here are some key applications of Digital Twins in smart healthcare:

- Personalized Medicine: Digital Twins create virtual representations of individual patients, incorporating their health data, genetic information, and medical history. This allows for highly personalized treatment plans, drug regimens, and medical interventions tailored to each patient's unique needs.

- Early Disease Detection: Digital Twins continuously monitor and analyze a patient's health data. They can detect subtle changes and anomalies, enabling the early detection of diseases, conditions, or deviations from normal health parameters. This early detection improves patient outcomes and reduces healthcare costs.

- Remote Patient Monitoring: Digital Twins facilitate remote patient monitoring by integrating data from wearable IoT devices. Healthcare providers can remotely track important signs, medication adherence, and overall health status, enabling timely interventions when abnormalities are detected.

- Treatment Optimization: Healthcare providers can use Digital Twins to simulate different treatment scenarios, considering an individual's unique health data. This leads to more informed treatment decisions, reducing trial-and-error approaches and enhancing treatment success rates.

- Drug Development and Testing: In pharmaceutical research, Digital Twins are employed to simulate the effects of new drugs on virtual patient avatars. This enables researchers to anticipate potential outcomes, side effects, and efficacy before undertaking expensive and time-consuming clinical trials.

- Chronic Disease Management: Digital Twins are employed in the management of chronic diseases such as diabetes, heart disease, and hypertension. They provide continuous monitoring, predict disease exacerbations, and enable timely interventions to prevent complications.

- Surgical Simulation and Training: Surgeons can use Digital Twins to practice and simulate complex surgical procedures. This enhances surgical precision, reduces the risk of complications, and improves surgical training and education.

- Interdisciplinary Collaboration: Digital Twins encourage collaboration among healthcare professionals and specialists from various fields. This enables a more integrated and holistic approach to patient care, particularly for complex cases and patient care coordination.

- Data Security and Privacy: Digital Twins prioritize data security and privacy by employing technologies like blockchain. Patients have greater control over their health data, knowing it is stored securely and can only be accessed with their consent.

- Population Health Management: Digital Twins aggregate and analyze data from a large group of patients, enabling healthcare organizations to identify health trends, allocate resources efficiently, and implement preventive measures at a population level.

- Mental Health Support: Digital Twins can monitor and provide support for individuals with mental health conditions by analyzing data related to mood, behavior, and other indicators. This enhances early intervention and personalized mental health care.

- Public Health and Epidemiology: Digital Twins play a role in public health by tracking disease outbreaks, monitoring health trends, and supporting epidemiological studies. They provide essential data for public health decision-making and emergency response.

- Maternal and Child Health: Digital Twins can be used to monitor the health of pregnant women and infants, providing early intervention and support to ensure safe pregnancies and healthy childbirth.

Hence, digital twins are at the forefront of healthcare innovation, provideing the potential to deliver more patient-centered, data-driven, and proactive care. However, their implementation requires careful consideration of data privacy, ethical issues, and regulatory compliance to ensure responsible and secure use in healthcare.

8. SECURITY AND DATA PRIVACY ISSUES IN DIGITAL TWINS BASED HEALTHCARE

Security and data privacy are important issues in Digital Twins based healthcare, as they involve sensitive patient information and healthcare data. Here are some of the primary issues and issues related to security and data privacy, as mentioned in Table 1.

Hence, addressing security and data privacy issues in Digital Twins based healthcare requires a comprehensive and proactive approach. It involves robust technical measures, adherence to regulations, and a commitment to ethical and responsible data use to maintain patient trust and ensure the confidentiality and integrity of healthcare data.

Table 1. Primary issues and issues related to security and data privacy

Types	Issues	Solutions
Data Breaches and Unauthorized Access:	Unauthorized access to Digital Twins can lead to data breaches, exposing patients' sensitive health information.	Enforce strong access controls, encryption, and multi-factor authentication to safeguard Digital Twins against unauthorized access.
Data Encryption	Patient data in Digital Twins must be securely transmitted and stored to prevent interception by malicious actors.	Use strong encryption protocols to protect data both in transit and at rest.
Consent and Patient Ownership:	Patients should have control over who can access their Digital Twins and how their data is used.	Implement clear consent mechanisms, allowing patients to specify who can access their data and for what purposes. Patients should own and have the ability to modify their data.
Data Integrity:	Ensuring the precision and integrity of patient data within Digital Twins is crucial for secure healthcare decision-making.	Implement data validation checks, regular audits, and tamper-evident technology to maintain data integrity.
Regulatory Compliance:	Healthcare organizations are obligated to adhere to data protection regulations, including HIPAA in the United States or GDPR in Europe.	Ensure that Digital Twins and related systems comply with relevant healthcare data privacy and security regulations. Regularly update policies and procedures to remain in compliance.
Secure Interoperability:	Sharing patient data between different healthcare systems and providers can introduce vulnerabilities.	Establish secure data exchange standards and protocols to ensure that data sharing is safe and compliant.
Insider Threats:	Healthcare employees or contractors may misuse or inappropriately access patient data.	Implement user access controls, employee training, and ongoing monitoring to mitigate insider threats.
Anonymization and De-Identification:	Anonymizing patient data is essential to protect individual privacy.	Use anonymization and de-identification techniques to eliminate personally identifiable information (PII) while retaining the data's usefulness for research and analysis.
Data Lifecycle Management:	Patient data must be securely managed throughout its lifecycle, including data retention and disposal.	Create data lifecycle management policies to establish the duration of data storage and secure procedures for its deletion when it is no longer required.

9. Challenges and Future opportunities towards Digital Twins based smart Healthcare

Digital Twins in smart healthcare provide several opportunities for enhancing patient care, clinical decision-making, and healthcare operations. However, they also pose several challenges that require attention to unlock their full potential. Here is an overview of the challenges and future opportunities in smart healthcare based on Digital Twins:

Challenges:
- ◦ Data Security and Privacy: Protecting patient data is a primary issue. Ensuring the security and privacy of patient information in Digital Twins is an ongoing challenge.
- ◦ Interoperability: Integrating Digital Twins with various healthcare systems, IoT devices, and EHRs can be complex. Ensuring interoperability is important for seamless data exchange.
- ◦ Data Quality: Ensuring the accuracy and reliability of data used to create and update Digital Twins is essential for their effectiveness.

- ○ Regulatory Compliance: Adhering to healthcare regulations, such as HIPAA or GDPR, while utilizing Digital Twins is challenging due to the complexity of healthcare data.
- ○ Ethical Issues: Ethical issues surrounding patient data use, informed consent, and responsible data handling must be addressed.
- ○ Data Overload: The abundance of data generated by IoT devices and continuous monitoring can lead to information overload for healthcare providers. It's essential to filter and prioritize relevant information.
- ○ Cost and Resource Constraints: Integrating and sustaining Digital Twins in healthcare systems can incur significant expenses and demand substantial resources, particularly for smaller healthcare providers.

Future Opportunities:

- ○ Personalized Medicine: Digital Twins will facilitate the creation of highly personalized treatment plans, utilizing a patient's unique health data and genetic information, ultimately resulting in more effective and efficient care.
- ○ Preventive Healthcare: Early disease detection and predictive analytics from Digital Twins will shift healthcare towards a preventive rather than reactive model.
- ○ Remote Patient Monitoring: Digital Twins will make remote patient monitoring more effective, allowing patients to receive care in the comfort of their homes and reducing the burden on healthcare facilities.
- ○ AI-Driven Clinical Decision Support: The integration with AI will furnish healthcare professionals with real-time, data-driven decision support, contributing to improved clinical outcomes.
- ○ Drug Discovery and Development: Digital Twins will expedite drug discovery by simulating drug effects on virtual patient avatars, reducing the time and cost of bringing new drugs to market.
- ○ Telemedicine and Virtual Consultations: Telehealth and virtual consultations will become more sophisticated, providing patients with convenient access to healthcare professionals.
- ○ Data-Driven Public Health: Data from Digital Twins will support public health initiatives, helping in the early detection of disease outbreaks and monitoring population health.
- ○ Enhanced Surgical Training: Digital Twins will improve surgical training, enabling more realistic simulations and reducing the learning curve for surgeons.
- ○ Improved Resource Allocation: Healthcare facilities will optimize resource allocation and bed management, leading to cost savings and better patient care.
- ○ Patient Empowerment: Patients will have greater access to and control over their health data, contributing to their active involvement in their healthcare.

Note that the future of Digital Twins in smart healthcare holds great promise, with the potential to revolutionize patient care and healthcare systems. As the challenges are addressed and technology advances, Digital Twins will play an increasingly integral role in delivering efficient, patient-centered, and data-driven healthcare services.

10. SUSTAINABILITY AND ETHICAL ISSUES

10.1 Sustainable Healthcare Practices for Next-Generation

Sustainable healthcare practices for the next generation aim to balance the provision of high-quality healthcare with environmental and economic sustainability. Implementing these practices can help reduce the ecological footprint of healthcare while maintaining or improving patient care. Here are some key sustainable healthcare practices for the next generation:

- Energy Efficiency: Healthcare facilities should invest in energy-efficient technologies, such as LED lighting, smart HVAC systems, and energy management systems, to reduce energy consumption and lower greenhouse gas emissions.
- Green Building Design: Construct healthcare facilities utilizing sustainable building materials and designs that comply with green building certifications, such as LEED (Leadership in Energy and Environmental Design). This practice minimizes resource consumption and improves energy efficiency.
- Waste Reduction: Incorporate waste reduction strategies, including recycling, reusing, and minimizing waste in healthcare settings. It is crucial to ensure proper disposal and recycling of medical equipment and supplies.
- Water Conservation: Healthcare facilities should use water-saving fixtures and implement water conservation practices to reduce water consumption. This includes the use of low-flow faucets, toilets, and rainwater harvesting.
- Sustainable Procurement: Healthcare organizations should embrace sustainable procurement policies that prioritize the acquisition of environmentally friendly, energy-efficient, and recyclable products and equipment.
- Telemedicine and Remote Monitoring: Employing telemedicine and remote monitoring technologies lessens the necessity for in-person healthcare visits, thereby mitigating greenhouse gas emissions resulting from patient travel and reducing the overall carbon footprint of healthcare facilities.
- Eco-friendly Transportation: Encourage the use of eco-friendly transportation options for healthcare staff and patients, such as public transportation, cycling, or carpooling.
- Renewable Energy Sources: Allocate resources to renewable energy sources, such as solar panels and wind turbines, for powering healthcare facilities, thereby diminishing dependence on fossil fuels.
- Sustainable Practices in Healthcare Waste Management: Implement sustainable waste management practices, including proper disposal of hazardous medical waste and adopting recycling programs for non-hazardous waste.
- Green Healthcare Supply Chains: Develop sustainable supply chains that prioritize responsible sourcing, minimize packaging waste, and reduce the carbon footprint of transportation.
- Education and Training: Educate healthcare professionals, staff, and patients about sustainable healthcare practices to promote awareness and behavioral changes.
- Efficient Healthcare Operations: Streamline healthcare operations to reduce resource consumption and promote operational efficiency. This includes optimizing appointment scheduling, reducing patient wait times, and minimizing paper-based processes.

- Resilience Planning: Prepare healthcare facilities for the impact of climate change by developing resilience plans that ensure continued service provision during extreme weather events and other emergencies.
- Environmental Accountability: Monitor and report on environmental performance, including carbon emissions and resource consumption, to set sustainability targets and track progress.
- Community Engagement: Involve the local community in sustainable healthcare initiatives, collaborating with consumers to create healthier and more environmentally friendly healthcare systems.

Hence, sustainable healthcare practices not only reduce the environmental impact of healthcare but also enhance healthcare resilience and cost-effectiveness. By incorporating these practices, healthcare systems can align with the principles of environmental stewardship and contribute to a healthier and more sustainable future for the next generation.

10.2 Ethical Implications of Healthcare Digital Twins

The utilization of healthcare Digital Twins presents several ethical implications that require thoughtful consideration and management to ensure responsible and ethical use of this technology. Here are some of the ethical issues associated with healthcare Digital Twins, as outlined in table 2.

Hence, managing these ethical issues requires a multi-pronged approach, including robust privacy policies, regulatory oversight, transparent communication with patients, and ongoing ethical evaluation of Digital Twin practices. Healthcare providers and organizations must balance the potential benefits of Digital Twins with their ethical responsibilities to patients.

10.3 Social and Cultural Factors in Next-Generation Healthcare

Social and cultural factors play a significant role in shaping the landscape of next-generation healthcare. Understanding and addressing these factors are important for delivering patient-centered, equitable, and effective healthcare services. Here are some key social and cultural issues in next-generation healthcare:

- Cultural Competence: Healthcare providers must possess cultural competence and be sensitive to the diverse backgrounds and beliefs of patients. Grasping cultural norms, values, and preferences is crucial for delivering respectful and effective care.
- Health Disparities: Social and cultural factors contribute to health disparities. Addressing these disparities is a priority for next-generation healthcare, aiming to reduce inequities in health outcomes among different population groups.
- Language Barriers: Language diversity can be a significant barrier to effective healthcare. Next-generation healthcare should incorporate language interpretation services and translation tools to ensure clear communication between patients and healthcare providers.
- Trust and Belief Systems: Building trust with patients is essential. Understanding patients' belief systems, including religious and spiritual beliefs, can help healthcare providers deliver care that aligns with a patient's values and preferences.

Table 2. Ethical issues associated with healthcare Digital Twins

Types	Issues	Ethical Solutions
Data Privacy and Informed Consent	Patients' personal health data is used to create and update Digital Twins, raising questions about informed consent and data privacy.	Patients should offer explicit and informed consent for the generation and utilization of their Digital Twins. Healthcare providers must uphold the utmost standards of data privacy and security to safeguard patient information.
Ownership and Control	Patients should have ownership and control over their Digital Twins and the data contained within them.	Patients should have the right to access, modify, and even delete their Digital Twins. They should be informed about how their data is used and have the ability to exercise control over it.
Algorithmic Bias and Fairness	Algorithms used in Digital Twins may inadvertently introduce bias, affecting patient care and outcomes.	Initiatives should be undertaken to guarantee the fairness and impartiality of algorithms. Regular audits and assessments of algorithms should be performed to identify and rectify any biases.
Transparency and Accountability	The complex of Digital Twins and the algorithms they employ can pose challenges in comprehending the decision-making processes.	Transparency is important. Healthcare providers and organizations must be transparent about how Digital Twins work, the data sources used, and the factors influencing recommendations. Accountability mechanisms should be in place to address errors or biases.
Security and Unauthorized Access	Digital Twins house highly sensitive patient data, rendering them enticing targets for cyberattacks and unauthorized access.	Rigorous security measures must be implemented to safeguard Digital Twins from unauthorized access. Employing cybersecurity protocols and encryption is essential to ensure the protection of patient information.
Informed Decision-Making	Healthcare providers should use Digital Twins as a tool for informed decision-making rather than blindly following their recommendations.	Healthcare professionals should maintain their clinical judgment and not solely rely on Digital Twins. The technology should be used as a support system to enhance decision-making, not replace it.
Use in Research and Education	Digital Twins can be used for research and educational purposes, potentially exposing patient data to a wider audience.	Research and educational uses of Digital Twins should follow strict ethical guidelines and require de-identification of patient data to protect privacy.
Equity and Accessibility	Not all patients may have equal access to Digital Twins or may be excluded from their benefits.	Efforts should be made to ensure that Digital Twins are accessible to all patients, regardless of socioeconomic status, geography, or other factors. This includes addressing the digital divide and ensuring healthcare equity.
Long-term Data Management	The long-term storage and management of Digital Twins and associated data can raise ethical questions about data retention and disposal.	Healthcare organizations must establish clear data management policies, including data retention and secure disposal procedures.

- Family and Community Involvement: Many cultures place a strong emphasis on the role of family and community in healthcare decision-making. Healthcare services should consider and respect these dynamics.
- Health Literacy: Health literacy varies among individuals and communities. Next-generation healthcare should prioritize health education and communication strategies that are accessible and understandable to all, regardless of literacy level.
- Socioeconomic Factors: Economic disparities have a profound impact on health outcomes. Healthcare should be designed to address socioeconomic factors, such as access to care, housing, and nutrition.
- Patient-Centered Care: Next-generation healthcare emphasizes patient-centered care, which tailors treatment plans and communication to individual preferences and needs, considering social and cultural factors.

- Ethical and Legal issues: Ethical and legal frameworks may differ across cultures. Healthcare providers should navigate these differences while upholding ethical standards and respecting local laws.
- Digital Divide: Access to technology and digital healthcare services varies across communities. Initiatives should be undertaken to narrow the digital divide and guarantee equitable access to healthcare technologies.
- End-of-Life and Palliative Care: Cultural beliefs and practices around death and end-of-life care vary significantly. Next-generation healthcare should accommodate cultural preferences in end-of-life care planning.
- Traditional and Alternative Medicine: Many cultures rely on traditional or alternative medicine practices. Healthcare providers should respect and, when appropriate, integrate these practices into patient care plans.
- Social Support and Mental Health: Next-generation healthcare should recognize the importance of social support networks and address mental health stigma, as both have a substantial impact on overall well-being.
- Community Health Programs: Culturally tailored community health programs can be effective in promoting healthy behaviors and addressing specific health issues within diverse populations.
- Crisis Response and Disaster Preparedness: Understanding cultural norms and practices can be important in responding to health crises and natural disasters, as they influence how communities react and seek help.

Hence, incorporating social and cultural factors into healthcare planning, delivery, and policies is essential for achieving healthcare equity, enhancing patient engagement, and providing care that respects the diversity and needs of the patient population. Next-generation healthcare must be sensitive to these factors to ensure it is inclusive and effective for all individuals and communities.

11. GOVERNMENT AND INDUSTRY INITIATIVES FOR SMART HEALTHCARE

Government and industry initiatives play an important role in advancing smart healthcare, promoting innovation, and addressing important healthcare challenges. These initiatives provide the framework, funding, and collaboration necessary for the development and deployment of smart healthcare solutions. Here are some examples of government and industry initiatives in the realm of smart healthcare:

Government Initiatives:
- National Health IT Initiatives: Governments worldwide are dedicating investments to health information technology (IT) infrastructure. As an example, the U.S. government's Meaningful Use program incentivized healthcare providers to embrace electronic health records (EHRs) and advance health IT interoperability.
- Healthcare Data Standards: Governments often set and promote healthcare data standards to ensure interoperability and data exchange among healthcare systems. The HL7 and SNOMED CT standards are examples of global initiatives.

- Telemedicine and Telehealth Programs: Many governments have expanded telemedicine and telehealth programs to improve healthcare access, particularly in rural or underserved areas. These initiatives support remote consultations and monitoring.
- Research Funding: Governments fund medical research initiatives that drive healthcare innovation. These investments support research into new treatments, technologies, and preventive measures.
- Healthcare Regulatory Frameworks: Governments establish healthcare regulations, privacy laws (e.g., HIPAA in the United States, GDPR in Europe), and patient rights protections to ensure responsible healthcare data management and use.
- Digital Health Adoption Incentives: Some governments provide financial incentives and subsidies to healthcare providers who adopt digital health technologies, including EHRs and telemedicine solutions.

Industry Initiatives:
- Collaborative Partnerships: Healthcare technology companies, pharmaceutical firms, and medical device manufacturers collaborate with healthcare providers to develop and implement smart healthcare solutions. These partnerships drive innovation and improve healthcare delivery.
- Interoperability Standards: Industry organizations such as the Healthcare Information and Management Systems Society (HIMSS) and Integrating the Healthcare Enterprise (IHE) develop interoperability standards and frameworks, facilitating the seamless integration of healthcare systems and devices.
- Health Tech Innovation Hubs: Many industry leaders establish innovation hubs or accelerators dedicated to healthcare technology. These hubs support startups and innovators in developing and scaling smart healthcare solutions.
- Big Data Analytics and AI: Tech companies invest in big data analytics and artificial intelligence (AI) research and development to provide data-driven information, predictive analytics, and decision support tools for healthcare providers.
- Wearables and IoT Integration: The consumer electronics and wearables industry integrate healthcare monitoring and data collection capabilities into consumer products. These wearable devices and IoT technologies are used to track health metrics, improve patient engagement, and enhance remote monitoring.
- Cybersecurity Solutions: Cybersecurity firms specializing in healthcare develop and provide solutions to protect healthcare systems and patient data from cyber threats and data breaches.
- Blockchain in Healthcare: Initiatives provide the use of blockchain technology to enhance the security and integrity of healthcare data, including patient records and drug supply chain management.
- Digital Twin Development: Tech companies and healthcare organizations collaborate to develop and implement Digital Twin technology to improve patient care, treatment planning, and drug development.

These government and industry initiatives are essential for shaping the future of smart healthcare, fostering innovation, ensuring regulatory compliance, and enhancing the quality of care provided to patients. They reflect the collaborative efforts required to drive healthcare transformation and meet the evolving needs of patients and healthcare systems.

12. CONCLUSION

Digital Twins represent a transformative force in the evolution of healthcare services for the next generation society. This innovative technology provides a promising avenue to deliver patient-centered, data-driven, and proactive healthcare solutions. With the power to create virtual replicas of individuals, combining their health data, genetics, and medical history, Digital Twins hold the potential to revolutionize healthcare in several ways. Smart healthcare services empowered by Digital Twins enable personalized medicine, early disease detection, virtual health consultations, optimized treatment plans, and streamlined drug development. Hence, these applications are redefining patient care and reshaping the healthcare landscape by placing greater emphasis on preventive and proactive measures, ultimately improving patient outcomes and reducing healthcare costs.

One of the primary advantages of Digital Twin-based healthcare services lies in their remote monitoring and telehealth capabilities. This allows patients to be continuously monitored from the comfort of their homes, thereby reducing the need for frequent hospital visits. The proactive intervention by healthcare providers in case of anomalies or deteriorating health conditions leads to timely and cost-effective interventions. Moreover, the integration of artificial intelligence and machine learning into Digital Twins facilitates predictive modeling and early disease detection, enabling the implementation of preventive healthcare strategies. This not only alleviates the burden on healthcare systems but also contributes to an overall improvement in population health.

In the next-generation society, the concept of Digital Twins is poised to redefine the healthcare ecosystem, elevating it to new levels of comfort. This innovative approach empowers individuals to take control of their health, enables healthcare providers to deliver proactive and personalized care, and supports groundbreaking research and drug development. However, the successful implementation of Digital Twins in healthcare necessitates addressing ethical, regulatory, and technical challenges.

However, the transition to a Digital Twin-based healthcare system brings forth various challenges, notably concerning data privacy, ethical considerations, security, and ensuring equitable distribution of benefits. Addressing these challenges is imperative to guarantee the responsible and ethical utilization of this transformative technology.

Government and industry initiatives play a crucial role in advancing smart healthcare, fostering innovation, and addressing key healthcare challenges. Collaborative partnerships, regulatory frameworks, and research funding initiatives between these sectors contribute to driving the adoption and integration of Digital Twins into healthcare systems worldwide.

Moving forward, the integration of Digital Twins into healthcare necessitates a comprehensive approach that considers technological advancements, ethical considerations, and societal impacts. This holistic approach will ultimately contribute to the establishment of a more sustainable, patient-centered, and data-driven healthcare system tailored to meet the needs of the next generation society. Smart healthcare services powered by Digital Twins are not merely the future; they are the present, and their potential for transformation is both exciting and promising.

In the last, Digital Twin-based smart healthcare services have the potential to transform healthcare delivery in the next generation society. By using real-time data, artificial intelligence, and collaborative approaches, We can see that Digital Twins provide personalized, data-driven healthcare solutions that enhance patient outcomes, reduce healthcare costs, and promote overall well-being.

REFERENCES

Abou-Nassar, E. M., Iliyasu, A. M., El-Kafrawy, P. M., Song, O.-Y., Kashif Bashir, A., & Abd El-Latif, A. A. (2020). DITrust chain: Towards blockchain-based trust models for sustainable healthcare IoT systems. *IEEE Access: Practical Innovations, Open Solutions, 8,* 111223–111238. doi:10.1109/AC-CESS.2020.2999468

Al-Marridi, A. Z., Mohamed, A., & Erbad, A. (2021). Reinforcement learning approaches for efficient and secure blockchain-powered smart health systems. *Computer Networks, 197,* 108279. doi:10.1016/j.comnet.2021.108279

Ali, A., Pasha, M. F., Fang, O. H., Khan, R., Almaiah, M. A., & Al Hwaitat, A. K. (2022). Big Data Based Smart Blockchain for Information Retrieval in Privacy-Preserving Healthcare System. In Big Data Intelligence for Smart Applications (pp. 279–296). Springer International Publishing. doi:10.1007/978-3-030-87954-9_13

Tyagi, A. (2020). Challenges of Applying Deep Learning in Real-World Applications. In Challenges and Applications for Implementing Machine Learning in Computer Vision. IGI Global. doi:10.4018/978-1-7998-0182-5.ch004

Chen, M., Malook, T., Rehman, A. U., Muhammad, Y., Alshehri, M. D., Akbar, A., Bilal, M., & Khan, M. A. (2021). Blockchain-Enabled healthcare system for detection of diabetes. *Journal of Information Security and Applications, 58,* 102771. doi:10.1016/j.jisa.2021.102771

Dasaklis, T. K., Casino, F., & Patsakis, C. (2018). Blockchain meets smart health: Towards next generation healthcare services. In *9th International conference on information, intelligence, systems and applications (IISA),* pp. 1-8. IEEE. doi:10.1109/IISA.2018.8633601

Gudeti, B., Mishra, S., Malik, S., Fernandez, T. F., Tyagi, A. K., & Kumari, S. (2020). A Novel Approach to Predict Chronic Kidney Disease using Machine Learning Algorithms. *2020 4th International Conference on Electronics, Communication and Aerospace Technology (ICECA),* Coimbatore. doi:10.1109/ICECA49313.2020.9297392

Hathaliya, J., Sharma, P., Tanwar, S., & Gupta, R. (2019). Blockchain-based remote patient monitoring in healthcare 4.0. In 2019 IEEE 9th international conference on advanced computing (IACC). IEEE., doi:10.1109/IACC48062.2019.8971593

Tyagi, A. (2021). Healthcare Solutions for Smart Era: An Useful Explanation from User's Perspective. In Recent Trends in Blockchain for Information Systems Security and Privacy. CRC Press.

Khatoon, A. (2020). A blockchain-based smart contract system for healthcare management. *Electronics (Basel), 9*(1), 94. doi:10.3390/electronics9010094

Khezr, S., Moniruzzaman, M., Yassine, A., & Benlamri, R. (2019). Blockchain technology in healthcare: A comprehensive review and directions for future research. *Applied Sciences (Basel, Switzerland), 9*(9), 1736. doi:10.3390/app9091736

Khubrani, M. M. (2021). A framework for blockchain-based smart health system. [TURCOMAT]. *Turkish Journal of Computer and Mathematics Education, 12*(9), 2609–2614.

Kumar, T., Ramani, V., Ahmad, I., Braeken, A., Harjula, E., & Ylianttila, M. (2018). Blockchain utilization in healthcare: Key requirements and challenges. In *2018 IEEE 20th International conference on e-health networking, applications and services (Healthcom)*. IEEE. doi:10.1109/HealthCom.2018.8531136

Kumari, S., & Muthulakshmi, P. (2022). Transformative Effects of Big Data on Advanced Data Analytics: Open Issues and Critical Challenges. *Journal of Computational Science*, *18*(6), 463–479. doi:10.3844/jcssp.2022.463.479

Kute, S. (2021). Building a Smart Healthcare System Using Internet of Things and Machine Learning. In Big Data Management in Sensing: Applications in AI and IoT. River Publishers.

Kute, S. S., Tyagi, A. K., & Aswathy, S. U. (2022). Industry 4.0 Challenges in e-Healthcare Applications and Emerging Technologies. In A. K. Tyagi, A. Abraham, & A. Kaklauskas (Eds.), *Intelligent Interactive Multimedia Systems for e-Healthcare Applications*. Springer., doi:10.1007/978-981-16-6542-4_14

Kute, S. S., Tyagi, A. K., & Aswathy, S. U. (2022). Security, Privacy and Trust Issues in Internet of Things and Machine Learning Based e-Healthcare. In A. K. Tyagi, A. Abraham, & A. Kaklauskas (Eds.), *Intelligent Interactive Multimedia Systems for e-Healthcare Applications*. Springer., doi:10.1007/978-981-16-6542-4_15

Le, H. T., Lam, N. T. T., Vo, H. K., Luong, H. H., Khoi, N. H. T., & Anh, T. D. (2022). Patient-chain: patient-centered healthcare system a blockchain-based technology in dealing with emergencies. In *Parallel and Distributed Computing, Applications and Technologies: 22nd International Conference, PDCAT 2021*. Springer International Publishing., doi:10.1007/978-3-030-96772-7_54

Madhav, A. V. S., & Tyagi, A. K. (2022). The World with Future Technologies (Post-COVID-19): Open Issues, Challenges, and the Road Ahead. In A. K. Tyagi, A. Abraham, & A. Kaklauskas (Eds.), *Intelligent Interactive Multimedia Systems for e-Healthcare Applications*. Springer., doi:10.1007/978-981-16-6542-4_22

Nair, M. M., Kumari, S., Tyagi, A. K., & Sravanthi, K. (2021). Deep Learning for Medical Image Recognition: Open Issues and a Way to Forward. In D. Goyal, A. K. Gupta, V. Piuri, M. Ganzha, & M. Paprzycki (Eds.), *Proceedings of the Second International Conference on Information Management and Machine Intelligence. Lecture Notes in Networks and Systems*. Springer., doi:10.1007/978-981-15-9689-6_38

Prabadevi, B. (2021). Toward blockchain for edge-of-things: A new paradigm, opportunities, and future directions. IEEE Internet of Things Magazine, 4(2), 102–108. doi:10.1109/IOTM.0001.2000191

Quasim, M. T., Algarni, F., Abd Elhamid Radwan, A., & Goram Mufareh, M. A. (2020). *A blockchain based secured healthcare framework. In 2020 International Conference on Computational Performance Evaluation (ComPE)*. IEEE., doi:10.1109/ComPE49325.2020.9200024

Ramani, V., Kumar, T., Bracken, A., Liyanage, M., & Ylianttila, M. (2018). Secure and efficient data accessibility in blockchain based healthcare systems. In *2018 IEEE Global Communications Conference (GLOBECOM)*. IEEE. doi:10.1109/GLOCOM.2018.8647221

Sai, G. H., Tripathi, K., & Tyagi, A. K. (2023). Internet of Things-Based e-Health Care: Key Challenges and Recommended Solutions for Future. In P. K. Singh, S. T. Wierzchoń, S. Tanwar, J. J. P. C. Rodrigues, & M. Ganzha (Eds.), *Proceedings of Third International Conference on Computing, Communications, and Cyber-Security. Lecture Notes in Networks and Systems*. Springer., doi:10.1007/978-981-19-1142-2_37

Shamila, M., & Vinuthna, K. (2023). Genomic privacy: performance analysis, open issues, and future research directions. In A. K. Tyagi & A. Abraham (eds.) Data Science for Genomics. Academic Press. doi:10.1016/B978-0-323-98352-5.00015-X

Sharma, A., Tomar, R., Chilamkurti, N., & Kim, B.-G. (2020). Blockchain based smart contracts for internet of medical things in e-healthcare. *Electronics (Basel)*, *9*(10), 1609. doi:10.3390/electronics9101609

Sharma, P., Moparthi, N. R., Namasudra, S., Shanmuganathan, V., & Hsu, C.-H. (2022). Blockchain-based IoT architecture to secure healthcare system using identity-based encryption. *Expert Systems: International Journal of Knowledge Engineering and Neural Networks*, *39*(10), e12915. doi:10.1111/exsy.12915

Singh, S., Sharma, S. K., Mehrotra, P., Bhatt, P., & Kaurav, M. (2022). Blockchain technology for efficient data management in healthcare system: Opportunity, challenges and future perspectives. *Materials Today: Proceedings*, *62*, 5042–5046. doi:10.1016/j.matpr.2022.04.998

Soltanisehat, L., Alizadeh, R., Hao, H., & Choo, K.-K. R. (2020). Technical, temporal, and spatial research challenges and opportunities in blockchain-based healthcare: A systematic literature review. *IEEE Transactions on Engineering Management*.

Son, H. X., Le, T. H., Nga, T. T. Q., Hung, N. D. H., Duong-Trung, N., & Luong, H. H. (2021). Toward a blockchain-based technology in dealing with emergencies in patient-centered healthcare systems. In *Mobile, Secure, and Programmable Networking: 6th International Conference, MSPN 2020*, Paris. doi:10.1007/978-3-030-67550-9_4

Tandon, A., Dhir, A., Islam, A. K. M. N., & Mäntymäki, M. (2020). Blockchain in healthcare: A systematic literature review, synthesizing framework and future research agenda. *Computers in Industry*, *122*, 103290. doi:10.1016/j.compind.2020.103290

Tripathi, G., Ahad, M. A., & Paiva, S. (2020). S2HS-A blockchain based approach for smart healthcare system. In *Healthcare, 8*. Elsevier., doi:10.1016/j.hjdsi.2019.100391

Tyagi, A. (2020). Artificial Intelligence and Machine Learning Algorithms. In Challenges and Applications for Implementing Machine Learning in Computer Vision. IGI Global. doi:10.4018/978-1-7998-0182-5.ch008

Tyagi, A. K., & Goyal, D. (2020). A Survey of Privacy Leakage and Security Vulnerabilities in the Internet of Things. *2020 5th International Conference on Communication and Electronics Systems (ICCES)*. IEEE. doi:10.1109/ICCES48766.2020.9137886

Tyagi, A. (2022). Using Multimedia Systems, Tools, and Technologies for Smart Healthcare Services. IGI Global. doi:10.4018/978-1-6684-5741-2

Wu, G., Wang, S., Ning, Z., & Zhu, B. (2021). Privacy-preserved electronic medical record exchanging and sharing: A blockchain-based smart healthcare system. *IEEE Journal of Biomedical and Health Informatics*, 26(5), 1917–1927. doi:10.1109/JBHI.2021.3123643 PubMed

Xu, J., Xue, K., Li, S., Tian, H., Hong, J., Hong, P., & Yu, N. (2019). Healthchain: A blockchain-based privacy preserving scheme for large-scale health data. *IEEE Internet of Things Journal*, 6(5), 8770–8781. doi:10.1109/JIOT.2019.2923525

Yaqoob, I., Salah, K., Jayaraman, R., & Al-Hammadi, Y. (2021). Blockchain for healthcare data management: Opportunities, challenges, and future recommendations. *Neural Computing & Applications*, 1–16.

Compilation of References

Abbas, H., Garberson, F., Glover, E., & Wall, D. P. (2018). Machine learning approach for early detection of autism by combining questionnaire and home video screening. *Journal of the American Medical Informatics Association : JAMIA*, *25*(8), 1000–1007. doi:10.1093/jamia/ocy039 PMID:29741630

Abdul-Kareem, S., Baba, S., Zubairi, Y. Z., Prasad, U., Ibrahim, M., & Wahid, A. (2002). Prognostic systems for NPC: A comparison of the multi layer perceptron model and the recurrent model. *Proceedings of the 9th International Conference on Neural Information Processing, 2002*. IEEE. 10.1109/ICONIP.2002.1202176

Abdullah, M. F., Sulaiman, S. N., Osman, M. K., Karim, N. K. A., Setumin, S., & Ani, A. I. C. (2023). Lung Lesion Identification Using Geometrical Feature and Optical Flow Method from Computed Tomography Scan Images. In Intelligent Multimedia Signal Processing for Smart Ecosystems (pp. 165–193). Springer International Publishing. doi:10.1007/978-3-031-34873-0_7

Abou-Nassar, E. M., Iliyasu, A. M., El-Kafrawy, P. M., Song, O.-Y., Kashif Bashir, A., & Abd El-Latif, A. A. (2020). DITrust chain: Towards blockchain-based trust models for sustainable healthcare IoT systems. *IEEE Access : Practical Innovations, Open Solutions*, 8, 111223–111238. doi:10.1109/ACCESS.2020.2999468

Abou-Nassar, E. M., Iliyasu, A. M., El-Kafrawy, P. M., Song, O.-Y., Kashif Bashir, A., & Abd El-Latif, A. A. (2020). DITrust chain: Towards blockchain-based trust models for sustainable healthcare IoT systems. *IEEE Access: Practical Innovations, Open Solutions*, 8, 111223–111238. doi:10.1109/ACCESS.2020.2999468

Abunasser, B., AL-Hiealy, M. R., Zaqout, I., & Abu-Naser, S. (2023). Convolution Neural Network for Breast Cancer Detection and Classification Using Deep Learning. *Asian Pacific Journal of Cancer Prevention*, *24*(2), 531–544. doi:10.31557/APJCP.2023.24.2.531 PMID:36853302

Adebiyi, M. O., Afolayan, J. O., Arowolo, M. O., Tyagi, A. K., & Adebiyi, A. A. (2023). Breast Cancer Detection Using a PSO-ANN Machine Learning Technique. In A. Tyagi (Ed.), *Using Multimedia Systems, Tools, and Technologies for Smart Healthcare Services* (pp. 96–116). IGI Global. doi:10.4018/978-1-6684-5741-2.ch007

Ahmed, F. M., & Mohammed, D. B. A. D. A. M. A. S. I. S. A. N. I. (2023). Feasibility of Breast Cancer Detection Through a Convolutional Neural Network in Mammographs. *Tamjeed Journal of Healthcare Engineering and Science Technology*, *1*(2), 36–43. doi:10.59785/tjhest.v1i2.24

Akhtar, M. M., & Rizvi, D. R. (2021). Traceability and detection of counterfeit medicines in pharmaceutical supply chain using blockchain-based architectures. In *EAI/Springer Innovations in Communication and Computing* (pp. 1–31). Springer Nature Switzerland. doi:10.1007/978-3-030-51070-1_1

Akter, T., Satu, M. S., Khan, M. I., Ali, M. H., Uddin, S., Lio, P., Quinn, J. M. W., & Moni, M. A. (2019). Machine learning-based models for early stage detection of autism spectrum disorders. *IEEE Access : Practical Innovations, Open Solutions*, 7, 166509–166527. doi:10.1109/ACCESS.2019.2952609

Alam, N., Hasan Tanvir, M. R., Shanto, S. A., Israt, F., Rahman, A., & Momotaj, S. (2021). Blockchain based counterfeit medicine authentication system. *ISCAIE 2021 - IEEE 11th Symposium on Computer Applications and Industrial Electronics*, 214–217. 10.1109/ISCAIE51753.2021.9431789

Alcañiz Raya, M., Chicchi Giglioli, I. A., Marín-Morales, J., Higuera-Trujillo, J. L., Olmos, E., Minissi, M. E., Teruel Garcia, G., Sirera, M., & Abad, L. (2020). Application of supervised machine learning for behavioral biomarkers of autism spectrum disorder based on electrodermal activity and virtual reality. *Frontiers in Human Neuroscience*, *14*, 90. doi:10.3389/fnhum.2020.00090 PMID:32317949

Alcaniz Raya, M., Marín-Morales, J., Minissi, M. E., Teruel Garcia, G., Abad, L., & Chicchi Giglioli, I. A. (2020). Machine learning and virtual reality on body movements' behaviors to classify children with autism spectrum disorder. *Journal of Clinical Medicine*, *9*(5), 1260. doi:10.3390/jcm9051260 PMID:32357517

Alcañiz, M. L., Olmos-Raya, E., & Abad, L. (2019). Uso de entornos virtuales para trastornos del neurodesarrollo: una revisión del estado del arte y agenda futura. *Medicina (Buenos Aires), 79*(1), 77–81.

Alcañiz, M., Chicchi-Giglioli, I. A., Carrasco-Ribelles, L. A., Marín-Morales, J., Minissi, M. E., Teruel-García, G., Sirera, M., & Abad, L. (2022). Eye gaze as a biomarker in the recognition of autism spectrum disorder using virtual reality and machine learning: A proof of concept for diagnosis. *Autism Research*, *15*(1), 131–145. doi:10.1002/aur.2636 PMID:34811930

Aldamaeen, O., Rashideh, W., & Obidallah, W. J. (2023). Toward Patient-Centric Healthcare Systems: Key Requirements and Framework for Personal Health Records Based on Blockchain Technology. *Applied Sciences (Basel, Switzerland)*, *13*(13), 7697. doi:10.3390/app13137697

Ali, A., Pasha, M. F., Fang, O. H., Khan, R., Almaiah, M. A., & Al Hwaitat, A. K. (2022). Big Data Based Smart Blockchain for Information Retrieval in Privacy-Preserving Healthcare System. In Big Data Intelligence for Smart Applications (pp. 279–296). Springer International Publishing. doi:10.1007/978-3-030-87954-9_13

Ali, A., Pasha, M. F., Fang, O. H., Khan, R., Almaiah, M. A., & Al Hwaitat, A. K. (2022). Big Data Based Smart Blockchain for Information Retrieval in Privacy-Preserving Healthcare System. In *Big Data Intelligence for Smart Applications* (pp. 279–296). Springer International Publishing. doi:10.1007/978-3-030-87954-9_13

Al-Marridi, A. Z., Mohamed, A., & Erbad, A. (2021). Reinforcement learning approaches for efficient and secure blockchain-powered smart health systems. *Computer Networks*, *197*, 108279. doi:10.1016/j.comnet.2021.108279

Almigdad, A., Al-Zoubi, A., Mustafa, A., Al-Qasaimeh, M., Azzam, E., Mestarihi, S., ... Almanasier, G. (2023). A review of scaphoid fracture, treatment outcomes, and consequences. *International Orthopaedics*, 1–8. doi:10.1007/s00264-023-06014-2 PMID:37880341

Alsuliman, M., & Al-Baity, H. H. (2022). Efficient Diagnosis of Autism with Optimized Machine Learning Models: An Experimental Analysis on Genetic and Personal Characteristic Datasets. *Applied Sciences (Basel, Switzerland)*, *12*(8), 3812. doi:10.3390/app12083812

Ameer, I., Arif, M., Sidorov, G., Gòmez-Adorno, H., & Gelbukh, A. (2022). *Mental Illness Classification on Social Media Texts using Deep Learning and Transfer Learning* (arXiv:2207.01012). arXiv. http://arxiv.org/abs/2207.01012

Amrami, K. K., Frick, M. A., & Matsumoto, J. M. (2019). Imaging for acute and chronic scaphoid fractures. *Hand Clinics*, *35*(3), 241–257. doi:10.1016/j.hcl.2019.03.001 PMID:31178083

Anand, R., & Khadheeja Niyas, S. G. and S. R. (. (2020). *Anti-Counterfeit on Medicine Detection Using Blockchain Technology* (pp. 1223–1238). *Springer Nature Singapore Pte Ltd., 2020.* doi:10.1007/978-981-15-0146-3_119

Anastas, Z. M., Jimerson, E., & Garolis, S. (2008). Comparison of noninvasive blood pressure measurements in patients with atrial fibrillation. *The Journal of Cardiovascular Nursing, 23*(6), 519–524. doi:10.1097/01.JCN.0000338935.71285.36 PMID:18953216

Angelovirgin, G., & Sangeetha, M. (2017). Conversion of ecg graph into digital format and detecting the disease. *Mathematics, A. Ijpam.Eu, 116*, 465–471.

Aruselvi, K. (2020). Digitization of ECG Trace and Classification. *International Journal of Emerging Technologies and Innovative Research*. www.jetir.org

Arya, R., Kumar, A., & Bhushan, M. (2021). Affect Recognition using Brain Signals: A Survey. In V. Singh, V. K. Asari, S. Kumar, & R. B. Patel (Eds.), *Computational Methods and Data Engineering* (pp. 529–552). Springer Singapore. doi:10.1007/978-981-15-7907-3_40

Arya, R., Kumar, A., Bhushan, M., & Samant, P. (2022). Big five personality traits prediction using brain signals. [IJFSA]. *International Journal of Fuzzy System Applications, 11*(2), 1–10. doi:10.4018/IJFSA.296596

Asfia, A., Novak, J. I., Mohammed, M. I., Rolfe, B., & Kron, T. (2020). A review of 3D printed patient specific immobilisation devices in radiotherapy. *Physics and Imaging in Radiation Oncology, 13*, 30–35. doi:10.1016/j.phro.2020.03.003 PMID:33458304

Asuntha, A., & Srinivasan, A. (2020). Deep learning for lung Cancer detection and classification. *Multimedia Tools and Applications, 79*(11–12), 7731–7762. doi:10.1007/s11042-019-08394-3

Ayalew, A. M., Bezabih, Y. A., Abuhayi, B. M., & Ayalew, A. Y. (2024). Atelectasis detection in chest X-ray images using convolutional neural networks and transfer learning with anisotropic diffusion filter. *Informatics in Medicine Unlocked, 45*, 101448. doi:10.1016/j.imu.2024.101448

Badhotiya, G. K., Sharma, V. P., Prakash, S., Kalluri, V., & Singh, R. (2021). Investigation and assessment of blockchain technology adoption in the pharmaceutical supply chain. *Materials Today: Proceedings, 46*(xxxx), 10776–10780. doi:10.1016/j.matpr.2021.01.673

Baker, P. D., Westenskow, D. R., & Kuck, K. (1997). Theoretical analysis of non-invasive oscillometric maximum amplitude algorithm for estimating mean blood pressure. Med. Biol. Eng. Comput, 35.

Baydoun, M., Safatly, L., Abou Hassan, O. K., Ghaziri, H., El Hajj, A., & Isma'eel, H. (2019, November 7). High Precision Digitization of Paper-Based ECG Records: A Step Toward Machine Learning. *IEEE Journal of Translational Engineering in Health and Medicine, 7*, 1900808. doi:10.1109/JTEHM.2019.2949784 PMID:32166049

Betts, K. S., Chai, K., Kisely, S., & Alati, R. (2023). Development and validation of a machine learning-based tool to predict autism among children. *Autism Research, 16*(5), 941–952. doi:10.1002/aur.2912 PMID:36899450

Bharti, U., Bajaj, D., Batra, H., Lalit, S., Lalit, S., & Gangwani, A. (2020). Medbot: Conversational artificial intelligence powered chatbot for delivering tele-health after covid-19. *2020 5th International Conference on Communication and Electronics Systems (ICCES)*, (pp. 870–875). IEEE. https://ieeexplore.ieee.org/abstract/document/9137944/

Bhashyam, A. R., & Mudgal, C. (2023). Scaphoid and Carpal Bone Fracture: The Difficult Cases and Approach to Management. *Hand Clinics, 39*(3), 265–277. Advance online publication. doi:10.1016/j.hcl.2023.02.003 PMID:37453756

Bhatia, S., Sinha, Y., & Goel, L. (2019). *Lung Cancer Detection: A Deep Learning Approach.*, doi:10.1007/978-981-13-1595-4_55

Bilandi, N., Verma, H. K., & Dhir, R. (2021). An intelligent and energy-efficient wireless body area network to control coronavirus outbreak. *Arabian Journal for Science and Engineering*, *46*(9), 1–20. doi:10.1007/s13369-021-05411-2 PMID:33680703

Biocca, F., Harms, C., & Gregg, J. (2001). *The networked minds measure of social presence: Pilot test of the factor structure and concurrent validity. 4th Annual International Workshop on Presence*, Philadelphia, PA.

Birjais, R., Mourya, A. K., Chauhan, R., & Kaur, H. (2019). Prediction and diagnosis of future diabetes risk: A machine learning approach. *SN Applied Sciences*, *1*(9), 1–8. doi:10.1007/s42452-019-1117-9

Bishnoi, V., Goel, N., & Tayal, A. (2023). Automated system-based classification of lung cancer using machine learning. *International Journal of Medical Engineering and Informatics*, *15*(5), 403–415. doi:10.1504/IJMEI.2023.133130

Bowman, D. A., Gabbard, J. L., & Hix, D. (2002). A survey of usability evaluation in virtual environments: Classification and comparison of methods. *Presence (Cambridge, Mass.)*, *11*(4), 404–424. doi:10.1162/105474602760204309

Bushara A. R., Vinod Kumar R. S., & Kumar S. S. (2023). Classification of Benign and Malignancy in Lung Cancer Using Capsule Networks with Dynamic Routing Algorithm on Computed Tomography Images. Journal of Artificial Intelligence and Technology. doi:10.37965/jait.2023.0218

Caronongan, A., Gorgui-Naguib, H., & Naguib, R. N. (2018). The development of intelligent patient-centric systems for health care. *Theories to Inform Superior Health Informatics Research and Practice*, 355-373.

Cattivelli, F. S., & Garudadri, H. (2009). Noninvasive cuffless estimation of blood pressure from pulse arrival time and heart rate with adaptive calibration. *Wearable and Implantable Body Sensor Networks*. IEEE. 10.1109/BSN.2009.35

Chalmers, K., Pearson, S. A., & Elshaug, A. G. (2017). *Quantifying low-value care: a patient-centric versus service-centric lens.*

Chang, M. T. K., Price, M., Furness, J., Kemp-Smith, K., Simas, V., Pickering, R., & Lenaghan, D. (2022). The current management of scaphoid fractures in the emergency department across an Australian metropolitan public health service: A retrospective cohort study. *Medicine*, *101*(28), e29659. doi:10.1097/MD.0000000000029659 PMID:35839014

Chartrand, G., Cheng, P. M., Vorontsov, E., Drozdzal, M., Turcotte, S., Pal, C. J., Kadoury, S., & Tang, A. (2017). Deep learning: A primer for radiologists. *Radiographics*, *37*(7), 2113–2131. doi:10.1148/rg.2017170077 PMID:29131760

Chen, D. (2021). Analysis of machine learning methods for COVID-19 detection using serum Raman spectroscopy. *Applied Artificial Intelligence*, *35*(14), 1147–1168. doi:10.1080/08839514.2021.1975379

Chen, M., Malook, T., Rehman, A. U., Muhammad, Y., Alshehri, M. D., Akbar, A., Bilal, M., & Khan, M. A. (2021). Blockchain-Enabled healthcare system for detection of diabetes. *Journal of Information Security and Applications*, *58*, 102771. doi:10.1016/j.jisa.2021.102771

Chen, Y., Hou, X., Yang, Y., Ge, Q., Zhou, Y., & Nie, S. (2022). A Novel Deep Learning Model Based on Multi-Scale and Multi-View for Detection of Pulmonary Nodules. *Journal of Digital Imaging*, *36*(2), 688–699. doi:10.1007/s10278-022-00749-x PMID:36544067

Chhabra, M. (2023). Implications of Cloud Computing for Health Care. In *Cloud-based Intelligent Informative Engineering for Society 5.0* (pp. 41–59). Chapman and Hall/CRC. doi:10.1201/9781003213895-3

Chong, H. H., Kulkarni, K., Shah, R., Hau, M. Y., Athanatos, L., & Singh, H. P. (2022). A meta-analysis of union rate after proximal scaphoid fractures: Terminology matters. *Journal of Plastic Surgery and Hand Surgery*, *56*(5), 298–309. doi:10.1080/2000656X.2021.1979016 PMID:34550858

Chu, L. F., Shah, A. G., Rouholiman, D., Riggare, S., & Gamble, J. G. (2018). Patient-centric strategies in digital health. *Digital Health: Scaling Healthcare to the World*, 43-54.

Chunara, M. H., McLeavy, C. M., Kesavanarayanan, V., Paton, D., & Ganguly, A. (2019). Current imaging practice for suspected scaphoid fracture in patients with normal initial radiographs: UK-wide national audit. *Clinical Radiology*, *74*(6), 450–455. doi:10.1016/j.crad.2019.02.016 PMID:30952360

Ciompi, F., Chung, K., van Riel, S. J., Setio, A. A. A., Gerke, P. K., Jacobs, C., Scholten, E. Th., Schaefer-Prokop, C., Wille, M. M. W., Marchianò, A., Pastorino, U., Prokop, M., & van Ginneken, B. (2017). Towards automatic pulmonary nodule management in lung cancer screening with deep learning. *Scientific Reports*, *7*(1), 46479. doi:10.1038/srep46479 PMID:28422152

Cipresso, P., Giglioli, I. A. C., Raya, M. A., & Riva, G. (2018). The past, present, and future of virtual and augmented reality research: A network and cluster analysis of the literature. *Frontiers in Psychology*, *9*, 2086. doi:10.3389/fpsyg.2018.02086 PMID:30459681

Clauson, K. A., Breeden, E. A., Davidson, C., & Mackey, T. K. (2018). Leveraging Blockchain Technology to Enhance Supply Chain Management in Healthcare. *Blockchain in Healthcare Today*, 1–12. doi:10.30953/bhty.v1.20

Conombo, B., Guertin, J. R., Tardif, P. A., Gagnon, M. A., Duval, C., Archambault, P., Berthelot, S., Lauzier, F., Turgeon, A. F., Stelfox, H. T., Chassé, M., Hoch, J. S., Gabbe, B., Champion, H., Lecky, F., Cameron, P., & Moore, L. (2022). Economic Evaluation of In-Hospital Clinical Practices in Acute Injury Care: A Systematic Review. *Value in Health*, *25*(5), 844–854. doi:10.1016/j.jval.2021.10.018 PMID:35500953

Cortes, C., & Vapnik, V. (1995). Support-vector networks. *Machine Learning*, *20*(3), 273–297. doi:10.1007/BF00994018

Coventry, L., Oldrini, I., Dean, B., Novak, A., Duckworth, A., & Metcalfe, D. (2023). Which clinical features best predict occult scaphoid fractures? A systematic review of diagnostic test accuracy studies. *Emergency Medicine Journal*, *40*(8), 576–582. Advance online publication. doi:10.1136/emermed-2023-213119 PMID:37169546

Crestani, F., Losada, D. E., & Parapar, J. (2022). *Early Detection of Mental Health Disorders by Social Media Monitoring: The First Five Years of the ERisk Project (Vol. 1018)*. Springer Nature. https://books.google.com/books?hl=en&lr=&id=03KJEAAAQBAJ&oi=fnd&pg=PR5&dq=Mental+Health+Monitoring+from+social+media+content&ots=imytRcJRhF&sig=66ToTnyQucKr9ulHSUQZA4Po-Hg

Cummings, J. J., & Bailenson, J. N. (2016). How immersive is enough? A meta-analysis of the effect of immersive technology on user presence. *Media Psychology*, *19*(2), 272–309. doi:10.1080/15213269.2015.1015740

D'Alfonso, S. (2020). AI in mental health. *Current Opinion in Psychology*, *36*, 112–117. doi:10.1016/j.copsyc.2020.04.005 PMID:32604065

da Silva, C. C., de Lima, C. L., da Silva, A. C. G., Silva, E. L., Marques, G. S., de Araújo, L. J. B., Albuquerque, L. A. Junior, de Souza, S. B. J., de Santana, M. A., & Gomes, J. C. (2021). Covid-19 dynamic monitoring and real-time spatio-temporal forecasting. *Frontiers in Public Health*, *9*, 641253. doi:10.3389/fpubh.2021.641253 PMID:33898377

Dangare, C., & Apte, S. (2012). A data mining approach for prediction of heart disease using neural networks. [IJCET]. *International Journal of Computer Engineering and Technology*, *3*(3).

Daniels, A. M., Bevers, M. S. A. M., Sassen, S., Wyers, C. E., Van Rietbergen, B., Geusens, P. P. M. M., Kaarsemaker, S., Hannemann, P. F. W., Poeze, M., van den Bergh, J. P., & Janzing, H. M. J. (2020). Improved detection of scaphoid fractures with high-resolution peripheral quantitative CT compared with conventional CT. *The Journal of Bone and Joint Surgery. American Volume*, *102*(24), 2138–2145. doi:10.2106/JBJS.20.00124 PMID:33079896

Dasaklis, T. K., Casino, F., & Patsakis, C. ().Blockchain meets smart health: Towards next generation healthcare services. In *2018 9th International conference on information, intelligence, systems and applications (IISA)*, pp. 1-8. IEEE. 10.1109/IISA.2018.8633601

Dasaklis, T. K., Casino, F., & Patsakis, C. (2018). Blockchain meets smart health: Towards next generation healthcare services. In *9th International conference on information, intelligence, systems and applications (IISA)*, pp. 1-8. IEEE. doi:10.1109/IISA.2018.8633601

Das, S., & Majumder, S. (2020). Lung Cancer Detection Using Deep Learning Network: A Comparative Analysis. *2020 Fifth International Conference on Research in Computational Intelligence and Communication Networks (ICRCICN)*, 30–35. 10.1109/ICRCICN50933.2020.9296197

Dawson, G., Jones, E. J. H., Merkle, K., Venema, K., Lowy, R., Faja, S., Kamara, D., Murias, M., Greenson, J., Winter, J., Smith, M., Rogers, S. J., & Webb, S. J. (2012). Early behavioral intervention is associated with normalized brain activity in young children with autism. *Journal of the American Academy of Child and Adolescent Psychiatry*, *51*(11), 1150–1159. doi:10.1016/j.jaac.2012.08.018 PMID:23101741

de Lurdes, P. M. M. (2022). *Surgical versus conservative treatment of undisplaced or minimally-displaced acute scaphoid waist fractures: a systematic review and meta-analysis.*

Dean, B. J.SUSPECT study group. (2021). The management of suspected scaphoid fractures in the UK: A national cross-sectional study. *Bone & Joint Open*, *2*(11), 997–1003. doi:10.1302/2633-1462.211.BJO-2021-0146 PMID:34839716

Deekshetha, H. R. (2023). Automated and intelligent systems for next-generation-based smart applications. Data Science for Genomics. Academic Press. doi:10.1016/B978-0-323-98352-5.00019-7

Deshmukh, A., Sreenath, N., Tyagi, A. K., & Eswara Abhichandan, U. V. (2022). Blockchain Enabled Cyber Security: A Comprehensive Survey. *2022 International Conference on Computer Communication and Informatics (ICCCI)*, (pp. 1-6). IEEE. 10.1109/ICCCI54379.2022.9740843

Devarapalli, D., Apparao, A., Narasinga Rao, M. R., Kumar, A., & Sridhar, G. R. (2012). A Multi-layer perceptron (MLP) neural network based diagnosis of diabetes using brain derived neurotrophic factor (BDNF) levels. *Int. J. Adv. Comput*, *35*(12), 2051–0845.

Di Giovanni, D., Enea, R., Di Micco, V., Benvenuto, A., Curatolo, P., & Emberti Gialloreti, L. (2023). Using Machine Learning to Explore Shared Genetic Pathways and Possible Endophenotypes in Autism Spectrum Disorder. *Genes*, *14*(2), 313. doi:10.3390/genes14020313 PMID:36833240

Di Martino, A., Yan, C.-G., Li, Q., Denio, E., Castellanos, F. X., Alaerts, K., Anderson, J. S., Assaf, M., Bookheimer, S. Y., Dapretto, M., Deen, B., Delmonte, S., Dinstein, I., Ertl-Wagner, B., Fair, D. A., Gallagher, L., Kennedy, D. P., Keown, C. L., Keysers, C., & Milham, M. P. (2014). The autism brain imaging data exchange: Towards a large-scale evaluation of the intrinsic brain architecture in autism. *Molecular Psychiatry*, *19*(6), 659–667. doi:10.1038/mp.2013.78 PMID:23774715

Di Noia, T., Ostuni, V. C., Pesce, F., Binetti, G., Naso, D., Schena, F. P., & Di Sciascio, E. (2013). An end stage kidney disease predictor based on an artificial neural networks ensemble. *Expert Systems with Applications*, *40*(11), 4438–4445. doi:10.1016/j.eswa.2013.01.046

Ding, X. R., Zhao, N., Yang, G. Z., Pettigrew, R., Lo, B., Miao, F., Li, Y., Liu, J., & Zhang, Y.-T. (2016). Continuous Blood Pressure Measurement from Invasive to Unobtrusive: Celebration of 200th Birth Anniversary of Carl Ludwig. *IEEE Journal of Biomedical and Health Informatics*, *20*(6), 1455–1465. doi:10.1109/JBHI.2016.2620995 PMID:28113184

Dodia, S. B. A., & Mahesh, P. A. (2022). Recent advancements in deep learning based lung cancer detection: A systematic review. *Engineering Applications of Artificial Intelligence*, *116*, 105490. doi:10.1016/j.engappai.2022.105490

Do, Q., Son, T. C., & Chaudri, J. (2017). Classification of asthma severity and medication using TensorFlow and multilevel databases. *Procedia Computer Science*, *113*, 344–351. doi:10.1016/j.procs.2017.08.343

Duda, M., Kosmicki, J. A., & Wall, D. P. (2014). Testing the accuracy of an observation-based classifier for rapid detection of autism risk. *Translational Psychiatry*, *4*(8), e424–e424. doi:10.1038/tp.2014.65 PMID:25116834

Edeh, M. O., Dalal, S., Dhaou, I. B., Agubosim, C. C., Umoke, C. C., Richard-Nnabu, N. E., & Dahiya, N. (2022). Artificial intelligence-based ensemble learning model for prediction of hepatitis C disease. *Frontiers in Public Health*, *10*, 892371. doi:10.3389/fpubh.2022.892371 PMID:35570979

Elshoky, B. R. G., Younis, E. M. G., Ali, A. A., & Ibrahim, O. A. S. (2022). Comparing automated and non-automated machine learning for autism spectrum disorders classification using facial images. *ETRI Journal*, *44*(4), 613–623. doi:10.4218/etrij.2021-0097

Eslami, T., Raiker, J. S., & Saeed, F. (2021). Explainable and scalable machine learning algorithms for detection of autism spectrum disorder using fMRI data. In *Neural engineering techniques for autism spectrum disorder* (pp. 39–54). Elsevier. doi:10.1016/B978-0-12-822822-7.00004-1

Esqueda-Elizondo, J. J., Juárez-Ramírez, R., López-Bonilla, O. R., García-Guerrero, E. E., Galindo-Aldana, G. M., Jiménez-Beristáin, L., Serrano-Trujillo, A., Tlelo-Cuautle, E., & Inzunza-González, E. (2022). Attention measurement of an autism spectrum disorder user using EEG signals: A case study. *Mathematical & Computational Applications*, *27*(2), 21. doi:10.3390/mca27020021

Fan, X., Wang, L., & Li, S. (2016). Predicting chaotic coal prices using a multi-layer perceptron network model. *Resources Policy*, *50*, 86–92. doi:10.1016/j.resourpol.2016.08.009

Fei, J., & Liu, R. (2016). Drug-laden 3D biodegradable label using QR code for anti-counterfeiting of drugs. *Materials Science and Engineering C*, *63*, 657–662. doi:10.1016/j.msec.2016.03.004 PMID:27040262

Fenikilé, T. S., Ellerbeck, K., Filippi, M. K., & Daley, C. M. (2015). Barriers to autism screening in family medicine practice: A qualitative study. *Primary Health Care Research and Development*, *16*(4), 356–366. doi:10.1017/S1463423614000449 PMID:25367194

Ferrante, E., Dokania, P. K., Marini, R., & Paragios, N. (2017) *Deformable registration through learning of context-specific metric aggregation*. Machine Learning in Medical Imaging Workshop. MLMI (MICCAI 2017), Quebec City, Canada. 10.1007/978-3-319-67389-9_30

Filip, R., Gheorghita Puscaselu, R., Anchidin-Norocel, L., Dimian, M., & Savage, W. K. (2022). Global challenges to public health care systems during the COVID-19 pandemic: A review of pandemic measures and problems. *Journal of Personalized Medicine*, *12*(8), 1295. doi:10.3390/jpm12081295 PMID:36013244

Fu, X., Bi, L., Kumar, A., Fulham, M., & Kim, J. (2022). An attention-enhanced cross-task network to analyse lung nodule attributes in CT images. *Pattern Recognition*, *126*, 108576. doi:10.1016/j.patcog.2022.108576

Gayap, H. T., & Akhloufi, M. A. (2024). Deep Machine Learning for Medical Diagnosis, Application to Lung Cancer Detection: A Review. *BioMedInformatics*, *4*(1), 236–284. doi:10.3390/biomedinformatics4010015

Gesche, H., Grosskurth, D., Küchler, G., & Patzak, A. (2012). Continuous blood pressure measurement by using the pulse transit time: Comparison to a cuff-based method. *European Journal of Applied Physiology*, *112*(1), 309–315. doi:10.1007/s00421-011-1983-3 PMID:21556814

Geselowitz, D. B. (1989). In the theory of the electrocardiogram. *Proceedings of the IEEE, 77*(6), 857–876. doi:10.1109/5.29327

Ghonge, N. P. (2019). Being a "Clinical Radiologist""Patient-centric approach" and "problem-solving attitude" in radiology. *The Indian Journal of Radiology & Imaging, 29*(03), 336–337. doi:10.4103/ijri.IJRI_173_19 PMID:31741608

Gkotsis, G., Oellrich, A., Velupillai, S., Liakata, M., Hubbard, T. J., Dobson, R. J., & Dutta, R. (2017). Characterisation of mental health conditions in social media using Informed Deep Learning. *Scientific Reports, 7*(1), 45141. doi:10.1038/srep45141 PMID:28327593

Gökalp, E.,, Mert Onuralp Gökalp, S. Ç., & Eren, P. E. (2018). Analysing Opportunities and Challenges of Integrated Blockchain Technologies in Healthcare. *Springer Nature Switzerland AG 2018, 174*–183. Springer. doi:10.1007/978-3-030-00060-8_13

Gomathi, L., Mishra, A. K., & Tyagi, A. K. (2023). *Industry 5.0 for Healthcare 5.0: Opportunities, Challenges and Future Research Possibilities.* 2023 7th International Conference on Trends in Electronics and Informatics (ICOEI), Tirunelveli, India. 10.1109/ICOEI56765.2023.10125660

Guazzaroni, G. (2018). *Virtual and augmented reality in mental health treatment.* IGI Global.

Gudeti, B., Mishra, S., Malik, S., Fernandez, T. F., Tyagi, A. K., & Kumari, S. (2020). *A Novel Approach to Predict Chronic Kidney Disease using Machine Learning Algorithms.* 2020 4th International Conference on Electronics, Communication and Aerospace Technology (ICECA), Coimbatore. 10.1109/ICECA49313.2020.9297392

Gudeti, B., Mishra, S., Malik, S., Fernandez, T. F., Tyagi, A. K., & Kumari, S. (2020). A Novel Approach to Predict Chronic Kidney Disease using Machine Learning Algorithms. *2020 4th International Conference on Electronics, Communication and Aerospace Technology (ICECA)*, Coimbatore. doi:10.1109/ICECA49313.2020.9297392

Gudur, R., Asif, D., Tamboli, I., Garg, A., & Sharma, M. (n.d.). International Journal of INTELLIGENT SYSTEMS AND APPLICATIONS IN ENGINEERING Optimizing Computed Tomography Image Reconstruction Parameters for Improved Lung Cancer Diagnosis with Grey Wolf Algorithm. In *Original Research Paper International Journal of Intelligent Systems and Applications in Engineering IJISA.* www.ijisae.org

Guidi, A., Lanata, A., Baragli, P., Valenza, G., & Scilingo, E. P. (2016). A wearable system for the evaluation of the human-horse interaction: A preliminary study. *Electronics (Basel), 5*(4), 63. doi:10.3390/electronics5040063

Guntuku, S. C., Yaden, D. B., Kern, M. L., Ungar, L. H., & Eichstaedt, J. C. (2017a). Detecting depression and mental illness on social media: An integrative review. *Current Opinion in Behavioral Sciences, 18*, 43–49. doi:10.1016/j.cobeha.2017.07.005

Guthrie, W., Wallis, K., Bennett, A., Brooks, E., Dudley, J., Gerdes, M., Pandey, J., Levy, S. E., Schultz, R. T., & Miller, J. S. (2019). Accuracy of autism screening in a large pediatric network. *Pediatrics, 144*(4), e20183963. doi:10.1542/peds.2018-3963 PMID:31562252

Han, S. M., Cao, L., Yang, C., Yang, H. H., Wen, J. X., Guo, Z., Wu, H.-Z., Wu, W.-J., & Gao, B. L. (2022). Value of the 45-degree reverse oblique view of the carpal palm in diagnosing scaphoid waist fractures. *Injury, 53*(3), 1049–1056. doi:10.1016/j.injury.2021.10.023 PMID:34809925

Haq, A. U., Li, J. P., Khan, J., Memon, M. H., Nazir, S., Ahmad, S., Khan, G. A., & Ali, A. (2020). Intelligent machine learning approach for effective recognition of diabetes in E-healthcare using clinical data. *Sensors (Basel), 20*(9), 2649. doi:10.3390/s20092649 PMID:32384737

Hasan, M. K., Alam, M. A., Das, D., Hossain, E., & Hasan, M. (2020). Diabetes prediction using ensembling of different machine learning classifiers. *IEEE Access : Practical Innovations, Open Solutions*, *8*, 76516–76531. doi:10.1109/ACCESS.2020.2989857

Hata, E., Seo, C., Nakayama, M., Iwasaki, K., Ohkawauchi, T., & Ohya, J. (2020). Classification of Aortic Stenosis Using ECG by Deep Learning and its Analysis Using Grad-CAM. *Proc. Annu. Int. Conf. IEEE Eng. Med. Biol. Soc.* IEEE. 10.1109/EMBC44109.2020.9175151

Hathaliya, J., Sharma, P., Tanwar, S., & Gupta, R. (2019). Blockchain-based remote patient monitoring in healthcare 4.0. In *2019 IEEE 9th international conference on advanced computing (IACC)*, (pp. 87-91). IEEE. 10.1109/IACC48062.2019.8971593

Hathaliya, J., Sharma, P., Tanwar, S., & Gupta, R. (2019). Blockchain-based remote patient monitoring in healthcare 4.0. In 2019 IEEE 9th international conference on advanced computing (IACC). IEEE., doi:10.1109/IACC48062.2019.8971593

He, D., Winokur E., & Sodini, C. (2015). An Ear-Worn Vital Signs Monitor. *IEEE Transactions on Biomedica Engineering, 62*(11), 2547-2552.

Hendrix, N., Scholten, E., Vernhout, B., Bruijnen, S., Maresch, B., de Jong, M., Diepstraten, S., Bollen, S., Schalekamp, S., de Rooij, M., Scholtens, A., Hendrix, W., Samson, T., Sharon Ong, L.-L., Postma, E., van Ginneken, B., & Rutten, M. (2021). Development and validation of a convolutional neural network for automated detection of scaphoid fractures on conventional radiographs. *Radiology. Artificial Intelligence, 3*(4), e200260. doi:10.1148/ryai.2021200260 PMID:34350413

Holloway, R., Fuchs, H., & Robinett, W. (1992). Virtual-worlds research at the University of North Carolina at Chapel Hill as of February 1992. *Visual Computing: Integrating Computer Graphics with Computer Vision*, 109–128.

Hossain, M. A., Islam, S. M. S., Quinn, J. M. W., Huq, F., & Moni, M. A. (2019). Machine learning and bioinformatics models to identify gene expression patterns of ovarian cancer associated with disease progression and mortality. *Journal of Biomedical Informatics*, *100*, 103313. doi:10.1016/j.jbi.2019.103313 PMID:31655274

HowladerK. C.SatuM. S.BaruaA.MoniM. A. (2018). Mining significant features of diabetes mellitus applying decision trees: A case study in bangladesh. BioRxiv, 481994. doi:10.1101/481994

Hyman, S. L., Levy, S. E., Myers, S. M., Kuo, D. Z., Apkon, S., Davidson, L. F., Ellerbeck, K. A., Foster, J. E. A., Noritz, G. H., Leppert, M. O., Saunders, B. S., Stille, C., Yin, L., Weitzman, C. C., Childers, D. O. Jr, Levine, J. M., Peralta-Carcelen, A. M., Poon, J. K., Smith, P. J., & Bridgemohan, C. (2020). Identification, evaluation, and management of children with autism spectrum disorder. *Pediatrics*, *145*(1), e20193447. doi:10.1542/peds.2019-3447

Ibrahim, B., Baker, P., Jeyakumar, G., & Ali, K. (2022). MRI as gold standard for scaphoid fracture diagnosis. *Clinical Radiology*, *77*, e28–e29. doi:10.1016/j.crad.2022.09.086

Iglesias, J. E., & Sabuncu, M. R. (2015). Multi-atlas segmentation of biomedical images: A survey. *Medical Image Analysis*, *24*(1), 205–219. doi:10.1016/j.media.2015.06.012 PMID:26201875

Jabarulla, M. Y., & Lee, H. N. (2021, August). A blockchain and artificial intelligence-based, patient-centric healthcare system for combating the COVID-19 pandemic: Opportunities and applications. In Healthcare, 9(8). MDPI.

Jabarulla, M. Y., & Lee, H. N. (2020). Blockchain-based distributed patient-centric image management system. *Applied Sciences (Basel, Switzerland)*, *11*(1), 196. doi:10.3390/app11010196

Jahmunah, V., Ng, E. Y. K., Tan, R. S., Oh, S. L., & Acharya, U. R. (2022). Explainable detection of myocardial infarction using deep learning models with Grad-CAM technique on ECG signals. *Computers in Biology and Medicine*, *146*, 105550. doi:10.1016/j.compbiomed.2022.105550 PMID:35533457

Compilation of References

Javaid, M., Sarfraz, M. S., Aftab, M. U., Zaman, Q., Rauf, H. T., & Alnowibet, K. A. (2023). WebGIS-Based Real-Time Surveillance and Response System for Vector-Borne Infectious Diseases. *International Journal of Environmental Research and Public Health*, *20*(4), 3740. doi:10.3390/ijerph20043740 PMID:36834443

Jin, T., Cui, H., Zeng, S., & Wang, X. (2017). Learning Deep Spatial Lung Features by 3D Convolutional Neural Network for Early Cancer Detection. *2017 International Conference on Digital Image Computing: Techniques and Applications (DICTA)*, (pp. 1–6). IEEE. 10.1109/DICTA.2017.8227454

Ji, S., Li, X., Huang, Z., & Cambria, E. (2022). Suicidal ideation and mental disorder detection with attentive relation networks. *Neural Computing & Applications*, *34*(13), 10309–10319. doi:10.1007/s00521-021-06208-y

Johny, S., & Priyadharsini, C. (2021). Investigations on the Implementation of Blockchain Technology in Supplychain Network. *2021 7th International Conference on Advanced Computing and Communication Systems, ICACCS 2021*, 1609–1614. 10.1109/ICACCS51430.2021.9441820

Jørgsholm, P., Ossowski, D., Thomsen, N., & Björkman, A. (2020). Epidemiology of scaphoid fractures and non-unions: A systematic review. *Handchirurgie· Mikrochirurgie· Plastische Chirurgie*, *52*(05), 374-381. doi:10.1055/a-1250-8190

Joshi, R. D., & Dhakal, C. K. (2021). Predicting type 2 diabetes using logistic regression and machine learning approaches. *International Journal of Environmental Research and Public Health*, *18*(14), 7346. doi:10.3390/ijerph18147346 PMID:34299797

Kachuee, M., Kiani, M. M., Mohammadzade, H., & Shabany, M. (2016). Cuffless blood pressure estimation algorithms for continuous health-care monitoring. *IEEE Transactions on Biomedical Engineering*, *64*(4), 859–869. doi:10.1109/TBME.2016.2580904 PMID:27323356

Kamiński, B., Jakubczyk, M., & Szufel, P. (2018). A framework for sensitivity analysis of decision trees. *Central European Journal of Operations Research*, *26*(1), 135–159. doi:10.1007/s10100-017-0479-6 PMID:29375266

Kansal, M., Singh, P., Shukla, S., & Srivastava, S. (2023). A Comparative Study of Machine Learning Models for House Price Prediction and Analysis in Smart Cities. In F. Ortiz-Rodríguez, S. Tiwari, P. Usoro Usip, & R. Palma (Eds.), Electronic Governance with Emerging Technologies (pp. 168–184). Springer Nature Switzerland. doi:10.1007/978-3-031-43940-7_14

Kansal, M., Singh, P., Srivastava, M., & Chaurasia, P. (2023). Empowering Agriculture With Conversational AI: An Application for Farmer Advisory and Communication. In Convergence of Cloud Computing, AI, and Agricultural Science (pp. 210–227). IGI Global. doi:10.4018/979-8-3693-0200-2.ch011

Kanzaria, H. K., McCabe, A. M., Meisel, Z. M., LeBlanc, A., Schaffer, J. T., Bellolio, M. F., Vaughan, W., Merck, L. H., Applegate, K. E., Hollander, J. E., Grudzen, C. R., Mills, A. M., Carpenter, C. R., & Hess, E. P. (2015). Advancing patient-centered outcomes in emergency diagnostic imaging: A research agenda. *Academic Emergency Medicine*, *22*(12), 1435–1446. doi:10.1111/acem.12832 PMID:26574729

Karmegam, D., Ramamoorthy, T., & Mappillairajan, B. (2020). A systematic review of techniques employed for determining mental health using social media in psychological surveillance during disasters. *Disaster Medicine and Public Health Preparedness*, *14*(2), 265–272. doi:10.1017/dmp.2019.40 PMID:31272518

Kaur, J. (2023, May). How is Robotic Process Automation Revolutionising the Way Healthcare Sector Works? In *International Conference on Information, Communication and Computing Technology* (pp. 1037-1055). Singapore: Springer Nature Singapore. 10.1007/978-981-99-5166-6_70

Kaur, J. (2023). Robotic Process Automation in Healthcare Sector. In *E3S Web of Conferences* (Vol. 391, p. 01008). EDP Sciences.

Kaur, N., & Sood, S. K. (2018). A trustworthy system for secure access to patient centric sensitive information. *Telematics and Informatics*, *35*(4), 790–800. doi:10.1016/j.tele.2017.09.008

Keerthi, A. M., Ramapriya, S., Kashyap, S. B., Gupta, P. K., & Rekha, B. S. (2021). Pharmaceutical management information systems: A sustainable computing paradigm in the pharmaceutical industry and public health management. In EAI/Springer Innovations in Communication and Computing. Springer. doi:10.1007/978-3-030-51070-1_2

Keikhosrokiani, P., Mustaffa, N., & Zakaria, N. (2018). Success factors in developing iHeart as a patient-centric healthcare system: A multi-group analysis. *Telematics and Informatics*, *35*(4), 753–775. doi:10.1016/j.tele.2017.11.006

Khanam, J. J., & Foo, S. Y. (2021). A comparison of machine learning algorithms for diabetes prediction. *ICT Express.*, *7*(4), 432–439. doi:10.1016/j.icte.2021.02.004

Khanna, S., & Srivastava, S. (2020). Patient-Centric Ethical Frameworks for Privacy, Transparency, and Bias Awareness in Deep Learning-Based Medical Systems. *Applied Research in Artificial Intelligence and Cloud Computing*, *3*(1), 16–35.

Khatoon, A. (2020). A blockchain-based smart contract system for healthcare management. *Electronics (Basel)*, *9*(1), 94. doi:10.3390/electronics9010094

Khezr, S., Moniruzzaman, M., Yassine, A., & Benlamri, R. (2019). Blockchain technology in healthcare: A comprehensive review and directions for future research. *Applied Sciences (Basel, Switzerland)*, *9*(9), 1736. doi:10.3390/app9091736

Khubrani, M. M. (2021). A framework for blockchain-based smart health system. [TURCOMAT]. *Turkish Journal of Computer and Mathematics Education*, *12*(9), 2609–2614.

Kim, J. I., Bang, S., Yang, J.-J., Kwon, H., Jang, S., Roh, S., Kim, S. H., Kim, M. J., Lee, H. J., & Lee, J.-M. (2022). Classification of preschoolers with low-functioning autism spectrum disorder using multimodal MRI data. *Journal of Autism and Developmental Disorders*, 1–13. PMID:34984638

Kim, J. K., Jung, S., Park, J., & Han, S. W. (2022). Arrhythmia detection model using modified DenseNet for comprehensible Grad-CAM visualization. *Biomedical Signal Processing and Control*, *73*, 103408. doi:10.1016/j.bspc.2021.103408

Kim, J., Lee, D., & Park, E. (2021). Machine learning for mental health in social media: Bibliometric study. *Journal of Medical Internet Research*, *23*(3), e24870. doi:10.2196/24870 PMID:33683209

Kim, J., Lee, J., Park, E., & Han, J. (2020). A deep learning model for detecting mental illness from user content on social media. *Scientific Reports*, *10*(1), 11846. doi:10.1038/s41598-020-68764-y PMID:32678250

Kim, K., Oh, S. J., Lee, J. H., & Chung, M. J. (2024). 3D unsupervised anomaly detection through virtual multi-view projection and reconstruction: Clinical validation on low-dose chest computed tomography. *Expert Systems with Applications*, *236*, 121165. doi:10.1016/j.eswa.2023.121165

Kim, N., Krasner, A., Kosinski, C., Wininger, M., Qadri, M., Kappus, Z., Danish, S., & Craelius, W. (2016). Trending autoregulatory indices during treatment for traumatic brain injury. *Journal of Clinical Monitoring and Computing*, *30*(6), 821–831. doi:10.1007/s10877-015-9779-3 PMID:26446002

Klabunde, R. E. (2005). *Cardiovascular Physiology Concepts*. Williams & Wilkins.

Knyazev, G. G., Slobodskaya, H. R., & Wilson, G. D. (2004). *Personality and brain oscillations in the developmental perspective.*

Kodumuri, P., McDonough, A., Lyle, V., Naqui, Z., & Muir, L. (2021). Reliability of clinical tests for prediction of occult scaphoid fractures and cost benefit analysis of a dedicated scaphoid pathway. [European Volume]. *The Journal of Hand Surgery*, *46*(3), 292–296. doi:10.1177/1753193420979465 PMID:33323009

Könneker, S., Krockenberger, K., Pieh, C., von Falck, C., Brandewiede, B., Vogt, P. M., Kirschner, M. H., & Ziegler, A. (2019). Comparison of SCAphoid fracture osteosynthesis by MAGnesium-based headless Herbert screws with titanium Herbert screws: Protocol for the randomized controlled SCAMAG clinical trial. *BMC Musculoskeletal Disorders*, *20*(1), 1–11. doi:10.1186/s12891-019-2723-9 PMID:31387574

Kopitar, L., Kocbek, P., Cilar, L., Sheikh, A., & Stiglic, G. (2020). Early detection of type 2 diabetes mellitus using machine learning-based prediction models. *Scientific Reports*, *10*(1), 1–2. doi:10.1038/s41598-020-68771-z PMID:32686721

Kraus, W. L. (2015). Editorial: Would you like a hypothesis with those data? Omics and the age of discovery science. *Molecular Endocrinology (Baltimore, Md.)*, *29*(11), 1531–1534. doi:10.1210/me.2015-1253 PMID:26524008

Kumar, D., Wong, A., & Clausi, D. A. (2015). Lung Nodule Classification Using Deep Features in CT Images. *2015 12th Conference on Computer and Robot Vision*, (pp. 133–138). IEEE. 10.1109/CRV.2015.25

Kumar, R., & Tripathi, R. (2019). Traceability of counterfeit medicine supply chain through Blockchain. *2019 11th International Conference on Communication Systems and Networks, COMSNETS 2019*, *2061*(1), 568–570. 10.1109/COMSNETS.2019.8711418

Kumar, T., Ramani, V., Ahmad, I., Braeken, A., Harjula, E., & Ylianttila, M. (2018). Blockchain utilization in healthcare: Key requirements and challenges. In *2018 IEEE 20th International conference on e-health networking, applications and services (Healthcom)*. IEEE. 10.1109/HealthCom.2018.8531136

Kumar, T., Ramani, V., Ahmad, I., Braeken, A., Harjula, E., & Ylianttila, M. (2018). Blockchain utilization in healthcare: Key requirements and challenges. In *2018 IEEE 20th International conference on e-health networking, applications and services (Healthcom)*. IEEE. doi:10.1109/HealthCom.2018.8531136

Kumari, S., & Muthulakshmi, P. (2022). Transformative Effects of Big Data on Advanced Data Analytics: Open Issues and Critical Challenges. *Journal of Computational Science*, *18*(6), 463–479. doi:10.3844/jcssp.2022.463.479

Kumari, S., Muthulakshmi, P., & Agarwal, D. (2022). Deployment of Machine Learning Based Internet of Things Networks for Tele-Medical and Remote Healthcare. In V. Suma, X. Fernando, K. L. Du, & H. Wang (Eds.), *Evolutionary Computing and Mobile Sustainable Networks. Lecture Notes on Data Engineering and Communications Technologies* (Vol. 116). Springer. doi:10.1007/978-981-16-9605-3_21

Kumar, N. (2014). Cuffless BP measurement using a correlation study of pulse transient time and heart rate. *Int. Conf. Adv. Comp. Info. (ICACCI)*. IEEE. 10.1109/ICACCI.2014.6968642

Kute, S. (2021). Building a Smart Healthcare System Using Internet of Things and Machine Learning. Big Data Management in Sensing: Applications in AI and IoT. River Publishers.

Kute, S. (2021). Building a Smart Healthcare System Using Internet of Things and Machine Learning. In Big Data Management in Sensing: Applications in AI and IoT. River Publishers.

Kute, S. (2021). Research Issues and Future Research Directions Toward Smart Healthcare Using Internet of Things and Machine Learning. Big Data Management in Sensing: Applications in AI and IoT. River Publishers.

Kute, S. S., Tyagi, A. K., & Aswathy, S. U. (2022). Industry 4.0 Challenges in e-Healthcare Applications and Emerging Technologies. In A. K. Tyagi, A. Abraham, & A. Kaklauskas (Eds.), *Intelligent Interactive Multimedia Systems for e-Healthcare Applications*. Springer. doi:10.1007/978-981-16-6542-4_14

Kute, S. S., Tyagi, A. K., & Aswathy, S. U. (2022). Security, Privacy and Trust Issues in Internet of Things and Machine Learning Based e-Healthcare. In A. K. Tyagi, A. Abraham, & A. Kaklauskas (Eds.), *Intelligent Interactive Multimedia Systems for e-Healthcare Applications*. Springer. doi:10.1007/978-981-16-6542-4_15

Lai, M., Lee, J., Chiu, S., Charm, J., So, W. Y., Yuen, F. P., Kwok, C., Tsoi, J., Lin, Y., & Zee, B. (2020). A machine learning approach for retinal images analysis as an objective screening method for children with autism spectrum disorder. *EClinicalMedicine*, *28*, 100588. doi:10.1016/j.eclinm.2020.100588 PMID:33294809

Lanjewar, M. G., Panchbhai, K. G., & Patle, L. B. (2024). Fusion of transfer learning models with LSTM for detection of breast cancer using ultrasound images. *Computers in Biology and Medicine*, *169*, 107914. doi:10.1016/j.comp-biomed.2023.107914 PMID:38190766

Le, H. T., Lam, N. T. T., Vo, H. K., Luong, H. H., Khoi, N. H. T., & Anh, T. D. (2022). Patient-chain: patient-centered healthcare system a blockchain-based technology in dealing with emergencies. In *Parallel and Distributed Computing, Applications and Technologies: 22nd International Conference, PDCAT 2021*. Cham: Springer International Publishing. 10.1007/978-3-030-96772-7_54

Leblanc, E., Washington, P., Varma, M., Dunlap, K., Penev, Y., Kline, A., & Wall, D. P. (2020). Feature replacement methods enable reliable home video analysis for machine learning detection of autism. *Scientific Reports*, *10*(1), 1–11. doi:10.1038/s41598-020-76874-w PMID:33277527

LeCun, Y., Bengio, Y., & Hinton, G. (2015). Deep learning. *Nature*, *521*(7553), 436–444. doi:10.1038/nature14539 PMID:26017442

LeDoux, J. E., & Pine, D. S. (2016). Using neuroscience to help understand fear and anxiety: A two-system framework. *The American Journal of Psychiatry*, *173*(11), 1083–1093. doi:10.1176/appi.ajp.2016.16030353 PMID:27609244

Le, H. T., Lam, N. T. T., Vo, H. K., Luong, H. H., Khoi, N. H. T., & Anh, T. D. (2022). Patient-chain: patient-centered healthcare system a blockchain-based technology in dealing with emergencies. In *Parallel and Distributed Computing, Applications and Technologies: 22nd International Conference, PDCAT 2021*. Springer International Publishing., doi:10.1007/978-3-030-96772-7_54

Liang, S., Sabri, A. Q. M., Alnajjar, F., & Loo, C. K. (2021). Autism spectrum self-stimulatory behaviors classification using explainable temporal coherency deep features and SVM classifier. *IEEE Access : Practical Innovations, Open Solutions*, *9*, 34264–34275. doi:10.1109/ACCESS.2021.3061455

Liu, D., Feng, X. L., Ahmed, F., Shahid, M., & Guo, J. (2022). Detecting and measuring depression on social media using a machine learning approach: Systematic review. *JMIR Mental Health*, *9*(3), e27244. doi:10.2196/27244 PMID:35230252

Liu, Y., Hsu, H. Y., Lin, T., Peng, B., Saqi, A., Salvatore, M. M., & Jambawalikar, S. (2024). Lung nodule malignancy classification with associated pulmonary fibrosis using 3D attention-gated convolutional network with CT scans. *Journal of Translational Medicine*, *22*(1), 51. doi:10.1186/s12967-023-04798-w PMID:38216992

Loch, A. A., Lopes-Rocha, A. C., Ara, A., Gondim, J. M., Cecchi, G. A., Corcoran, C. M., Mota, N. B., & Argolo, F. C. (2022). Ethical implications of the use of language analysis technologies for the diagnosis and prediction of psychiatric disorders. *JMIR Mental Health*, *9*(11), e41014. doi:10.2196/41014 PMID:36318266

Lorenzo, G., Lledó, A., Arráez-Vera, G., & Lorenzo-Lledó, A. (2019). The application of immersive virtual reality for students with ASD: A review between 1990–2017. *Education and Information Technologies*, *24*(1), 127–151. doi:10.1007/s10639-018-9766-7

Losada, D. E., Crestani, F., & Parapar, J. (2018). Overview of eRisk: Early Risk Prediction on the Internet. In P. Bellot, C. Trabelsi, J. Mothe, F. Murtagh, J. Y. Nie, L. Soulier, E. SanJuan, L. Cappellato, & N. Ferro (Eds.), Experimental IR Meets Multilinguality, Multimodality, and Interaction (Vol. 11018, pp. 343–361). Springer International Publishing. doi:10.1007/978-3-319-98932-7_30

Compilation of References

Lu, W. Z., Fan, H. Y., Leung, A. Y. T., & Wong, J. C. K. (2002). Analysis of pollutant levels in central Hong Kong applying neural network method with particle swarm optimization. *Environmental Monitoring and Assessment*, *79*(3), 217–230. doi:10.1023/A:1020274409612 PMID:12392160

Madhav, A. V. S., & Tyagi, A. K. (2022). The World with Future Technologies (Post-COVID-19): Open Issues, Challenges, and the Road Ahead. In A. K. Tyagi, A. Abraham, & A. Kaklauskas (Eds.), *Intelligent Interactive Multimedia Systems for e-Healthcare Applications*. Springer. doi:10.1007/978-981-16-6542-4_22

Mallee, W. H., Walenkamp, M. M. J., Mulders, M. A. M., Goslings, J. C., & Schep, N. W. L. (2020). Detecting scaphoid fractures in wrist injury: A clinical decision rule. *Archives of Orthopaedic and Trauma Surgery*, *140*(4), 575–581. doi:10.1007/s00402-020-03383-w PMID:32125528

Mao, K., Tang, R., Wang, X., Zhang, W., & Wu, H. (2018). Feature Representation Using Deep Autoencoder for Lung Nodule Image Classification. *Complexity*, *2018*, 1–11. doi:10.1155/2018/3078374

Mariappan, M. B., Devi, K., Venkataraman, Y., & Fosso Wamba, S. (2022). A large-scale real-world comparative study using pre-COVID lockdown and post-COVID lockdown data on predicting shipment times of therapeutics in e-pharmacy supply chains. *International Journal of Physical Distribution & Logistics Management*, *52*(7), 512–537. doi:10.1108/IJPDLM-05-2021-0192

Masood, A., Sheng, B., Li, P., Hou, X., Wei, X., Qin, J., & Feng, D. (2018). Computer-Assisted Decision Support System in Pulmonary Cancer detection and stage classification on CT images. *Journal of Biomedical Informatics*, *79*, 117–128. doi:10.1016/j.jbi.2018.01.005 PMID:29366586

Mastrovito, D., Hanson, C., & Hanson, S. J. (2018). Differences in atypical resting-state effective connectivity distinguish autism from schizophrenia. *NeuroImage. Clinical*, *18*, 367–376. doi:10.1016/j.nicl.2018.01.014 PMID:29487793

Matsuyama, E., & Tsai, D.-Y. (2018). Automated Classification of Lung Diseases in Computed Tomography Images Using a Wavelet Based Convolutional Neural Network. *Journal of Biomedical Science and Engineering*, *11*(10), 263–274. doi:10.4236/jbise.2018.1110022

McClellan, C., Ali, M. M., Mutter, R., Kroutil, L., & Landwehr, J. (2017). Using social media to monitor mental health discussions- evidence from Twitter. *Journal of the American Medical Informatics Association : JAMIA*, *24*(3), 496–502. doi:10.1093/jamia/ocw133 PMID:27707822

McCombie, D. B. (2006). Adaptive blood pressure estimation from wearable PPG sensors using peripheral artery pulse wave velocity measurements and multi-channel blind identification of local arterial dynamics. *Annu. Int. Conf. Eng. Med. Bio. (EMBS)*. IEEE. 10.1109/IEMBS.2006.260590

Meghriche, S., Boulemden, M., & Draa, A. (2008). Agreement between multi-layer perceptron and a compound neural network on ECG diagnosis of aatrioventricular blocks. *WSEAS Trans. Biol. Biomed*, *5*(1), 12–22.

Mellema, C. J., Nguyen, K. P., Treacher, A., & Montillo, A. (2022). Reproducible neuroimaging features for diagnosis of autism spectrum disorder with machine learning. *Scientific Reports*, *12*(1), 3057. doi:10.1038/s41598-022-06459-2 PMID:35197468

Mettler, M. (2016). Blockchain technology in healthcare: The revolution starts here. *Blockchain Technology in Healthcare, 2016 IEEE 18th International Conference on e-Health Networking, Applications and Services, Healthcom 2016*, (pp. 1–3). IEEE. 10.1109/HealthCom.2016.7749510

Mir, A., & Dhage, S. N. Diabetes disease prediction using machine learning on big data of healthcare. In *2018 fourth international conference on computing communication control and automation (ICCUBEA)* (pp. 1-6). IEEE. 10.1109/ICCUBEA.2018.8697439

Mishra, S., Khatwani, G., Patil, R., Sapariya, D., Shah, V., Parmar, D., Dinesh, S., Daphal, P., & Mehendale, N. (2021). ECG Paper Record Digitization and Diagnosis Using Deep Learning. *Journal of Medical and Biological Engineering*, *41*(4), 422–432. doi:10.1007/s40846-021-00632-0 PMID:34149335

Mohsan, S. A. H., Razzaq, A., Ghayyur, S. A. K., Alkahtani, H. K., Al-Kahtani, N., & Mostafa, S. M. (2022). Decentralized Patient-Centric Report and Medical Image Management System Based on Blockchain Technology and the Inter-Planetary File System. *International Journal of Environmental Research and Public Health*, *19*(22), 14641. doi:10.3390/ijerph192214641 PMID:36429351

Monteiro, S. A., Dempsey, J., Berry, L. N., Voigt, R. G., & Goin-Kochel, R. P. (2019). Screening and referral practices for autism spectrum disorder in primary pediatric care. *Pediatrics*, *144*(4), e20183326. doi:10.1542/peds.2018-3326 PMID:31515298

Moody, B., Moody, G., Villarroel, M., Clifford, G. D., & Silva, I. (2020). MIMIC-III Waveform Database (version 1.0). *PhysioNet*. doi:10.13026/c2607m

Nafisah, S. I., & Muhammad, G. (2024). Tuberculosis detection in chest radiograph using convolutional neural network architecture and explainable artificial intelligence. *Neural Computing & Applications*, *36*(1), 111–131. doi:10.1007/s00521-022-07258-6 PMID:35462630

Nair, M. M., & Tyagi, A. K. (2023). AI, IoT, blockchain, and cloud computing: The necessity of the future. Rajiv Pandey, Sam Goundar, Shahnaz Fatima (eds.), Distributed Computing to Blockchain. Academic Press. doi:10.1016/B978-0-323-96146-2.00001-2

Nair, M. M., Kumari, S., Tyagi, A. K., & Sravanthi, K. (2021) Deep Learning for Medical Image Recognition: Open Issues and a Way to Forward. In: Goyal D., Gupta A.K., Piuri V., Ganzha M., Paprzycki M. (eds) *Proceedings of the Second International Conference on Information Management and Machine Intelligence. Lecture Notes in Networks and Systems*. Springer, Singapore. /10.1007/978-981-15-9689-6_38

Nair, M. M., Kumari, S., Tyagi, A. K., & Sravanthi, K. (2021). Deep Learning for Medical Image Recognition: Open Issues and a Way to Forward. In D. Goyal, A. K. Gupta, V. Piuri, M. Ganzha, & M. Paprzycki (Eds.), *Proceedings of the Second International Conference on Information Management and Machine Intelligence. Lecture Notes in Networks and Systems*. Springer., doi:10.1007/978-981-15-9689-6_38

Nam, J. G., Park, S., Hwang, E. J., Lee, J. H., Jin, K.-N., Lim, K. Y., Vu, T. H., Sohn, J. H., Hwang, S., Goo, J. M., & Park, C. M. (2019). Development and Validation of Deep Learning–based Automatic Detection Algorithm for Malignant Pulmonary Nodules on Chest Radiographs. *Radiology*, *290*(1), 218–228. doi:10.1148/radiol.2018180237 PMID:30251934

Naresh, V. S., Reddi, S., & Allavarpu, V. D. (2021). Blockchain-based patient centric health care communication system. *International Journal of Communication Systems*, *34*(7), e4749. doi:10.1002/dac.4749

Nasrullah, N., Sang, J., Alam, M. S., Mateen, M., Cai, B., & Hu, H. (2019). Automated Lung Nodule Detection and Classification Using Deep Learning Combined with Multiple Strategies. *Sensors (Basel)*, *19*(17), 3722. doi:10.3390/s19173722 PMID:31466261

Nickel, P., & Nachreiner, F. (2003). Sensitivity and diagnosticity of the 0.1-Hz component of heart rate variability as an indicator of mental workload. *Human Factors*, *45*(4), 575–590. doi:10.1518/hfes.45.4.575.27094 PMID:15055455

Nikula, R. (1991). Psychological correlates of nonspecific skin conductance responses. *Psychophysiology*, *28*(1), 86–90. doi:10.1111/j.1469-8986.1991.tb03392.x PMID:1886966

Norimoto, M., Yamashita, M., Yamaoka, A., Yamashita, K., Abe, K., Eguchi, Y., Furuya, T., Orita, S., Inage, K., Shiga, Y., Maki, S., Umimura, T., Sato, T., Sato, M., Enomoto, K., Takaoka, H., Hozumi, T., Mizuki, N., Kim, G., & Ohtori, S. (2021). Early mobilization reduces the medical care cost and the risk of disuse syndrome in patients with acute osteoporotic vertebral fractures. *Journal of Clinical Neuroscience*, *93*, 155–159. doi:10.1016/j.jocn.2021.09.011 PMID:34656240

Nosek, B. A., Hawkins, C. B., & Frazier, R. S. (2011). Implicit social cognition: From measures to mechanisms. *Trends in Cognitive Sciences*, *15*(4), 152–159. doi:10.1016/j.tics.2011.01.005 PMID:21376657

Ofori-Parku, S. S., & Park, S. E. (2022). I (Don't) want to consume counterfeit medicines: Exploratory study on the antecedents of consumer attitudes toward counterfeit medicines. *BMC Public Health*, *22*(1), 1–13. doi:10.1186/s12889-022-13529-7 PMID:35650557

Okada, T., Linguraru, M. G., Hori, M., Summers, R. M., Tomiyama, N., & Sato, Y. (2015). Abdominal multi-organ segmentation from CT images using conditional shape-location and unsupervised intensity priors. *Medical Image Analysis*, *26*(1), 1–18. doi:10.1016/j.media.2015.06.009 PMID:26277022

Omar, K. S., Mondal, P., Khan, N. S., Rizvi, M. R. K., & Islam, M. N. (2019). A machine learning approach to predict autism spectrum disorder. *2019 International Conference on Electrical, Computer and Communication Engineering (ECCE)*, (pp. 1–6). IEEE. 10.1109/ECACE.2019.8679454

Pandey, P., & Litoriya, R. (2021). Securing E-health Networks from Counterfeit Medicine Penetration Using Blockchain. *Wireless Personal Communications*, *117*(1), 7–25. doi:10.1007/s11277-020-07041-7

Park, G. W., Kim, Y., Park, K., & Agarwal, A. (2016). Patient-centric quality assessment framework for healthcare services. *Technological Forecasting and Social Change*, *113*, 468–474. doi:10.1016/j.techfore.2016.07.012

Park, H., Bland, P. H., & Meyer, C. R. (2003). Construction of an abdominal probabilistic atlas and its application in segmentation. *IEEE Transactions on Medical Imaging*, *22*(4), 483–492. doi:10.1109/TMI.2003.809139 PMID:12774894

Parry, D. A., Fisher, J. T., Mieczkowski, H., Sewall, C. J., & Davidson, B. I. (2022). Social media and well-being: A methodological perspective. *Current Opinion in Psychology*, *45*, 101285. doi:10.1016/j.copsyc.2021.11.005 PMID:35008029

Parsons, T. D. (2011). Neuropsychological assessment using virtual environments: enhanced assessment technology for improved ecological validity. *Advanced Computational Intelligence Paradigms in Healthcare 6. Virtual Reality in Psychotherapy, Rehabilitation, and Assessment*, 271–289.

Parsons, S., Mitchell, P., & Leonard, A. (2004). The use and understanding of virtual environments by adolescents with autistic spectrum disorders. *Journal of Autism and Developmental Disorders*, *34*(4), 449–466. doi:10.1023/B:JADD.0000037421.98517.8d PMID:15449520

Parsons, T. D., Rizzo, A. A., Rogers, S., & York, P. (2009). Virtual reality in paediatric rehabilitation: A review. *Developmental Neurorehabilitation*, *12*(4), 224–238. doi:10.1080/17518420902991719 PMID:19842822

Pastorelli, E., & Herrmann, H. (2013). A small-scale, low-budget semi-immersive virtual environment for scientific visualization and research. *Procedia Computer Science*, *25*, 14–22. doi:10.1016/j.procs.2013.11.003

Pathak, R., Gaur, V., Sankrityayan, H., & Gogtay, J. (2023). Tackling Counterfeit Drugs: The Challenges and Possibilities. *Pharmaceutical Medicine*, *37*(4), 281–290. doi:10.1007/s40290-023-00468-w PMID:37188891

Pathan, S., Bhushan, M., & Bai, A. (2020). A study on health care using data mining techniques. *Journal of Critical Reviews*, *7*(19), 7877–7890.

Patil, P., & Karthikeyan, A. (2020). A survey on K-means clustering for analyzing variation in data. In Lecture Notes in Networks and Systems (Vol. 89). doi:10.1007/978-981-15-0146-3_29

Peral, J., Gil, D., Rotbei, S., Amador, S., Guerrero, M., & Moradi, H. (2020). A machine learning and integration based architecture for cognitive disorder detection used for early autism screening. *Electronics (Basel)*, *9*(3), 516. doi:10.3390/electronics9030516

Pessana, F. M., Lev, G., Mirada, M., Ramirez, A. J., Mendiz, O., & Fischer, E. I. C. (2019). *Central Blood Pressure Waves Assessment: A Validation Study of Non-Invasive Aortic Pressure Measurement in Human Beings*. Global Medical Engineering Physics Exchanges.

Peter, L., Noury, N., & Cerny, M. (2014). A review of methods for non-invasive and continuous blood pressure monitoring: Pulse transit time method is promising? *Ingénierie et Recherche Biomédicale : IRBM = Biomedical Engineering and Research*, *35*(5), 271–282. doi:10.1016/j.irbm.2014.07.002

Pham, H. L., Tran, T. H., & Nakashima, Y. (2019). Practical Anti-Counterfeit Medicine Management System Based on Blockchain Technology. *TIMES-ICON 2019 - 2019 4th Technology Innovation Management and Engineering Science International Conference*, 1–5. IEEE. 10.1109/TIMES-iCON47539.2019.9024674

Pickering, T. G., Hall, J. E., Appel, L. J., Falkner, B. E., Graves, J., Hill, M. N., Jones, D. W., Kurtz, T., Sheps, S. G., & Roccella, E. J. (2005). Recommendations for blood pressure measurement in humans and experimental animals—Part 1: Blood pressure measurement in humans: A statement for professionals from the subcommittee of professional and public education of the American Heart Association Council on high blood pressure research. *Hypertension*, *45*(1), 142–161. doi:10.1161/01.HYP.0000150859.47929.8e PMID:15611362

Piryonesi, S. M., & El-Diraby, T. E. (2020). Role of data analytics in infrastructure asset management: Overcoming data size and quality problems. *Journal of Transportation Engineering. Part B, Pavements*, *146*(2), 04020022. doi:10.1061/JPEODX.0000175

Pitros, P., O'Connor, N., Tryfonos, A., & Lopes, V. (2020). A systematic review of the complications of high-risk third molar removal and coronectomy: Development of a decision tree model and preliminary health economic analysis to assist in treatment planning. *British Journal of Oral & Maxillofacial Surgery*, *58*(9), e16–e24. doi:10.1016/j.bjoms.2020.07.015 PMID:32800608

Ploug, T., & Holm, S. (2020). The four dimensions of contestable AI diagnostics-A patient-centric approach to explainable AI. *Artificial Intelligence in Medicine*, *107*, 101901. doi:10.1016/j.artmed.2020.101901 PMID:32828448

Polo Simón, F., García Medrano, B., & Delgado Serrano, P. J. (2020). Diagnostic and Therapeutic Approach to Acute Scaphoid Fractures. *Revista Iberoamericana de Cirugía de la Mano*, *48*(02), 109–118. doi:10.1055/s-0040-1718457

Poon, C., & Zhang, Y. (2006). Cuff-less and noninvasive measurements of arterial blood pressure by pulse transit time. *Annu. Int. Conf. Eng. Med. Bio. (EMBS)*. IEEE.

Poonkodi, S., & Kanchana, M. (2024). Lung cancer segmentation from CT scan images using modified mayfly optimization and particle swarm optimization algorithm. *Multimedia Tools and Applications*, *83*(2), 3567–3584. doi:10.1007/s11042-023-15688-0

Powers, D. M. (2020). *Evaluation: from precision, recall and F-measure to ROC, informedness, markedness and correlation*. arXiv preprint arXiv:2010.16061. Oct 11.

Prabadevi, B. (2021). Toward blockchain for edge-of-things: A new paradigm, opportunities, and future directions. *IEEE Internet of Things Magazine*, *4*(2), 102–108. doi:10.1109/IOTM.0001.2000191

Prabadevi, B. (2021). Toward blockchain for edge-of-things: A new paradigm, opportunities, and future directions. IEEE Internet of Things Magazine, 4(2), 102–108. doi:10.1109/IOTM.0001.2000191

Prabu Shankar, K. C., & Deeba, K. (2023). *Machine Learning-Based Big Data Analytics for IoT-Enabled Smart Healthcare Systems, in the book: AI-Based Digital Health Communication for Securing Assistive Systems*. IGI Global. doi:10.4018/978-1-6684-8938-3.ch004

Price, M. (2016). Circle of care modelling: An approach to assist in reasoning about healthcare change using a patient-centric system. *BMC Health Services Research*, *16*(1), 1–10. doi:10.1186/s12913-016-1806-7 PMID:27716188

Qian, L., Bai, J., Huang, Y., Zeebaree, D. Q., Saffari, A., & Zebari, D. A. (2024). Breast cancer diagnosis using evolving deep convolutional neural network based on hybrid extreme learning machine technique and improved chimp optimization algorithm. *Biomedical Signal Processing and Control*, *87*, 105492. doi:10.1016/j.bspc.2023.105492

Qteat, H., & Awad, M. (2021). Using Hybrid Model of Particle Swarm Optimization and Multi-Layer Perceptron Neural Networks for Classification of Diabetes. *International Journal of Intelligent Engineering & Systems*, *14*(3), 11–22. doi:10.22266/ijies2021.0630.02

Quasim, M. T., Algarni, F., Abd Elhamid Radwan, A., & Goram Mufareh, M. A. (2020). A blockchain based secured healthcare framework. In *2020 International Conference on Computational Performance Evaluation (ComPE)*, (pp. 386-391). IEEE. 10.1109/ComPE49325.2020.9200024

Quasim, M. T., Algarni, F., Abd Elhamid Radwan, A., & Goram Mufareh, M. A. (2020). *A blockchain based secured healthcare framework. In 2020 International Conference on Computational Performance Evaluation (ComPE)*. IEEE., doi:10.1109/ComPE49325.2020.9200024

Rahman, M. M., Islam, M. M., Manik, M. M. H., Islam, M. R., & Al-Rakhami, M. S. (2021). Machine learning approaches for tackling novel coronavirus (COVID-19) pandemic. *SN Computer Science*, *2*(5), 1–10. doi:10.1007/s42979-021-00774-7 PMID:34308367

Rajamhoana, S. P., Devi, C. A., Umamaheswari, K., Kiruba, R., Karunya, K., & Deepika, R. (2018). Analysis of neural networks based heart disease prediction system. *2018 11th International Conference on Human System Interaction (HSI)*, (pp. 233–239). IEEE.

Raj, S., & Masood, S. (2020). Analysis and detection of autism spectrum disorder using machine learning techniques. *Procedia Computer Science*, *167*, 994–1004. doi:10.1016/j.procs.2020.03.399

Ramachandran, S., George, J., Skaria, S., & V.V., V. (2018). Using YOLO based deep learning network for real time detection and localization of lung nodules from low dose CT scans. In K. Mori & N. Petrick (Eds.), *Medical Imaging 2018: Computer-Aided Diagnosis* (p. 53). SPIE. doi:10.1117/12.2293699

Ramani, V., Kumar, T., Bracken, A., Liyanage, M., & Ylianttila, M. (2018). Secure and efficient data accessibility in blockchain based healthcare systems. In *2018 IEEE Global Communications Conference (GLOBECOM)*. IEEE. doi:10.1109/GLOCOM.2018.8647221

Ramani, V., Kumar, T., Bracken, A., Liyanage, M., & Ylianttila, M. (2018). Secure and efficient data accessibility in blockchain based healthcare systems. In *2018 IEEE Global Communications Conference (GLOBECOM)*. IEEE. 10.1109/GLOCOM.2018.8647221

Randazzo, V., Puleo, E., Paviglianiti, A., Vallan, A., & Pasero, E. (2022). Development and Validation of an Algorithm for the Digitization of ECG Paper Images. *Sensors (Basel)*, *22*(19), 7138. doi:10.3390/s22197138 PMID:36236237

Rani, K. V., & Jawhar, S. J. (2020). Superpixel with nanoscale imaging and boosted deep convolutional neural network concept for lung tumor classification. *International Journal of Imaging Systems and Technology*, *30*(4), 899–915. doi:10.1002/ima.22422

Rao, G. V. E., B, R., Srinivasu, P. N., Ijaz, M. F., & Woźniak, M. (2024). Hybrid framework for respiratory lung diseases detection based on classical CNN and quantum classifiers from chest X-rays. *Biomedical Signal Processing and Control*, *88*, 105567. doi:10.1016/j.bspc.2023.105567

Reno, S., Sadi, I., Karmakar, J., & Abir, M. (2021). Counterfeit medicine identification using hyperledger based private blockchain. *2021 2nd International Conference for Emerging Technology, INCET 2021*, (pp. 1–7). IEEE. 10.1109/INCET51464.2021.9456418

Rhoades, R. A., Scarpa, A., & Salley, B. (2007). The importance of physician knowledge of autism spectrum disorder: Results of a parent survey. *BMC Pediatrics*, *7*(1), 1–10. doi:10.1186/1471-2431-7-37 PMID:18021459

Rodionova, Y., & Pomerantsev, A. L. (2010). NIR-based approach to counterfeit-drug detection. *Trends in Analytical Chemistry*, *29*(8), 795–803. doi:10.1016/j.trac.2010.05.004

Roy, S., Prasanna Venkatesan, S., & Goh, M. (2021). Healthcare services: A systematic review of patient-centric logistics issues using simulation. *The Journal of the Operational Research Society*, *72*(10), 2342–2364. doi:10.1080/01605682.2020.1790306

Rua, T., Gidwani, S., Malhotra, B., Vijayanathan, S., Hunter, L., Peacock, J., Turville, J., Razavi, R., Goh, V., McCrone, P., & Shearer, J. (2020). Cost-effectiveness of immediate magnetic resonance imaging in the management of patients with suspected scaphoid fracture: Results from a randomized clinical trial. *Value in Health*, *23*(11), 1444–1452. doi:10.1016/j.jval.2020.05.020 PMID:33127015

Sabbagh, M. D., Morsy, M., & Moran, S. L. (2019). Diagnosis and management of acute scaphoid fractures. *Hand Clinics*, *35*(3), 259–269. doi:10.1016/j.hcl.2019.03.002 PMID:31178084

Sahu, A., Kuek, D. K., MacCormick, A., Gozzard, C., Ninan, T., Fullilove, S., & Suresh, P. (2023). Prospective comparison of magnetic resonance imaging and computed tomography in diagnosing occult scaphoid fractures. *Acta Radiologica*, *64*(1), 201–207. doi:10.1177/02841851211064595 PMID:34918571

Sai Dhakshan, Y. (2023). Introduction to Smart Healthcare: Healthcare Digitization. 6G-Enabled IoT and AI for Smart Healthcare. CRC Press.

Sai, G. H., Tripathi, K., & Tyagi, A. K. (2023). Internet of Things-Based e-Health Care: Key Challenges and Recommended Solutions for Future. In: Singh, P.K., Wierzchoń, S.T., Tanwar, S., Rodrigues, J.J.P.C., Ganzha, M. (eds) *Proceedings of Third International Conference on Computing, Communications, and Cyber-Security*. Springer, Singapore. 10.1007/978-981-19-1142-2_37

Sai, G. H., Tripathi, K., & Tyagi, A. K. (2023). Internet of Things-Based e-Health Care: Key Challenges and Recommended Solutions for Future. In P. K. Singh, S. T. Wierzchoń, S. Tanwar, J. J. P. C. Rodrigues, & M. Ganzha (Eds.), *Proceedings of Third International Conference on Computing, Communications, and Cyber-Security. Lecture Notes in Networks and Systems*. Springer., doi:10.1007/978-981-19-1142-2_37

Sailaja, N. V., Yelamarthi, M., Chandana, Y. H., Karadi, P., & Yedla, S. (2021). Early detection of sepsis on clinical data using multi-layer perceptron. Machine Learning Technologies and Applications. *Proceedings of ICACECS, 2020*, 223–233.

Sajidha, S. A. (2023). Robust and Secure Evidence Management in Digital Forensics Investigations Using Blockchain Technology. AI-Based Digital Health Communication for Securing Assistive Systems. IGI Global. doi:10.4018/978-1-6684-8938-3.ch010

Sala, C., Santin, E., Rescaldani, M., Cuspidi, C., & Magrini, F. (2005). What is the accuracy of clinic blood pressure measurement? *American Journal of Hypertension*, *18*(2), 244–248. doi:10.1016/j.amjhyper.2004.09.006 PMID:15752953

Salas-Zárate, R., Alor-Hernández, G., Salas-Zárate, M. del P., Paredes-Valverde, M. A., Bustos-López, M., & Sánchez-Cervantes, J. L. (2022). Detecting depression signs on social media: A systematic literature review. *Health Care*, *10*(2), 291. https://www.mdpi.com/2227-9032/10/2/291 PMID:35206905

Sartorius, N. (2022, April 1). Depression and diabetes. *Dialogues in Clinical Neuroscience*. PMID:29946211

Sasaki Y. (2007). The truth of the F-measure. *Teach tutor mater, 1*(5), 1-5.

Satu, M. S., Sathi, F. F., Arifen, M. S., Ali, M. H., & Moni, M. A. (2019). Early detection of autism by extracting features: a case study in Bangladesh. *2019 International Conference on Robotics, Electrical and Signal Processing Techniques (ICREST)*, (pp. 400–405). IEEE. 10.1109/ICREST.2019.8644357

Sawhney, R., Malik, A., Sharma, S., & Narayan, V. (2023). A comparative assessment of artificial intelligence models used for early prediction and evaluation of chronic kidney disease. *Decision Analytics Journal*, *6*, 100169. doi:10.1016/j.dajour.2023.100169

Saydah, S. H., Geiss, L. S., Tierney, E. D., Benjamin, S. M., Engelgau, M., & Brancati, F. (2004). Review of the performance of methods to identify diabetes cases among vital statistics, administrative, and survey data. *Annals of Epidemiology*, *14*(7), 507–516. doi:10.1016/j.annepidem.2003.09.016 PMID:15301787

Schöner, M. M., Kourouklis, D., Sandner, P., Gonzalez, E., & Förster, J. (2017). Blockchain Technology in the Pharmaceutical Industry. *FSBC Working Paper, July*, 1–9. https://philippsandner.medium.com/blockchain-technology-in-the-pharmaceutical-industry-3a3229251afd

Self, T. L., Parham, D. F., & Rajagopalan, J. (2015). Autism spectrum disorder early screening practices: A survey of physicians. *Communication Disorders Quarterly*, *36*(4), 195–207. doi:10.1177/1525740114560060

Setio, A. A. A., Ciompi, F., Litjens, G., Gerke, P., Jacobs, C., van Riel, S. J., Wille, M. M. W., Naqibullah, M., Sanchez, C. I., & van Ginneken, B. (2016). Pulmonary Nodule Detection in CT Images: False Positive Reduction Using Multi-View Convolutional Networks. *IEEE Transactions on Medical Imaging*, *35*(5), 1160–1169. doi:10.1109/TMI.2016.2536809 PMID:26955024

Shabnam Kumari, P. (2023). *Muthulakshmi, Effective Deep Learning-Based Attack Detection Methods for the Internet of Medical Things, in the book: AI-Based Digital Health Communication for Securing Assistive Systems*. IGI Global. doi:10.4018/978-1-6684-8938-3.ch008

Shah, S. N. A., & Parveen, R. (2023). An Extensive Review on Lung Cancer Diagnosis Using Machine Learning Techniques on Radiological Data: State-of-the-art and Perspectives. *Archives of Computational Methods in Engineering*, *30*(8), 4917–4930. doi:10.1007/s11831-023-09964-3

Shamila, M., & Vinuthna, K. (2023). Genomic privacy: performance analysis, open issues, and future research directions. Amit Kumar Tyagi, Ajith Abraham (eds.) Data Science for Genomics. Academic Press. doi:10.1016/B978-0-323-98352-5.00015-X

Shamila, M., & Vinuthna, K. (2023). Genomic privacy: performance analysis, open issues, and future research directions. In A. K. Tyagi & A. Abraham (eds.) Data Science for Genomics. Academic Press. doi:10.1016/B978-0-323-98352-5.00015-X

Shannon, H., Bush, K., Villeneuve, P. J., Hellemans, K. G., & Guimond, S. (2022). Problematic social media use in adolescents and young adults: Systematic review and meta-analysis. *JMIR Mental Health*, *9*(4), e33450. doi:10.2196/33450 PMID:35436240

Sharif, H., & Khan, R. A. (2022). A novel machine learning based framework for detection of autism spectrum disorder (ASD). *Applied Artificial Intelligence*, *36*(1), 2004655. doi:10.1080/08839514.2021.2004655

Sharma, S. K., Sharma, N. K., & Potter, P. P. (2020). Fusion Approach for Document Classification using Random Forest and SVM. *Proceeding of SMART-2020, IEEE Conference ID: 50582, 9th IEEE Scopus Indexed International Conference on System Modelling & Advancement on Research Trends (SMART-2020).* IEEE. 10.1109/SMART50582.2020.9337131

Sharma, A., Tomar, R., Chilamkurti, N., & Kim, B.-G. (2020). Blockchain based smart contracts for internet of medical things in e-healthcare. *Electronics (Basel), 9*(10), 1609. doi:10.3390/electronics9101609

Sharma, P., Moparthi, N. R., Namasudra, S., Shanmuganathan, V., & Hsu, C.-H. (2022). Blockchain-based IoT architecture to secure healthcare system using identity-based encryption. *Expert Systems: International Journal of Knowledge Engineering and Neural Networks, 39*(10), e12915. doi:10.1111/exsy.12915

Sharma, S. K., & Sharma, N. K. (2019). Text Classification using Ensemble of Non-Linear Support Vector Machines. [IJITEE]. *International Journal of Innovative Technology and Exploring Engineering, 8*(10), 3170–3174. doi:10.35940/ijitee.J9520.0881019

Sharma, S. K., & Sharma, N. K. (2019). Text Classification using LSTM based Deep Neural Network Architecture. *International Journal on Emerging Technologies., 10*(4), 38–42.

Sharma, S. K., & Sharma, N. K. (2019). Text Document Categorization using Modified K-Means Clustering Algorithm. [IJRTE]. *International Journal of Recent Technology and Engineering, 8*(2), 508–511.

Sharma, S. K., & Sharma, N. K. (2019). Unified Framework for Deep Learning based Text Classification. *INTERNATIONAL JOURNAL OF SCIENTIFIC & TECHNOLOGY RESEARCH, 8*(10), 1479–1483.

Shen, W., Zhou, M., Yang, F., Yang, C., & Tian, J. (2015). *Multi-scale Convolutional Neural Networks for Lung Nodule Classification.*, doi:10.1007/978-3-319-19992-4_46

Sheridan, R. P., Wang, W. M., Liaw, A., Ma, J., & Gifford, E. M. (2016). Extreme gradient boosting as a method for quantitative structure–activity relationships. *Journal of Chemical Information and Modeling, 56*(12), 2353–2360. doi:10.1021/acs.jcim.6b00591 PMID:27958738

Sheth, H. S. K., & Tyagi, A. K. (2022). Mobile Cloud Computing: Issues, Applications and Scope in COVID-19. In A. Abraham, N. Gandhi, T. Hanne, T. P. Hong, T. Nogueira Rios, & W. Ding (Eds.), *Intelligent Systems Design and Applications. ISDA 2021. Lecture Notes in Networks and Systems* (Vol. 418). Springer. doi:10.1007/978-3-030-96308-8_55

Simjanoska, M. (2018). Non-invasive blood pressure estimation from ECG using machine learning techniques. *Sensors, 18*(4), 1160.

Simmons, J. P., Nelson, L. D., & Simonsohn, U. (2011). False-positive psychology: Undisclosed flexibility in data collection and analysis allows presenting anything as significant. *Psychological Science, 22*(11), 1359–1366. doi:10.1177/0956797611417632 PMID:22006061

Singh, P., Kansal, M., Srivastava, M., & Gupta, M. (2023). Smart Agriculture Resource Allocation and Cost Optimization Using ML in Cloud Computing Environment. In Convergence of Cloud Computing, AI, and Agricultural Science (pp. 152–163). IGI Global. doi:10.4018/979-8-3693-0200-2.ch008

Singh, A. (2023). Combating Counterfeit and Substandard Medicines in India: Legal Framework and the Way Ahead. *Current Research Journal of Social Sciences and Humanities, 6*(1), 101–111. doi:10.12944/CRJSSH.6.1.08

Singh, A. P., Pradhan, N. R., Luhach, A. K., Agnihotri, S., Jhanjhi, N. Z., Verma, S., Kavita, Ghosh, U., & Roy, D. S. (2020). A novel patient-centric architectural framework for blockchain-enabled healthcare applications. *IEEE Transactions on Industrial Informatics, 17*(8), 5779–5789. doi:10.1109/TII.2020.3037889

Singh, A., Raj, K., Kumar, T., Verma, S., & Roy, A. M. (2023). Deep learning-based cost-effective and responsive robot for autism treatment. *Drones (Basel)*, *7*(2), 81. doi:10.3390/drones7020081

Singh, S., Sharma, S. K., Mehrotra, P., Bhatt, P., & Kaurav, M. (2022). Blockchain technology for efficient data management in healthcare system: Opportunity, challenges and future perspectives. *Materials Today: Proceedings*, *62*, 5042–5046. doi:10.1016/j.matpr.2022.04.998

Singh, V. J., Bhushan, M., Kumar, V., & Bansal, K. L. (2015). Optimization of segment size assuring application perceived QoS in healthcare. *Proceedings of the World Congress on Engineering, 1*, (pp. 1–3). IEEE.

Sisodia, D., & Sisodia, D. S. (2018). Prediction of diabetes using classification algorithms. *Procedia Computer Science*, *132*, 1578–1585. doi:10.1016/j.procs.2018.05.122

Siyal, A. A., Junejo, A. Z., Zawish, M., Ahmed, K., Khalil, A., & Soursou, G. (2019). Applications of blockchain technology in medicine and healthcare: Challenges and future perspectives. *Cryptography*, *3*(1), 1–16. doi:10.3390/cryptography3010003

Skalski, P., & Tamborini, R. (2007). The role of social presence in interactive agent-based persuasion. *Media Psychology*, *10*(3), 385–413. doi:10.1080/15213260701533102

Slater, M. (2009). Place illusion and plausibility can lead to realistic behaviour in immersive virtual environments. *Philosophical Transactions of the Royal Society of London. Series B, Biological Sciences*, *364*(1535), 3549–3557. doi:10.1098/rstb.2009.0138 PMID:19884149

Snaith, B., Walker, A., Robertshaw, S., Spencer, N. J. B., Smith, A., & Harris, M. A. (2021). Has NICE guidance changed the management of the suspected scaphoid fracture: A survey of UK practice. *Radiography*, *27*(2), 377–380. doi:10.1016/j.radi.2020.09.014 PMID:33011069

Soltanisehat, L., Alizadeh, R., Hao, H., & Choo, K.-K. R. (2020). Technical, temporal, and spatial research challenges and opportunities in blockchain-based healthcare: A systematic literature review. *IEEE Transactions on Engineering Management*.

Son, H. X., Le, T. H., Nga, T. T. Q., Hung, N. D. H., Duong-Trung, N., & Luong, H. H. (2021). *Toward a blockchain-based technology in dealing with emergencies in patient-centered healthcare systems.* In Mobile, Secure, and Programmable Networking: 6th International Conference, MSPN 2020, Paris. 10.1007/978-3-030-67550-9_4

Son, H. X., Le, T. H., Nga, T. T. Q., Hung, N. D. H., Duong-Trung, N., & Luong, H. H. (2021). Toward a blockchain-based technology in dealing with emergencies in patient-centered healthcare systems. In *Mobile, Secure, and Programmable Networking: 6th International Conference, MSPN 2020*, Paris. doi:10.1007/978-3-030-67550-9_4

Spruit, M., & Lytras, M. (2018). Applied data science in patient-centric healthcare: Adaptive analytic systems for empowering physicians and patients. *Telematics and Informatics*, *35*(4), 643–653. doi:10.1016/j.tele.2018.04.002

Stehman, S. V. (1997). Selecting and interpreting measures of thematic classification accuracy. *Remote Sensing of Environment*, *62*(1), 77–89. doi:10.1016/S0034-4257(97)00083-7

Stirling, P. H., Strelzow, J. A., Doornberg, J. N., White, T. O., McQueen, M. M., & Duckworth, A. D. (2021). Diagnosis of suspected scaphoid fractures. *JBJS Reviews*, *9*(12), e20. doi:10.2106/JBJS.RVW.20.00247 PMID:34879033

Summers, R. M. (2016). Progress in fully automated abdominal CT interpretation. *AJR. American Journal of Roentgenology*, *207*(1), 67–79. doi:10.2214/AJR.15.15996 PMID:27101207

Suroto, H., Antoni, I., Siyo, A., Steendam, T. C., Prajasari, T., Mulyono, H. B., & De Vega, B. (2021). Traumatic brachial plexus injury in Indonesia: An experience from a developing country. *Journal of Reconstructive Microsurgery*, *38*(07), 511–523. doi:10.1055/s-0041-1735507 PMID:34470060

Swärd, E. M., Schriever, T. U., Franko, M. A., Björkman, A. C., & Wilcke, M. K. (2019). The epidemiology of scaphoid fractures in Sweden: A nationwide registry study. [European Volume]. *The Journal of Hand Surgery*, *44*(7), 697–701. doi:10.1177/1753193419849767 PMID:31106681

Sylim, P., Liu, F., Marcelo, A., & Fontelo, P. (2018). Blockchain technology for detecting falsified and substandard drugs in distribution: Pharmaceutical supply chain intervention. *JMIR Research Protocols*, *7*(9), 1–13. doi:10.2196/10163 PMID:30213780

Tandon, A., Dhir, A., Islam, A. K. M. N., & Mäntymäki, M. (2020). Blockchain in healthcare: A systematic literature review, synthesizing framework and future research agenda. *Computers in Industry*, *122*, 103290. doi:10.1016/j.comp-ind.2020.103290

Tandon, A., Dhir, A., Islam, A. K. M. N., & Mäntymäki, M. (2020). Blockchain in healthcare: A systematic literature review, synthesizing framework and future research agenda. *Computers in Industry*, *122*, 103290. doi:10.1016/j.comp-ind.2020.103290

Tang, A., Tam, R., Cadrin-Chênevert, A., Guest, W., Chong, J., Barfett, J., Chepelev, L., Cairns, R., Mitchell, J. R., Cicero, M. D., Poudrette, M. G., Jaremko, J. L., Reinhold, C., Gallix, B., Gray, B., Geis, R., O'Connell, T., Babyn, P., Koff, D., & Shabana, W.Canadian Association of Radiologists (CAR) Artificial Intelligence Working Group. (2018). Canadian Association of Radiologists white paper on artificial intelligence in radiology. *Canadian Association of Radiologists Journal*, *69*(2), 120–135. doi:10.1016/j.carj.2018.02.002 PMID:29655580

Tao, X., & Fisher, C. B. (2022). Exposure to Social Media Racial Discrimination and Mental Health among Adolescents of Color. *Journal of Youth and Adolescence*, *51*(1), 30–44. doi:10.1007/s10964-021-01514-z PMID:34686952

Tariq, S., Akhtar, N., Afzal, H., Khalid, S., Mufti, M. R., Hussain, S., Habib, A., & Ahmad, G. (2019). A novel co-training-based approach for the classification of mental illnesses using social media posts. *IEEE Access : Practical Innovations, Open Solutions*, *7*, 166165–166172. doi:10.1109/ACCESS.2019.2953087

Tartarisco, G., Cicceri, G., Di Pietro, D., Leonardi, E., Aiello, S., Marino, F., Chiarotti, F., Gagliano, A., Arduino, G. M., Apicella, F., Muratori, F., Bruneo, D., Allison, C., Cohen, S. B., Vagni, D., Pioggia, G., & Ruta, L. (2021). Use of machine learning to investigate the quantitative checklist for autism in toddlers (Q-CHAT) towards early autism screening. *Diagnostics (Basel)*, *11*(3), 574. doi:10.3390/diagnostics11030574 PMID:33810146

Teague, S. J., Shatte, A. B., Weller, E., Fuller-Tyszkiewicz, M., & Hutchinson, D. M. (2022). Methods and applications of social media monitoring of mental health during disasters: Scoping review. *JMIR Mental Health*, *9*(2), e33058. doi:10.2196/33058 PMID:35225815

Thabtah, F. (2017). Autism spectrum disorder screening: machine learning adaptation and DSM-5 fulfillment. *Proceedings of the 1st International Conference on Medical and Health Informatics 2017*, (pp. 1–6). IEEE. 10.1145/3107514.3107515

Thabtah, F. (2019). Machine learning in autistic spectrum disorder behavioral research: A review and ways forward. *Informatics for Health & Social Care*, *44*(3), 278–297. doi:10.1080/17538157.2017.1399132 PMID:29436887

Thabtah, F., Kamalov, F., & Rajab, K. (2018). A new computational intelligence approach to detect autistic features for autism screening. *International Journal of Medical Informatics*, *117*, 112–124. doi:10.1016/j.ijmedinf.2018.06.009 PMID:30032959

Thabtah, F., & Peebles, D. (2020). A new machine learning model based on induction of rules for autism detection. *Health Informatics Journal*, *26*(1), 264–286. doi:10.1177/1460458218824711 PMID:30693818

Thamilarasi, V., & Roselin, R. (2021). Automatic Classification and Accuracy by Deep Learning Using CNN Methods in Lung Chest X-Ray Images. *IOP Conference Series. Materials Science and Engineering*, *1055*(1), 012099. doi:10.1088/1757-899X/1055/1/012099

Tripathi, G., Ahad, M. A., & Paiva, S. (2020). S2HS-A blockchain based approach for smart healthcare system. In Healthcare, 8. Elsevier. doi:10.1016/j.hjdsi.2019.100391

Tripathi, G., Ahad, M. A., & Paiva, S. (2020). S2HS-A blockchain based approach for smart healthcare system. In *Healthcare, 8*. Elsevier., doi:10.1016/j.hjdsi.2019.100391

Tseng, J. H., Liao, Y. C., Chong, B., & Liao, S. W. (2018). Governance on the drug supply chain via gcoin blockchain. *International Journal of Environmental Research and Public Health*, *15*(6), 1055. Advance online publication. doi:10.3390/ijerph15061055 PMID:29882861

Tyagi, A. (2020). Artificial Intelligence and Machine Learning Algorithms. Challenges and Applications for Implementing Machine Learning in Computer Vision. IGI Global. doi:10.4018/978-1-7998-0182-5.ch008

Tyagi, A. (2020). Artificial Intelligence and Machine Learning Algorithms. In Challenges and Applications for Implementing Machine Learning in Computer Vision. IGI Global. doi:10.4018/978-1-7998-0182-5.ch008

Tyagi, A. (2020). Challenges of Applying Deep Learning in Real-World Applications. Challenges and Applications for Implementing Machine Learning in Computer Vision. IGI Global. doi:10.4018/978-1-7998-0182-5.ch004

Tyagi, A. (2020). Challenges of Applying Deep Learning in Real-World Applications. In Challenges and Applications for Implementing Machine Learning in Computer Vision. IGI Global. doi:10.4018/978-1-7998-0182-5.ch004

Tyagi, A. (2021). Healthcare Solutions for Smart Era: An Useful Explanation from User's Perspective. In Recent Trends in Blockchain for Information Systems Security and Privacy. CRC Press.

Tyagi, A. (2021). Healthcare Solutions for Smart Era: An Useful Explanation from User's Perspective. Recent Trends in Blockchain for Information Systems Security and Privacy. CRC Press.

Tyagi, A. (2021, October). AARIN: Affordable, Accurate, Reliable and INnovative Mechanism to Protect a Medical Cyber-Physical System using Blockchain Technology. *IJIN*, *2*, 175–183.

Tyagi, A. (2021, October). Aswathy S U, G Aghila, N Sreenath "AARIN: Affordable, Accurate, Reliable and INnovative Mechanism to Protect a Medical Cyber-Physical System using Blockchain Technology". *IJIN*, *2*, 175–183.

Tyagi, A. (2022). Using Multimedia Systems, Tools, and Technologies for Smart Healthcare Services. IGI Global. doi:10.4018/978-1-6684-5741-2

Tyagi, A. (2022). Using Multimedia Systems, Tools, and Technologies for Smart Healthcare Services. IGI Global., doi:10.4018/978-1-6684-5741-2

Tyagi, A. (2023). Decentralized everything: Practical use of blockchain technology in future applications. Distributed Computing to Blockchain. Academic Press. doi:10.1016/B978-0-323-96146-2.00010-3

Tyagi, A. (2023). Digital Twin Technology: Opportunities and Challenges for Smart Era's Applications. In *Proceedings of the 2023 Fifteenth International Conference on Contemporary Computing (IC3-2023)*. Association for Computing Machinery. 10.1145/3607947.3608015

Tyagi, A. (2023). Hemamalini, Gulshan Soni, Digital Health Communication With Artificial Intelligence-Based Cyber Security, in the book: AI-Based Digital Health Communication for Securing Assistive Systems. IGI Global. doi:10.4018/978-1-6684-8938-3.ch009

Tyagi, A. K., & Goyal, D. (2020). A Survey of Privacy Leakage and Security Vulnerabilities in the Internet of Things. 2020 5th International Conference on Communication and Electronics Systems (ICCES). IEEE. 10.1109/IC-CES48766.2020.9137886

Tyagi, A. K., & Goyal, D. (2020). A Survey of Privacy Leakage and Security Vulnerabilities in the Internet of Things. *2020 5th International Conference on Communication and Electronics Systems (ICCES)*. IEEE. doi:10.1109/IC-CES48766.2020.9137886

Tyagi, A. K., Chandrasekaran, S., & Sreenath, N. (2022). Blockchain Technology:– A New Technology for Creating Distributed and Trusted Computing Environment. 2022 International Conference on Applied Artificial Intelligence and Computing (ICAAIC), (pp. 1348-1354). IEEE.10.1109/ICAAIC53929.2022.9792702

Tyagi, A., Kukreja, S., Nair, M. M., & Tyagi, A. K. (2022). Machine Learning: Past, Present and Future. *NeuroQuantology: An Interdisciplinary Journal of Neuroscience and Quantum Physics*, *20*(8). doi:10.14704/nq.2022.20.8.NQ44468

Upadhyay, P., & Chhabra, M. (2023). Personality Analysis using Edge Detection. In *International Conference on Artificial Intelligence and Smart Communication (AISC)* (pp. 151-155). IEEE.

Vabalas, A., Gowen, E., Poliakoff, E., & Casson, A. J. (2020). Applying machine learning to kinematic and eye movement features of a movement imitation task to predict autism diagnosis. *Scientific Reports*, *10*(1), 1–13. doi:10.1038/s41598-020-65384-4 PMID:32433501

van Delft, E. A., van Gelder, T. G., de Vries, R., Vermeulen, J., & Bloemers, F. W. (2019). Duration of cast immobilization in distal radial fractures: A systematic review. *Journal of Wrist Surgery*, *8*(05), 430–438. doi:10.1055/s-0039-1683433 PMID:31579555

Van Leemput, K., Maes, F., Vandermeulen, D., Colchester, A., & Suetens, P. (2001). Automated segmentation of multiple sclerosis lesions by model outlier detection. *IEEE Transactions on Medical Imaging*, *20*(8), 677–688. doi:10.1109/42.938237 PMID:11513020

van't Hof, M., Tisseur, C., van Berckelear-Onnes, I., van Nieuwenhuyzen, A., Daniels, A. M., Deen, M., Hoek, H. W., & Ester, W. A. (2021). Age at autism spectrum disorder diagnosis: A systematic review and meta-analysis from 2012 to 2019. *Autism*, *25*(4), 862–873. doi:10.1177/1362361320971107 PMID:33213190

Verma, G., Bhardwaj, A., Aledavood, T., De Choudhury, M., & Kumar, S. (2022). Examining the impact of sharing COVID-19 misinformation online on mental health. *Scientific Reports*, *12*(1), 8045. doi:10.1038/s41598-022-11488-y PMID:35577820

Viergever, M. A., Maintz, J. B. A., Klein, S., Murphy, K., Staring, M., & Pluim, J. P. W. (2016). A survey of medical image registration - under review. *Medical Image Analysis*, *33*, 140–144. doi:10.1016/j.media.2016.06.030 PMID:27427472

Voinsky, I., Fridland, O. Y., Aran, A., Frye, R. E., & Gurwitz, D. (2023). Machine Learning-Based Blood RNA Signature for Diagnosis of Autism Spectrum Disorder. *International Journal of Molecular Sciences*, *24*(3), 2082. doi:10.3390/ijms24032082 PMID:36768401

Wallace, S., Parsons, S., Westbury, A., White, K., White, K., & Bailey, A. (2010). Sense of presence and atypical social judgments in immersive virtual environments: Responses of adolescents with Autism Spectrum Disorders. *Autism*, *14*(3), 199–213. doi:10.1177/1362361310363283 PMID:20484000

Wang, R. Y., Guo, T. Q., Li, L. G., Jiao, J. Y., & Wang, L. Y. (2020). Predictions of COVID-19 infection severity based on co-associations between the SNPs of co-morbid diseases and COVID-19 through machine learning of genetic data. *2020 IEEE 8th International Conference on Computer Science and Network Technology (ICCSNT),* (pp. 92–96).

Wang, C., Xiao, Z., Wang, B., & Wu, J. (2019). Identification of autism based on SVM-RFE and stacked sparse auto-encoder. *IEEE Access : Practical Innovations, Open Solutions, 7,* 118030–118036. doi:10.1109/ACCESS.2019.2936639

Wang, H., Chi, L., & Zhao, Z. (2022). ASDPred: An End-to-End Autism Screening Framework Using Few-Shot Learning. *Proceedings of the 31st ACM International Conference on Information & Knowledge Management,* (pp. 5004–5008). ACM. 10.1145/3511808.3557210

Wang, M., Doenyas, C., Wan, J., Zeng, S., Cai, C., Zhou, J., Liu, Y., Yin, Z., & Zhou, W. (2021). Virulence factor-related gut microbiota genes and immunoglobulin A levels as novel markers for machine learning-based classification of autism spectrum disorder. *Computational and Structural Biotechnology Journal, 19,* 545–554. doi:10.1016/j.csbj.2020.12.012 PMID:33510860

Wani, N. A., Kumar, R., & Bedi, J. (2024). DeepXplainer: An interpretable deep learning based approach for lung cancer detection using explainable artificial intelligence. *Computer Methods and Programs in Biomedicine, 243,* 107879. doi:10.1016/j.cmpb.2023.107879 PMID:37897989

Warfield, S. K., Zou, K. H., & Wells, W. M. (2004). Simultaneous truth and performance level estimation (STAPLE): An algorithm for the validation of image segmentation. *IEEE Transactions on Medical Imaging, 23*(7), 903–921. doi:10.1109/TMI.2004.828354 PMID:15250643

Wawer, A., & Chojnicka, I. (2022). Detecting autism from picture book narratives using deep neural utterance embeddings. *International Journal of Language & Communication Disorders, 57*(5), 948–962. doi:10.1111/1460-6984.12731 PMID:35555933

Wijetunga, A. R., Tsang, V. H., & Giuffre, B. (2019). The utility of cross-sectional imaging in the management of suspected scaphoid fractures. *Journal of Medical Radiation Sciences, 66*(1), 30–37. doi:10.1002/jmrs.302 PMID:30160062

Wilczyński, S., Koprowski, R., Stolecka-Warzecha, A., Duda, P., Deda, A., Ivanova, D., Kiselova-Kaneva, Y., & Błońska-Fajfrowska, B. (2019). The use of microtomographic imaging in the identification of counterfeit medicines. *Talanta, 195*(October 2018), 870–875. doi:10.1016/j.talanta.2018.12.009

Wolff, N., Kohls, G., Mack, J. T., Vahid, A., Elster, E. M., Stroth, S., Poustka, L., Kuepper, C., Roepke, S., Kamp-Becker, I., & Roessner, V. (2022). A data driven machine learning approach to differentiate between autism spectrum disorder and attention-deficit/hyperactivity disorder based on the best-practice diagnostic instruments for autism. *Scientific Reports, 12*(1), 18744. doi:10.1038/s41598-022-21719-x PMID:36335178

Wu, A. M., Bisignano, C., James, S. L., Abady, G. G., Abedi, A., Abu-Gharbieh, E., Alhassan, R. K., Alipour, V., Arabloo, J., Asaad, M., Asmare, W. N., Awedew, A. F., Banach, M., Banerjee, S. K., Bijani, A., Birhanu, T. T. M., Bolla, S. R., Cámera, L. A., Chang, J.-C., & Vos, T. (2021). Global, regional, and national burden of bone fractures in 204 countries and territories, 1990-2019: A systematic analysis from the Global Burden of Disease Study 2019. *The Lancet. Healthy Longevity, 2*(9), e580–e592. doi:10.1016/S2666-7568(21)00172-0 PMID:34723233

Wuerich, C. (2022). Blood Pressure Estimation based on Electrocardiograms. Current Directions in Biomedical Engineering, 8(2). doi:10.1515/cdbme-2022-1015

Wu, G., Wang, S., Ning, Z., & Zhu, B. (2021). Privacy-preserved electronic medical record exchanging and sharing: A blockchain-based smart healthcare system. *IEEE Journal of Biomedical and Health Informatics*, 26(5), 1917–1927. doi:10.1109/JBHI.2021.3123643 PMID:34714757

Wu, H., Patel, K. H. K., Li, X., Zhang, B., Galazis, C., Bajaj, N., Sau, A., Shi, X., Sun, L., Tao, Y., Al-Qaysi, H., Tarusan, L., Yasmin, N., Grewal, N., Kapoor, G., Waks, J. W., Kramer, D. B., Peters, N. S., & Ng, F. S. (2022). A fully-automated paper ECG digitisation algorithm using deep learning. *Scientific Reports*, 12(1), 20963. doi:10.1038/s41598-022-25284-1 PMID:36471089

Xie, Z., Nikolayeva, O., Luo, J., & Li, D. (2019). Peer reviewed: Building risk prediction models for type 2 diabetes using machine learning techniques. *Preventing Chronic Disease*, 16.

Xu, J., Xue, K., Li, S., Tian, H., Hong, J., Hong, P., & Yu, N. (2019). Healthchain: A blockchain-based privacy preserving scheme for large-scale health data. *IEEE Internet of Things Journal*, 6(5), 8770–8781. doi:10.1109/JIOT.2019.2923525

Yahyaoui, A., Jamil, A., Rasheed, J., & Yesiltepe, M. (2019). A decision support system for diabetes prediction using machine learning and deep learning techniques. *2019 1st International Informatics and Software Engineering Conference (UBMYK)* (pp. 1-4). IEEE. 10.1109/UBMYK48245.2019.8965556

Yang, X., Zhang, N., & Schrader, P. (2022). A study of brain networks for autism spectrum disorder classification using resting-state functional connectivity. *Machine Learning with Applications*, 8, 100290. doi:10.1016/j.mlwa.2022.100290

Yaqoob, I., Salah, K., Jayaraman, R., & Al-Hammadi, Y. (2021). Blockchain for healthcare data management: Opportunities, challenges, and future recommendations. *Neural Computing & Applications*, 1–16.

Yassin, W., Nakatani, H., Zhu, Y., Kojima, M., Owada, K., Kuwabara, H., Gonoi, W., Aoki, Y., Takao, H., Natsubori, T., Iwashiro, N., Kasai, K., Kano, Y., Abe, O., Yamasue, H., & Koike, S. (2020). Machine-learning classification using neuroimaging data in schizophrenia, autism, ultra-high risk and first-episode psychosis. *Translational Psychiatry*, 10(1), 278. doi:10.1038/s41398-020-00965-5 PMID:32801298

Yoon, A. P., Lee, Y. L., Kane, R. L., Kuo, C. F., Lin, C., & Chung, K. C. (2021). Development and validation of a deep learning model using convolutional neural networks to identify scaphoid fractures in radiographs. *JAMA Network Open*, 4(5), e216096–e216096. doi:10.1001/jamanetworkopen.2021.6096 PMID:33956133

Zeberga, K., Attique, M., Shah, B., Ali, F., Jembre, Y. Z., & Chung, T.-S. (2022). A novel text mining approach for mental health prediction using Bi-LSTM and BERT model. *Computational Intelligence and Neuroscience*, 2022, 1–18. https://www.hindawi.com/journals/cin/2022/7893775/. doi:10.1155/2022/7893775 PMID:35281185

Zhang, B., Qi, S., Monkam, P., Li, C., Yang, F., Yao, Y.-D., & Qian, W. (2019). Ensemble Learners of Multiple Deep CNNs for Pulmonary Nodules Classification Using CT Images. *IEEE Access : Practical Innovations, Open Solutions*, 7, 110358–110371. doi:10.1109/ACCESS.2019.2933670

Zhang, T., Schoene, A. M., Ji, S., & Ananiadou, S. (2022). Natural language processing applied to mental illness detection: A narrative review. *NPJ Digital Medicine*, 5(1), 46. doi:10.1038/s41746-022-00589-7 PMID:35396451

Zhao, Z., Zhu, Z., Zhang, X., Tang, H., Xing, J., Hu, X., Lu, J., & Qu, X. (2021). Identifying autism with head movement features by implementing machine learning algorithms. *Journal of Autism and Developmental Disorders*, 1–12. PMID:34250557

Zheng, A., & Casari, A. (2018). *Feature engineering for machine learning: Principles and techniques for data scientists.* O'Reilly Media, Inc. https://books.google.com/books?hl=en&lr=&id=sthSDwAAQBAJ&oi=fnd&pg=PT24&dq=Zheng,+A.,+%26+Casari,+A.+(2018).+Feature+engineering+for+machine+learning:+principles+and+techniques+for+data+scientists.+%22+O%27Reilly+Media,+Inc.%22.&ots=ZPWan_4mu1&sig=nt-jerAemDWDZvj07gudiPkwd_4

Zhuang, Y., Sheets, L. R., Chen, Y. W., Shae, Z. Y., Tsai, J. J., & Shyu, C. R. (2020). A patient-centric health information exchange framework using blockchain technology. *IEEE Journal of Biomedical and Health Informatics, 24*(8), 2169–2176. doi:10.1109/JBHI.2020.2993072 PMID:32396110

Zimmet, P., Alberti, K. G., Magliano, D. J., & Bennett, P. H. (2016). Diabetes mellitus statistics on prevalence and mortality: Facts and fallacies. *Nature Reviews. Endocrinology, 12*(10), 616–622. doi:10.1038/nrendo.2016.105 PMID:27388988

Zou, Q., Qu, K., Luo, Y., Yin, D., Ju, Y., & Tang, H. (2018). Predicting diabetes mellitus with machine learning techniques. *Frontiers in Genetics, 9*, 515. doi:10.3389/fgene.2018.00515 PMID:30459809

About the Contributors

Megha Bhushan is Associate Professor in the School of Computing, and Assistant Dean, Research & Consultancy at DIT University, Dehradun, India. She has received her ME and Ph.D. degrees from Thapar University, Punjab, India. She was awarded with a fellowship by UGC, Government of India, in 2014. In 2017, she was a recipient of Grace Hopper Celebration India (GHCI) fellowship. She has published 5 national patents and 1 international patent has been granted. She has published many research articles in international journals and conferences of repute. Further, she is the editor of many edited books with different publishers such as CRC Press, Taylor & Francis Group, Wiley-Scrivener and Bentham Science. Her research interests include Artificial Intelligence, Knowledge representation, Expert systems, and Software quality. She is also the reviewer and editorial board member of many international journals.

Hocine Chebi is a teacher and researcher in the Department of Automatique (Faculty of Electrical Engineering), Djillali Liabes University of Sidi Bel Abbes, Algeria. He obtained his baccalaureate in electrical engineering in 2007 from the Technical School of Tizi-ouzou, Algeria. He then obtained his State Engineer's degree in control of industrial processesing in 2013, from the Faculty of Hydrocarbons and Chemistry at the University of Boumerdès, Algeria. He obtained a Magister in electrical engineering/automatic option controls and order in 2015 at the Polytechnic Military Academy of Bordj El Bahri, Algeria. He obtained a doctorate degree of University Boumerdes Faculty of Hydrocarbons and Chemistry in 2019. His research area is oriented toward computer vision and the detection of automatic and control anomalies.

Fellag Sid Ali currently professor at boumedes university (Algeria) and, director of research laboratory LIST (ingenierie of systems and telecommunications) at faculty of technology. Got his phd from tashkent polytechnical institut in 2000 in the topic of automation of electro technical complexes-long belt conveyers. Joined Algerian university since 2000- up today. Worked on multirotor systems, wind energy, solar energy and recently working in biomedical engineering field supervising a phd thesis on ecg signal detection and classification.

Preeti Jaidka is of JSS Academy of Technical Education Noida (JSSATEN) is one of the leading Technical Institutions in the National Capital Region in the State of Uttar Pradesh. Established in the year 1998 by JSS Mahavidyapeetha, Noida, the Institution has set bench marks every year, and grown into an Institution of Excellence in Technical Education. Located in the central part of NOIDA, JSSATEN has become a household name for its excellence in Discipline, Teaching, Training and Placement. Today, JSSATEN has total student strength of over 4000, who are mentored by more than 250 Faculty Members. The Campus has finest accommodation for girls and boys.

A. Rajiv Kannan is working as a Professor and Head of the Department of Computer Science and Engineering, K.S.R. College of Engineering, Tiruchengode. He published more than 50 research publications in International Journal and Conferences with Citation -160, h-index - 07, i10 index-05. His research specializations are Artificial Intelligence, Machine Learning, Data Mining. Under his guidance, 13 Ph.D., scholars have completed their Ph.D., while 12 are pursuing their doctoral degrees. He received many grants from various funding agencies such as ICMR, SERB, DST, AICTE, etc. He has been credited with publishing 5 patents covering diverse domains.

Hemalatha Karnan pursued B.Tech. Bioengineering in SASTRA University during 2002-2006. She received her ME Applied Electronics degree from Anna University, BIT campus, Tiruchirappalli in the year 2012 and Ph.D. from the Department of Instrumentation & Control Engineering in National Institute of Technology, Tiruchirappalli. Her research areas are Bio- signal processing and machine learning techniques for clinical data analysis. She has also interests in image processing and its usage in point-of-care device design. She has over 15 years of research experience. She has presented her research findings in 15 different International and 3 National Conferences. Her publications are on learning model development and optimization with publishers like CRC press, Wiley and etc. She has submitted a patent on her recent research work on the design of wearable system for geriatric care.

Jaspreet Kaur is currently working as an Assistant Professor in University Business School,Chandigarh University,Mohali,Punjab.She is a post graduate (MBA-H.R) from Panjab University,Chandigarh.She has also qualified UGC NET JRF in Human Resource Management/Labour and Social Welfare and has completed PhD in Business Management from Chandigarh University,Mohali. She has over 8 years of experience in academic and administrative assignments.She also received "Best Teacher of the Department Award " in the year 2019 and 2021 in the field of imparting quality education.Her research interests include Employee Engagement, Management of Organizational Change and Organization Development. She has published several research papers and articles in reputed international and national journals and has presented papers in various national and international conferences.She also contributed one edited book and 10 book chapters on various topics.

Rita Komalasari is a lecturer at YARSI University. Her current work is focused on Advancing Healthcare: Economic Implications of Immediate MRI in Suspected Scaphoid Fractures - A Comprehensive Exploration. Please direct correspondence to rita.komalasari161@gmail.com.

Kuldeep Kumar received his Ph.D. degree from the School of Computing, National University of Singapore, Singapore in 2016. Currently, he is working as an Assistant Professor in the Department of Computer Engineering at the National Institute of Technology, Kurukshetra. Before that, he worked at the Birla Institute of Technology and Science Pilani and the National Institute of Technology Jalandhar for more than six years. His research interests include Software Engineering, Machine Learning, and Data Analytics. He has published more than 50 papers in peer-reviewed journals and international conferences, along with several book chapters.

Harsh Vardhan Kumar is doing his B Tech from NIT Hamirpur. His current research area is Medical Mining.

Vijay Kumar is Associate Professor in Department of Information Technology, Dr B R Ambedkar NIT Jalandhar. He received his Ph.D. degree from NIT Kuruksherta. Previously, he received M.Tech. and B.Tech. degrees from GJUS&T, Hisar and M.M. Engineering College, Mullana, respectively. Prior, he has 15 years of teaching experience in various reputed institutes such as Manipal University Jaipur, Thapar Institute of Engineering & Technology, Patiala and NIT Hamirpur. He completed 2 DST SERB and 1 CSIR sponsored research projects. He has published more than 180 research papers in International Journals/Conferences. He has many book chapters in international repute publishers. He has supervised many Ph.D. and M.Tech. thesis on Metaheuristics, Image Mining, and Data Clustering. He is the reviewer of several reputed SCI journals. He is member of ACM, CSI, International Association of Engineers, International Association of Computer Science and Information Technology, Singapore. His current research area is Soft Computing, Data Mining, Deep Learning, Steganography, and Pattern Recognition.

Siham Moussaoui is a doctoral student at the Electrical Systems Engineering Department (Faculty of Technology), M'hemed Bougara Boumerdes University, Algeria. She obtained her bachelor's degree in natural science in 2014 at the Naciria School in Boumerdes, Algeria. She then obtained her master's degree in Biomedical Instrumentation in 2019, at the Faculty of Technology of the University of Boumerdes, Algeria. His field of research is oriented toward artificial intelligence, biomedical instrumentation, medical signals, and data analysis.

Arun Negi is currently a Manager at Deloitte USI, Hyderabad, India. He has completed a course in Business Management from IIM, Ahmedabad and has obtained B. Tech degree from Jawaharlal Nehru University, New Delhi, India. He has 13+ years of diverse experience in cyber risk services. He has worked on various network security technologies and platforms for Fortune 500 clients. His experience includes cyber security audits, gap assessments, network security audits, cloud migrations and project management. He is currently oriented towards developing multi cloud skills and has achieved certifications in Oracle Cloud and AWS. He has published one national patent and one international patent has been granted. He has published many research articles in international journals and conferences of repute. His research areas include Artificial Intelligence, Software Product Line, Cloud Computing, and Cyber Security.

Raghuraj Singh is working as an Assistant Professor at the Department of Computer Science & Engineering, Sharda University, Greater Noida. He has done B.Tech and M.Tech in CSE & Pursuing Ph.D from B.R. Ambedkar National Institute of Technology, Jalandhar (Punjab), India. His area of research includes Software Fault Prediction, Software Engineering, Machine Learning and Deep Learning. He has 18+ years of Teaching Experience in various technical Universities/ Institutions. He has published several paper in SCI and Scopus Journal. He is Mentor and guiding research investigations for undergraduate, post-graduate engineering students in the areas including, Software Fault Prediction, Software Engineering, Machine Learning, Deep Learning, Artificial Intelligence, Soft Computing, and Image Processing. He has expertise in Salesforce and AWS.

Shrikant Tiwari (Senior Member, IEEE) received his Ph.D. in the Department of Computer Science & Engineering (CSE) from the Indian Institute of Technology (Banaras Hindu University), Varanasi (India) in 2012 and M. Tech. in Computer Science and Technology from University of Mysore (India) in 2009. Currently, he is working as an Associate Professor in the Department of Computer Science & Engineering (CSE) School of Computing Science and Engineering (SCSE) at Galgotias University, Greater Noida, Uttar Pradesh (India). He has authored or co-authored more than 75 national and international journal publications, book chapters, and conference articles. He has five patents filed to his credit. His research interests include machine learning, deep learning, computer vision, medical image analysis, pattern recognition, and biometrics. Dr. Tiwari is a member of ACM, IET, FIETE, CSI, ISTE, IAENG, SCIEI. He is also a guest editorial board member and a reviewer for many international journals of repute.

Amit Kumar Tyagi is working as Assistant Professor, at National Institute of Fashion Technology, 110016, New Delhi, India. Previously he has worked as Assistant Professor (Senior Grade 2), and Senior Researcher at Vellore Institute of Technology (VIT), Chennai Campus, 600127, Chennai, Tamilandu, India for the period of 2019-2022. He received his Ph.D. Degree (Full-Time) in 2018 from Pondicherry Central University, 605014, Puducherry, India. About his academic experience, he joined the Lord Krishna College of Engineering, Ghaziabad (LKCE) for the periods of 2009-2010, and 2012-2013. He was an Assistant Professor and Head- Research, Lingaya's Vidyapeeth (formerly known as Lingaya's University), Faridabad, Haryana, India for the period of 2018-2019. His supervision experience includes more than 10 Masters' dissertations and one PhD thesis. He has contributed to several projects such as "AARIN" and "P3- Block" to address some of the open issues related to the privacy breaches in Vehicular Applications (such as Parking) and Medical Cyber Physical Systems (MCPS). He has published over 200 papers in refereed high impact journals, conferences and books.

Hemamalini Venkatesan received her B.E degree in CSE from Sri Balaji Chockalingam Engineering College, Arni, affiliated to University of Madras, Chennai in 2004, her M.E degree in CSE from S.A Engineering College, Chennai, affiliated to Anna University, Chennai in 2008 and her Ph.D degree in Wireless Security on January 2018 from Puducherry Technological University (formerly called as Pondicherry Engineering College) affiliated under Pondicherry University, Puducherry. She is currently working as Assistant Professor in Department of Networking and Communications, School of Computing, SRM Institute of Science and Technology, Kattankulathur, Chengalpattu Dt., TN, India from November 2020. She is in teaching profession for more than 19 years and she had published 19 international journals/book chapters/conference paper and presented works in more than 15 regional conferences. She has also produced 4 patent publication and received 1 grant from IPR, Delhi. She has published a book on "Introduction to Cyber Security- A guide for Naive users " under Scientific International Publishing House, and Wireless Network And LANS published by AGPH. Her research interests include Networking, Wireless Security, Cyber Security, Mobile Computing, Wireless Communication, Cryptography & Security and Artificial Intelligence. She is currently guiding two Ph.d candidate in Cyber Security and ML.

Index

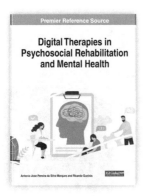
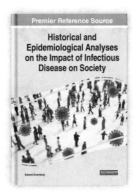
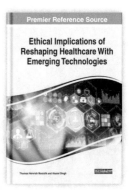
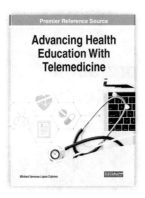
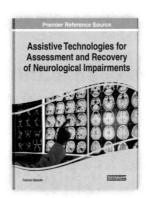
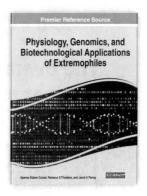
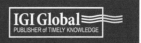 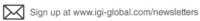

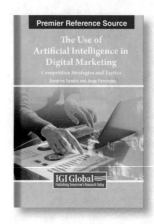 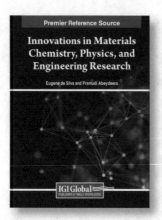 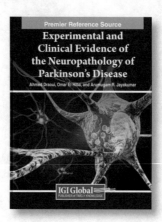 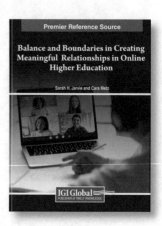

Submit an Open Access Book Proposal

Have Your Work Fully & Freely Available Worldwide After Publication

Seeking the Following Book Classification Types:

Authored & Edited Monographs • Casebooks • Encyclopedias • Handbooks of Research

Gold, Platinum, & Retrospective OA Opportunities to Choose From

Easily Track Your Work in Our Advanced Manuscript Submission System With **Rapid Turnaround Times**

Double-Blind Peer Review by Notable Editorial Boards (*Committee on Publication Ethics* (COPE) Certified

Publications Adhere to All **Current OA Mandates & Compliances**

Affordable APCs *(Often 50% Lower Than the Industry Average)* Including Robust Editorial Service Provisions

Direct Connections with **Prominent Research Funders** & OA Regulatory Groups

Institution Level OA Agreements Available (Recommend or Contact Your Librarian for Details)

Join a **Diverse Community of 150,000+ Researchers Worldwide** Publishing With IGI Global

Content Spread Widely to Leading Repositories (AGOSR, ResearchGate, CORE, & More)

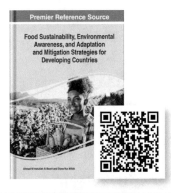

Premier Reference Source
Food Sustainability, Environmental Awareness, and Adaptation and Mitigation Strategies for Developing Countries

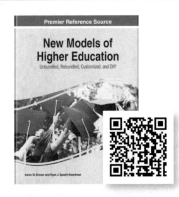

Premier Reference Source
New Models of Higher Education
Unbundled, Rebundled, Customized, and DIY

Handbook of Research on
The Global View of Open Access and Scholarly Communications

 DID YOU KNOW? ## Retrospective Open Access Publishing

You Can Unlock Your Recently Published Work, Including Full Book & Individual Chapter Content to Enjoy All the Benefits of Open Access Publishing

Learn More

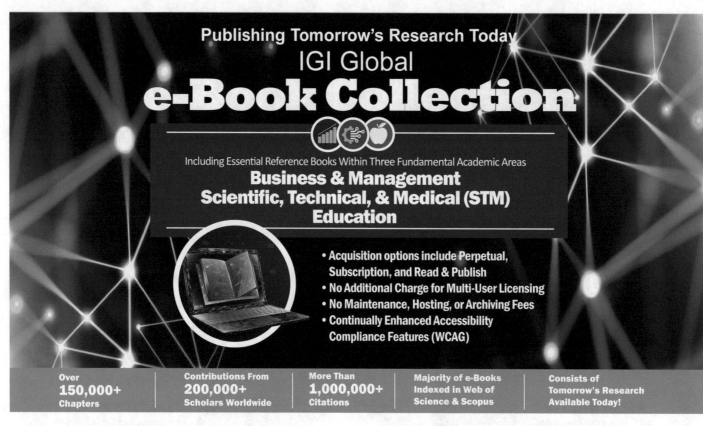

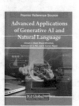
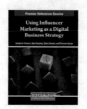
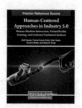
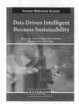
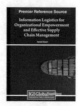
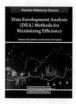

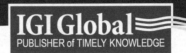
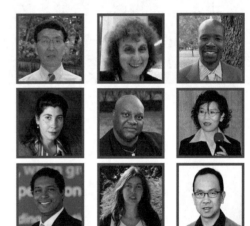
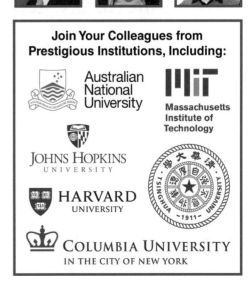

Individual Article & Chapter Downloads

US$ 37.50/each

Easily Identify, Acquire, and Utilize Published Peer-Reviewed Findings in Support of Your Current Research

- Browse Over *170,000+ Articles & Chapters*
- *Accurate & Advanced* Search
- Affordably Acquire *International Research*
- *Instantly Access* Your Content
- Benefit from the *InfoSci® Platform Features*

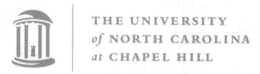

THE UNIVERSITY
of NORTH CAROLINA
at CHAPEL HILL

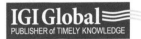
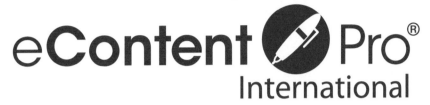

Printed in the United States
by Baker & Taylor Publisher Services